994-1995

Florida Health Care Reference

y **Richard F. Polangin & Ernest Feigenbaum, M.D., M.P.H.**

eston Nelson-Morrill, editor

This book is dedicated to the hope that a way will be found
to make quality health care available to everyone and to
those working to acheive that goal.

1994-95 Florida Health Care Reference
Richard F. Polangin and Ernest Feigenbaum, M.D., M.P.H.
Edited by Creston Nelson-Morrill

Published by HealthTrac Books, Tallahassee

Copyright © 1994 by HealthTrac Books

ISBN 1-879919-95-8 (hard cover)
ISBN 1-879919-88-5 (paper back)

Manufactured in the United States of America
Erdmann's Printing, Grand Rapids, Michigan
Second Edition, June 1994

10 9 8 7 6 5 4 3 2 1

☑Health*trac*
BOOKS

Post Office Box 13599
Tallahassee, FL 32317

This book is not intended as a substitute for the medical advice of physicians. Readers should consult
a physician regularly in matters relating to their health, particularly when there are symptoms that may
require diagnosis and treatment. The listing of a facility in this book does not in any way constitute an
endorsement or recommendation. Although the authors use sources they consider reliable, the authors and
the publisher disclaim any liability for errors and omissions, or for any actions taken by users of the
information in this book and no endorsement by any government agency is intended or implied.

In a book this large and complex, there will be inaccuracies. Health care facilities may have reported
incorrect information, government agencies may have made an error in compiling information, or the authors
may have inadvertently made an error in transcribing data. For these reasons, the accuracy of the data in this
book cannot be guaranteed. The inclusion of research studies in this book does not suggest an endorsement
of their content, a validation of their conclusions, or an assurance of accuracy. The authors appreciate
comments and notification of errors.

Contents

PREFACE ix

FOREWORD xi

INTRODUCTION xv

1. STATE-OF-THE-ART MEDICINE:
MEDICAL KNOWLEDGE EXPANDS 1

VARIATIONS IN MEDICAL TREATMENT 2
  Research findings 3
  Reducing the incidence of unnecessary medicine 5
  Experience and quality of care 6
  Other determinants of quality medical care 7
RESEARCHING MEDICAL PROBLEMS 7
  The National Cancer Institute 8
    Physician Data Query System 9
    CancerFax 9
  American Cancer Society 10
  Clinical practice guidelines 10
    AHCPR clinical practice guidelines 10
    RAND/AMA clinical practice guidelines 11
  National Institutes of Health Medical Consensus Statements 12
    Cancer 13
    Mental health 13
    Women and children 13
    The elderly 13
    Dentistry 13
    Other medical problems 14
    Medical specialty society practice guidelines 14
    AMA directory of practice parameters 16
  MEDLINE and the National Library of Medicine 16
  Special medical data bases 19
  AHCPR health technology assessment reports 19
  InfoTrac Health Reference Center Database 20
  National Institute on Aging 21
  Institutes in the National Institutes of Health 21
STATE AND NATIONAL SOURCES OF HEALTH CARE INFORMATION 22

2. CHOOSING A PHYSICIAN 29

RESEARCH STUDIES ON PHYSICIANS AND QUALITY OF CARE 29
QUALIFICATIONS AND PROFESSIONAL EXPERTISE 30
OTHER CONSIDERATIONS 32

SECOND OPINIONS 32

3. FLORIDA HOSPITALS 35

SELECTING A HOSPITAL 35
    Hospital accreditation 36
    Hospital characteristics and quality of care.....................................37
    Individual hospital mortality data 39
TEACHING AND RESEARCH HOSPITALS 40
OSTEOPATHIC HOSPITALS 41
HOSPITAL COMMUNITY BENEFITS STANDARDS PROGRAM 42
EMERGENCY ROOMS AND TRAUMA CENTERS 42
COMPREHENSIVE REHABILITATION 43
OBSTETRICAL CARE..47
    Hospital Cesarean Sections 51
OPEN HEART SURGERY 53
ANGIOPLASTY AND CARDIAC CATHETERIZATION 56
ORGAN TRANSPLANTAITON 57
    Becoming An Organ Donor 59
EYE, HEART, AND HAND SURGERY 59
CHILDREN'S HOSPITALS 60
CANCER TREATMENT 60
    National Cancer Institute-affiliated hospitals 60
    American College of Surgeons Cancer Programs 61
BURN TREATMENT 63
    Long-termAcute Care 63
SPECIAL DIAGNOSTIC AND THERAPEUTIC EQUIPMENT 64
JCAHO ACCREDITED HOSPITALS 65
LIST OF ACUTE CARE HOSPITALS 65

4. FLORIDA NURSING HOMES...77

CHARACTERISTICS OF NURSING HOME RESIDENTS 77
SERVICES PROVIDED BY NURSING HOMES 79
RESEARCH AND QUALITY OF CARE 80
VISITING A NURSING HOME RESIDENT 80
SELECTING A NURSING HOME 80
    Determining Which Nursing Homes to Visit....................................81
    Inspecting A Nursing Home 82
        Nursing Home Visit Checklist 82
    Determining Reputation for Providing Good Care 83
    Other Sources of Information..84
NURSING HOME RESIDENTS' RIGHTS 85
PAYING FOR NURSING HOME CARE 87
    Long-Term Care Insurance 87
    Medicaid Eligibility 87
    Medicare Eligibility 88
    Supplemental Security Income Medically Needy Program 89
COMPLAINTS 89
NURSING HOME CHARACTERISTICS AND RATINGS 90
JCAHO-ACCREDITED LONG-TERM CARE FACILITIES 90

5. RETIREMENT HOMES AND COMMUNITIES 91

CONTINUING CARE RETIREMENT COMMUNITIES 91
    Continuing Care Contracts 91
    Continuing Care Resident Organizations 92
    Quarterly Meetings 93
RETIREMENT COMMUNITIES LICENSED AS ACLFs 93
    ACLF Residents and Admission Requirements 94
    Services Provided by ACLFs 94
    Paying for Care in an ACLF 95
    ACLF Contracts 95
    Resident Rights 96
HOW TO CHOOSE AN ACLF 97
    Retirement Community Visit Checklist 97
RETIREMENT COMMUNITY INFORMATION SOURCES 99
COMPLAINTS 100
LIST OF CONTINUING CARE FACILITIES 101
LIST OF ACLFS WITH LIMITED NURSING SERVICES 108

6. BIRTH CENTERS, HOSPICES AND
HOME HEALTH AGENCIES 113

BIRTH CENTERS 113
    Sources of Information on Birth Centers 114
    List of Birth Centers 114
HOSPICE CARE 115
    Hospice Services 116
    Hospice Benefits Under Medicare 117
    Research on Care for Persons with Terminal Illnesses 117
    Sources of Information on Hospice Care 118
    Licensed Hospice Programs 119
HOME HEALTH CARE 121
    Selecting a Home Health Agency 122
    Sources of Information on Home Health Care 123
    Accredited Home Health Agencies 124
        Community Health Accreditation Program 124
        JCAHO 125

7. MENTAL HEALTH & SUBSTANCE ABUSE TREATMENT 133

PREVALENCE OF MENTAL DISORDERS 133
TREATMENT METHODS 135
    Biomedical Therapies 136
    Behavioral Therapy 136
    Psychotherapy 136
ALZHEIMER'S DISEASE 137
    Memory Disorder Clinics 138
    Suncoast Gerontology Center 138
    The Florida Brain Bank Program 139
    Other Sources of Information on Alzheimer's Disease 139
    Florida Chapters of the Alzheimer's Disease and Related Disorder Association 140

COMMUNITY MENTAL HEALTH CENTERS 141
HOSPITAL AND RESIDENTIAL TREATMENT 142
SOURCES OF INFORMATION 143
   Professional Organizations..143
   Self-Help Organizations...144
JCAHO- ACCREDITED MENTAL HEALTH AND ALCOHOL/DRUG
   TREATMENT PROGRAMS 145
SUBSTANCE ABUSE TREATMENT 151
   CARF-Accredited Outpatient Substance Abuse Programs 151
LIST OF PSYCHIATRIC AND
   SUBSTANCE ABUSE SPECIALTY HOSPITALS 152

8. VETERANS ADMINISTRATION HEALTH CARE SERVICES 157

ELIGIBILITY FOR VA HOSPITAL AND NURSING HOME CARE 157
   Mandatory 157
   Discretionary 157
ELIGIBILITY FOR VA OUTPATIENT CARE 158
VA NURSING HOMES 159
VA DOMICILIARY CARE 160
OTHER VA HEALTH CARE BENEFITS 160
NAMES AND ADDRESSES OF VA FACILITIES AND VET CENTERS 160
ADDITIONAL SOURCES OF INFORMATION 162

9. HEALTH CARE OPTIONS AND DECISION-MAKING
   N THE LAST YEARS OF LIFE 163

HOME CARE, ACLF, CONTINUING CARE FACILITY
   OR NURSING HOME? 163
   Option 1—Living at Home 164
   Option 2—Living in an ACLF 165
   Option 3—Living in a Continuing Care Retirement Community 166
   Option 4—Living in a Nursing Home 166
LIFE EXPECTANCY AND DISABILITY AFTER AGE 65 166
NURSING HOME USE AFTER AGE 65 168
AGING 169
THE YEAR BEFORE DEATH 173
LIVING WILLS AND FINAL DECISIONS 173
   Life-Sustaining Treatment in Hospitals 173
   Federal Law—The Patient Self-Determination Act 174
   Florida Law and the Browning Decision 174
      Advanced Medical Directive Check List 175
   Sources of Information on Advance Directives 175
   Euthanasia and Assisted Suicide 176

10. ENVIRONMENTAL HEALTH CARE PROBLEMS 179

POISONS IN FLORIDA'S ENVIRONMENT AND
THE FLORIDA POISON INFORMATION CENTER 179
MARINE LIFE 179

SEABATHER'S ERUPTION 180
SKIN CANCER 181
PRECAUTIONS IN HOT WEATHER 182

**11. HEALTH INSURANCE, ACCREDITATION
INFORMATION RESOURCES** 183

PUBLIC AND PRIVATE HEALTH INSURANCE 183
   Medicare 183
   Private Health Insurance 185
   Long-Term Care Insurance 186
   Medigap Insurance 187
   Medicaid 187
ACCREDITATION ORGANIZATIONS 188
LEGAL ADVICE 190
LOCAL HEALTH COUNCILS 190
AREA OFFICES OF HEALTH FACILITY REGULATION 192
NURSING HOME AND LONG-TERM CARE OMBUDSMAN COUNCILS 193
SOURCES OF INFORMATION ON SERVICES FOR THE ELDERLY 194
   Area Agencies on Aging 194
   Nationwide Eldercare Locator 196
NEWSLETTERS, RESEARCH SERVICES, AND ASSOCIATIONS 196
   Newsletters and Research Services 196
   Florida Associations of Medical Professionals 197
   Florida Health Care Facility Associations 197
   Other Florida Health Care Organizations 198
NATIONAL PROFESSIONAL ORGANIZATIONS 199

12. REFORM, MALPRACTICE, FRAUD AND COMPLAINTS 201

HEALTH CARE REFORM 201
PERSONAL HEALTH CARE REFORM STRATEGIES 203
MEDICAL MALPRACTICE 203
   The Extent of Medical Malpractice 204
   Medical Injury Risk Factors 205
   Malpractice Litigation 205
   Malpractice and Florida Physicians 206
HEALTH CARE FRAUD 207
   Reporting Health Care Fraud 207
HOSPITAL BILLING ERRORS 208
AGENCIES THAT INVESTIGATE AND RESOLVE HEALTH CARE
COMPLAINTS 209

BIBLIOGRAPHY 211

APPENDIX A—1991 HOSPITAL STATISTICAL TABLES 221

APPENDIX B—1992 HOSPITAL CESAREAN SECTION RATES 237

APPENDIX C—1993 HOSPITAL HEART SURGERY PROGRAMS 243

**APPENDIX D—1993 HOSPITAL CARDIAC CATHETERIZATION
PROGRAMS** 247

APPENDIX E—1992 NURSING HOME STATISTICS 251

Preface

The 1994-95 Florida Health Care Reference is a revised and expanded version of Health Care in Florida—A Handbook and Reference, published in 1991 by Pineapple Press in Sarasota. This new HealthTrac edition contains six new chapters and was extensively revised and updated. Ernest Feigenbaum, M.D., M.P.H., and Creston Nelson-Morrill are new contributors. Dr. Feigenbaum has a background in clinical medicine, health care research, and health policy analysis. Ms. Nelson-Morrill brings expert editing and a comprehensive knowledge of health care policy and the Florida Legislature to this book.

Making health care decisions in today's technologically advanced, high-cost, and complicated system requires much more effort than in the past.

Many factors are improving the quality of health care. Diagnostic and treatment breakthroughs are being made at faster and faster rates. State-of-the-art practice guidelines increasingly are becoming available to help physicians and patients make appropriate treatment decisions. Medical effectiveness research is helping to improve the quality of health care, and an extraordinary electronic information explosion is making medical research findings readily available to anyone. Yet, rising health care costs have made adequate health insurance unaffordable for far too many people, and are causing severe economic problems for both government and industry. All of these factors make it increasingly necessary to better understand our rapidly changing system, and to become more informed in making health care decisions.

This edition was written for everyone involved in the health care decision-making process: health care professionals, health care administrators, health care policymakers, and the public. Included are the findings of many recently published studies that have analyzed medical effectiveness and the quality of care provided by physicians and hospitals. Also included are sources of medical information, including diagnosis and treatment guidelines for many medical and surgical procedures. A new chapter discusses health care options for the elderly, research on life expectancy and aging, and living wills.

Research findings on many different aspects of health care are included throughout the book in non-technical, understandable language. It is important to emphasize, however, that when reviewing the findings of this research, readers should be aware that while many of these studies have found statistically "significant" differences in patient care, these differences can be relatively small in actual practice. The inclusion of these studies does not suggest an endorsement of their content, a validation of their conclusions, or an assurance of their accuracy. Readers with an interest in a particular study should consult the bibliography and obtain and review the study themselves.

Listings of accredited health care facilities also are included. Although research has not shown that accredited facilities offer better care than facilities that are not accredited, the federal Office of Technology Assessment states that accredited facilities have been recognized by independent experts as having, "the appropriate resources to provide care, either overall or for specific conditions." Accreditation also indicates that the facility has sought verification from impartial experts that it meets certain staffing, equipment, and other standards. Some health care experts, however, believe that accreditation is not a useful indicator of quality health care.

The inclusion of a health care facility is not a recommendation that the facility be used. Analyzing the quality of care in specific facilities is well beyond the scope of this book. It is the physicians, nurses, and other health care professionals that determine the quality of care that patients receive.

Richard F. Polangin

Foreword

As the debate intensifies over the structuring, financing, and evaluation of health services delivery in the nation, both laymen and health care professionals face a host of social, economic, political, and technologic opinions, facts, and sometimes contradictory analyses.

Change has come to the health care field in many ways; sometimes abruptly and sometimes through a process of gradual transition. Health care providers and facilities have been obliged to restructure the manner in which they work to deliver care. Meanwhile, consumers are confronted by a multitude of alternatives for gaining access to and paying for care. Many of these changes have been a source of anxiety for all concerned, despite a pace of technologic advancement that permits more to be done for—and to—the patient, albeit at increasing costs.

A recent article addressing the public policy implications of health system reform, which appeared in the *Journal of the American Medical Association*, identified significant trends in American health care (Friedman 1993). These trends were felt to be inevitable in the movement of health care reform from the *theoretical* to the *political*:

- Growth in managed care;
- Growth in group practice;
- Salaried practice;
- Shortages of key health professions;
- Data-based quality assessment; and
- Cost containment.

On the other hand, the layman must navigate a world in which objective consumer health data are scarce and price sensitivity is most likely to be based on the composite cost of insurance premiums and copayments rather than the discrete price of specific therapeutic modalities and services. Interstate differences in health care costs and variations in medical treatment patterns from region to region compound the difficulty in making knowledgeable consumer choices among alternative providers and systems of care.

The key dimensions of health care system reform were concisely listed in a 1991 Urban Institute publication (Holahan et al. 1991). The six questions that any proposal for change must address are:

- Who is covered? To what extent will access be expanded?
- How are costs controlled?
- Who pays? How is the system financed?
- What benefits are covered?
- Who administers and ultimately oversees the day-to-day management of the system?
- Is the system politically feasible?

Responses to these questions ultimately must face a "reality test" when they are measured against the fundamental policy issues of how much is enough and what really works. It is doubtful that sufficient resources currently exist within the health sector to fulfill the promise that "universal access" to care implies unless the system undergoes radical change. The assessment of technologies, treatments, and strategies for care with respect to efficiency and safety in health care also is problematic.

The governance of health system models now being discussed under the policy of "managed competition" is, in my view, dependent on modification of antitrust statutes and regulations that limit the ability of providers to form integrated health care systems capable of negotiating group contracts and prices. Some of the more promising models bear a closer resemblance to franchising arrangements than to conventional programs of health insurance coverage. The governing bodies of these models may be hospitals, coalitions of physicians, local government, proprietary and non-profit corporations, as well as insurance companies or industry groups seeking coverage for their employees.

The social adjustment required of both providers and patients in accessing and adapting to a changing universe of health care institutions and their interrelationships forms a significant counterpoint to the orchestration of health system reform. A recent commentary in *Health Affairs* addressed the instability of the relationship between hospitals and physicians, as well as the unsettling impact of evolving strategies that favor an integrated institutional approach to care over a system that has long depended on loose alliances of autonomous practitioners (Goldsmith, 1993).

It is precisely because of these social aspects in the culture of caregiving that "universal coverage" of health care is not the same as "universal access" to care. Access to care invariably will suffer if the match between patient and provider is socially flawed, despite the adequacy of health insurance coverage.

To facilitate the examination of existing and proposed health care systems, Soffel and Luft have suggested that two basic features must be considered (Soffel and Luft, 1993). The first is enrollment and eligibility functions, which involve how people enter the system and obtain coverage for health services. The second significant feature involves the provision of health care, including organization of physician services, payment mechanisms, quality assurance, degree of formal structure, and oversight. By using these building blocks, a plan to compare health system reform proposals can be developed.

The concept of "outcome accountability" slowly has come to light because of these concerns. A puzzling disparity exists between the diverse methodologies that are followed when coverage policies are developed for pharmaceuticals, medical devices, treatment modalities, and surgical procedures. There have been unexpected health outcomes, as well, when expanded health insurance coverage became available to those previously uninsured.

A recent Massachusetts study revealed that the provision of health insurance, alone, to low-income, uninsured pregnant women increased the rate of cesarean section without any discernible improvement in maternal health (Haes Udvarholy, and Epstein 1993). Because of the costs attributable to emerging technologies, the insurance coverage of new medical devices is approached with great care. Pharmaceuticals are a close second in the time and expense required for labelling and marketing approval. Surgical procedures require less formal assessment methods to achieve coverage status.

In contrast, the scenarios for health care reform currently being proposed represent major organizational interventions that will affect the "fit" between our existing framework of caregivers and the patients whom they serve. No organized process exists to gauge the community health status impact of these interventions. Structural shifts are occurring in health care delivery which appear to parallel the early evolution of the supermarket, discount store, and franchised business. Without local health outcome accountability, the cost of health insurance premiums will be the principal indicator used to evaluate health system reform.

The basis of current reform strategies remains economic. If we don't strive to identify the beneficial or adverse effects of these strategies on community health status, our policy choices will lack a fundamental element of validity. Those wishing to pursue this topic may refer to *Access To Health Care In America,* a publication of the National Institute of Medicine, which proposes an interesting system of health status indicators that parallel economic indicators (Millman 1993).

It is my great hope that this book will serve as a starting point for the health care professional or consumer to approach the topic of health care delivery policy, practices, and outcomes in an organized manner with insight and guidance toward sources of information on the past, present, and future of Florida's health system. As such it represents both a road map and an owner's manual for those who use it to make their way through our rapidly changing health care delivery system.

Ernest Feigenbaum, M.D., M.P.H.

Introduction

Florida has taken the lead nationally in the health care reform movement. In 1993, Florida lawmakers embraced "managed competition" as the model for reform and set into motion a bold, largely untested reordering of the health care system.

The linchpin of managed competition is the formation of private, non-profit community health purchasing alliances (CHPAs), which serve as information brokers on health care services available in each of 11 geographic regions. By May 1994, the CHPAs were expected to distribute to their members comparative information on available health insurance and health maintenance organization (HMO) plans including price, and coverage terms and limitations. Eventually, the CHPAs will issue provider "report cards" reflective of patient outcomes and satisfaction. The goal: to increase competition among participating providers and insurance companies (dubbed accountable health partnerships, or AHPs, in the new scheme) through informed consumerism and by focusing the buying power of many small businesses, the State of Florida, and the Medicaid program, for low-income Floridians, in one place.

As the start-up date approached, it appeared that as many as 50 AHPs would be offering a variety of plans in one or more of the CHPA regions. A number of plans appeared to be priced well below comparable products offered outside the CHPAs. The state Agency for Health Care Administration (AHCA) was quick to declare victory.

Will managed competition really work?

That's the billion dollar question.

In the 1994 regular legislative session, the debate over continued health care reform became mired in politics. Gov. Lawton Chiles proposed expanding the CHPAs' negotiating authority and membership base. The membership expansion would have involved allowing the enrollment of individuals, public schools and local government employers, and larger "small" businesses. He also unveiled an ambitious plan, Florida Health Security, to provide subsidized health care coverage to 1.2 million low- and middle-income uninsured Floridians. The subsidized coverage would have been available exclusively through the CHPAs and their AHPs. A special legislative session was pending as the *1994-95 Florida Health Care Reference* went to press.

One irony of the health care reform debate was the absence of any discussion of long-term care. With 270,000 Floridians expected to be over age 85 by 1995, the omission could prove costly, both in tax dollars and in terms of quality of life for the elderly. In Florida, nearly 70,000 persons are receiving care through community-based programs. Almost 68,000 older Floridians live in nursing homes, with nearly half over age 85. The *Florida Caregivers Handbook, Second Edition*, reported that estimates of the number of persons over age 85 who suffer from Alzheimer's disease or related dementia range from one in four to nearly half. E. Bentley Lipscomb, secretary of the Florida Department of Elder Affairs, terms Alzheimer's disease a "coming epidemic."

If managed competition and related reforms are to be successful, the business community, insurers, health care providers and the public will need solid information upon which to base crucial decisions. This book is intended to assist them in their quest for understanding of the system.

The Florida health care marketplace—and patient access and quality of care—bears close watching as the managed competition experiment gets under way.

Creston Nelson-Morrill

CHAPTER 1
State-of-the-art medicine: medical knowledge expands

Medical knowledge is expanding at a rapid pace and improvements in diagnosis and treatment are enhancing the quality of health care. More care is being provided on an outpatient basis because of new, less invasive diagnostic and treatment procedures. Research on medical effectiveness is shedding more light on factors influencing quality health care, and many state-of-the art medical treatment guidelines are now readily available to both physicians and patients. These guidelines cover many different medical and surgical problems, including cancer and heart surgery.

Although increasingly more powerful and less expensive technologies are making information more readily available to both physicians and patients, the availability of new medical knowledge does not mean that this knowledge will be applied. Two leading quality of care researchers, Glenn L. Laffel, M.D., and Donald M. Berwick, M.D., report that there is a "fragile connection" between the new knowledge generated by medical research and the care given to patients at the bedside (Laffel and Berwick 1993). "Physicians may not hear about or accept new findings; they may not know how or when to use them; and the health systems in which they practice may not support the implementation of new knowledge," they said.

Researchers have found problems in the timely application of new medical knowledge and in the delivery of appropriate medical care. Laffel and Berwick cite studies which have found that:

- Forty percent of patients at a tertiary-care hospital did not receive preventive antibiotics at a time that is known to minimize surgical infections;
- There was a 3.5 percent to 21.2 percent unexplained variation between states in the proportion of women with breast cancer who received breast-conserving treatment;
- Eighty percent of patients who were referred for a second opinion regarding the need for coronary angiography were advised that the procedure was not immediately necessary; and
- In response to the publication of the findings of a key trial, aspirin use after myocardial infarction increased from 39 percent to 72 percent.

High quality in medical care occurs when the treatment is needed, appropriate, reflects state-of-the-art medical practice, and results in patient satisfaction. Yet, studies that have examined the quality of care received by patients often have found that sizeable proportions of patients receive care that is either inappropriate or ineffective.

Many studies, particularly those that have examined heart surgery, hysterectomies, and cesarean sections, have found that there are substantial and unexplained differences in how physicians practice medicine. One well-known study found that patients in Boston were much more likely to have carotid endarterectomies than patients in New Haven, while patients in New Haven were much more likely to have coronary bypass operations than those in Boston (Wennberg, Freeman and Culp 1987). Many other studies also have found wide geographic differences in medical practice.

The principal author of the Boston-New Haven study, John E. Wennberg, M.D., is one of the nation's leading medical effectiveness researchers and is the director of the Center for Evaluative Clinical Sciences at Dartmouth Medical School. Dr. Wennberg says that it is very important to involve patients in making health care decisions. In addition, he believes that patient decision making should be an integral part of health care plans. According to Wennberg, "Once you liberate the patient to participate in decision-making, the amount of care demanded by the patient is likely to be different from the amount supplied when the physician prescribed it," (Lumsdon 1993).

Robert H. Brook, M.D., the director of the Health Sciences Program at the RAND Corporation, also suggests that patients should be involved in medical decision-making, and that they should be given the specific medical facts that are considered when a treatment decision is made (Brook 1993).

State-of-the-art medical treatment guidelines, or "practice parameters" are developed by experts to improve the scientific basis for medical decision making and to accelerate the application of new medical knowledge. Practice guidelines also can be used to involve patients in medical decision-making as recommended by Wennberg and Brook. Medical treatment guidelines often are readily available to patients. The National Cancer Institute and the U.S. Agency for Health Care Policy Research publish less technical versions of treatment guidelines intended for use by the general public. Many health care experts believe that practice guidelines will improve medical effectiveness and that unnecessary medicine will decline because patients will be more informed when making health care decisions.

This chapter discusses research that has examined the quality of medical care. Practice guidelines are discussed, and information is provided on how to obtain them. In addition, researching medical problems is discussed, including the new CD-ROM computer technology that has made it a very simple matter to search the National Library of Medicine's MEDLINE system, the most extensive medical data base in the world.

It is important to note that while practice guidelines and the application of medical research can certainly improve the practice of medicine, much of the practice of medicine remains an art. What medical treatment should be provided is not always clear, and patients often have unrealistic expectations as to what modern medicine can deliver. According to one physician, "There is so much in medicine that is absolutely unknown to us, and doctors are very uncomfortable talking to one another about these things. Even at the cutting edge of medical science, we're only scratching the surface of what human life is all about," (Pekkanen 1988).

VARIATIONS IN MEDICAL TREATMENT

"Is this treatment or surgery necessary?" That, often times, is a difficult question to answer. A frequently-used estimate in the medical research literature is that 20 percent of all medical care provided is unnecessary. Researchers also have found that the rates of unnecessary procedures vary dramatically for different medical and surgical conditions. In addition, researchers have found large geographic variations in the rates at which certain surgical procedures are performed. Experts attribute these differences to the fact that physicians have individual practice styles and because physicians in one community may practice very differently from those in another.

In addition to differing practice styles, other factors can influence a physician's decision to perform a medical procedure. According to the authors of the Medical Outcomes Study, these other factors include, "uncertainty about the most effective practice, response to regulations, legal concerns such as malpractice, patient and societal expectations to apply more and more technology, method of patient payment to physician, and type of patient insurance coverage," (Greenfield et al. 1992). Another factor that may explain a sizeable portion of unnecessary medicine is that when there is doubt, physicians may sometimes find it "better to be on the safe side" and perform a procedure.

To develop criteria that are used in determining if a procedure is appropriate, researchers analyze medical literature and obtain expert opinions. Robert H. Brook, M.D., classifies a procedure as appropriate for a patient if "the health benefits of a procedure exceed its health risk by a sufficiently wide margin to make the procedure worth doing," (Brook 1989). He adds, "Because the scientific basis on which medical decisions are made will always be incomplete, we must determine how we can validly combine what is contained in the medical literature with expert judgement to arrive at a judgement of appropriateness."

David A. Grimes, M.D., who has published several articles on the medical effectiveness of obstetrical practices, also points to weakness in the scientific foundation of medicine. He writes that, "Much, if not most, of contemporary medical practice still lacks a scientific foundation," (Grimes 1993). Grimes recommends that new medical technologies be rigorously examined to prove that they are both safe and effective. He cites sperm penetration assay infertility tests, electronic fetal monitoring during labor, laparoscopically assisted vaginal hysterectomies, and radial keratotomies, as examples of widely used tests and procedures that have not been proven to be desirable or effective by research. Grimes writes that, " 'Doing everything for everyone' is neither tenable nor desirable. What is done should be inspired by compassion and guided by science—and not merely reflect what the market will bear. As physicians, we are ethically bound to be sure that the tests, procedures, and treatments we provide are worth the money, pain, and inconvenience that they cost."

Research findings

More and more studies are being conducted to analyze the effectiveness of preventing, diagnosing, and treating medical conditions. The findings of this research are used to improve the quality of medical care, to develop clinical practice guidelines, and to hold down health care costs. A number of studies have examined whether certain medical procedures were necessary or appropriate. These studies often have found higher rates of "uncertain" or "equivocal" medical practice compared with inappropriate practice.

A 1991 national Blue Cross and Blue Shield study found that 27 percent of the tonsillectomy procedures studied were found to be inappropriate (Blue Cross and Blue Shield Association 1991). In addition, 23 percent of hysterectomies, 13 percent of laminectomies, 11 percent of hemorrhoidectomies, 9 percent of septo/rhinoplasty procedures, and 8 percent of knee arthroscopies were found to be inappropriate. On average, 11 percent of all cases reviewed were judged to have received surgery inappropriately.

A RAND study of the appropriateness of hysterectomy procedures examined 642 patients in seven managed care plans, one of them located in Florida (Bernstein et al. 1993). The researchers found that 58 percent of patients underwent hysterectomies for "appropriate" reasons, 25 percent for "uncertain" reasons, and 16 percent for "inappropriate" reasons. Among the seven plans, the "inappropriate" rate ranged from 10 percent to 27 percent. The researchers also found that younger women were more likely to have inappropriate hysterectomies than older women. The inappropriate rate for women 60 and older was only 5 percent, while the inappropriate rate for women age 21 to 40 was 28 percent. Other studies of hysterectomies also have found large variations in hysterectomy rates (Finkel and Finkel 1990; Banta and Thacker 1990).

High rates of inappropriate medicine also have been found in other areas. A large national study (Chassin et al. 1987) of Medicare patients in eight states was conducted by the RAND corporation and the University of California at Los Angles (UCLA). The study found that for carotid endarterectomies, 35 percent were appropriate, 32 percent equivocal, and 32 percent inappropriate. For coronary angiographies, 74 percent were judged to be appropriate, 9 percent equivocal, and 17 percent inappropriate. For upper gastrointestinal tract endoscopies, 72 percent were judged to be appropriate, 11 percent equivocal, and 17 percent inappropriate. Geographic differences were found. The authors, however, concluded that, "Differences in appropriateness cannot explain geographic variations in the use of these procedures."

Although many studies have shown that the likelihood of a favorable outcome increases when certain surgeries are performed by physicians who perform high volumes of those surgeries, this may not always be the case. For example, a subsequent RAND/UCLA study found that, "Physicians who performed high numbers of carotid endarterectomies were more likely to perform unnecessary surgery by operating on less sick, asymptomatic patients," (Brook et al. 1990). Relationships between high volume and inappropriate medicine were not found for coronary angiography or gastrointestinal endoscopy, however. In fact, in the case of coronary angiography, higher volume was found to be associated with "more appropriate decision making." None of the hospital, patient, or physician variables that were studied were found to predict inappropriate care.

The RAND/UCLA study concluded that very detailed studies of patients, physicians, and hospitals are needed to determine whether the care patients receive is appropriate. According to the study,

> *"Appropriateness of care cannot be closely predicted from many easily determined characteristics of patients, physicians, or hospitals. Thus, for the present, if appropriateness is to be improved it will have to be assessed directly at the level of each patient, hospital, and physician,"* (Brook et al. 1990).

A 1989 study by the U.S. General Accounting Office replicated the research conducted by RAND and UCLA for coronary angiography (U.S. General Accounting Office, December 1989). The GAO study findings were very similar to those found by RAND and UCLA, showing that 70 percent of the coronary angiographies were appropriate, 10 percent were equivocal, and 20 percent were inappropriate.

Another RAND/UCLA study examined the appropriateness of performing coronary artery bypass surgery (Winslow et al. 1988). The study, which analyzed patients in three hospitals located in a western state, found that 56 percent of the surgeries were appropriate, 30 percent were equivocal, and 14 percent were inappropriate.

A study of patients hospitalized in Massachusetts compared hospitalization rates in New Haven with those in Boston and found that there were dramatic differences between the two cities in the utilization rates for certain procedures. Patients in Boston hospitals were 2.3 times more likely to have carotid endarterectomies than were patients in New Haven hospitals, while patients in New Haven hospitals were twice as likely to have coronary bypass operations as patients in Boston hospitals (Wennberg, Freeman and Culp 1987).

Other studies also have found sharp differences in practice styles between geographic areas. For example, in Florida during 1992 there were wide variations in c-section rates between hospitals, with rates ranging from 13 percent to 44 percent.

In contrast to many earlier studies, three RAND studies conducted in the state of New York during 1990 found very low rates of inappropriate cardiac procedures. These very encouraging studies, which are discussed more fully in Chapter 3, found very low rates

(4 percent or less) of inappropriate coronary artery bypass graft surgery, percutaneous transluminal coronary angioplasty (PTCA), and coronary angiography. Although the 1990 studies are not directly comparable to earlier studies, the RAND authors cited several reasons why these rates of inappropriate care were so low:
- Improvements in medical practices and in medical technology;
- The development of alternative procedures;
- Changes in the types of patients on which the procedures were performed; and
- The regulatory environment in the state of New York.

High rates of inappropriate medical care have been found by researchers in other countries. For example, studies found that in the United Kingdom 51 percent of coronary angiographies and 42 percent of coronary artery bypass surgeries were inappropriate, and in four Israeli hospitals 29 percent of cholecystectomies were inappropriate (Brook 1993).

Reducing the incidence of unnecessary medicine

What reduces unnecessary medicine? Practice guidelines were developed specifically to reduce unnecessary medicine and improve medical decision-making. Some health care experts maintain that the fee-for-service system of paying for physician care encourages unnecessary medicine. RAND, however, maintains that clinical approaches, not changes in how physicians are paid, are needed to reduce inappropriate or equivocal care (Brook 1993). Clinical approaches include practice guidelines and quality assurance programs. In addition, studies have found that second opinions and physician review conferences can reduce the incidence of unnecessary c-sections. The Blue Cross and Blue Shield study found that inappropriate surgery decreased as "medical control" increased. Persons in health maintenance organizations (HMOs), which "control" access to medical specialists and health care services, had the lowest incidence of inappropriate surgery.

A Canadian study of methods to implement practice guidelines found that physician "opinion leaders" were very effective in reducing c-section rates (Lomas et al. 1991). Physicians practicing in hospitals in Ontario were surveyed to identify "opinion leaders"—physicians who were educationally influential with their peers. The opinion leaders then were trained, using techniques developed for sales persons in the pharmaceutical industry, in a practice guideline developed by the Society of Obstetricians and Gynecologists of Canada, which addressed indications for c-sections. The hospitals in the study were divided into three groups: a control group; a group of hospitals where audit and feedback programs were used to implement the practice guidelines; and a group of hospitals where the opinion leaders practiced. The study, which spanned 24 months during 1988 and 1989, found that c-section rates were 85 percent higher in both the control and audit and feedback hospitals than in the hospitals where the opinion leaders practiced.

Although there have been tremendous advances in medical science, the research literature repeatedly emphasizes that medical decisions are not always clear cut. Medicine is not an exact science and much in the practice of medicine is uncertain. Physicians have differing perspectives on uncertainty, and how it influences the practice of medicine.

"Uncertainty is the common enemy of the physician and the patient. A great deal of medical care is undertaken to reduce uncertainty, especially in the United States where most physicians are specialists trained to avoid "missing" something at all costs," (Fuchs 1993).

"Early in our training ... we learn to live and deal with uncertainty; and although we talk about primum non nocere (first do no harm), we clearly have a bias toward action. The fabric of our world seems to be opinion and uncertainty," (Schoenbaum 1993).

Experience and quality of care

Many studies published in our leading medical journals have found a relationship between greater experience in treating patients (high patient volume) and good patient outcomes. Likewise, other studies have found relationships between less experience (low volume) and poor outcomes. There appears to be a growing consensus that for certain surgical procedures, high volume leads to better outcomes. There are two principal theories that explain why high volume may be related to better patient outcomes:

- The "practice makes perfect" theory, which assumes a relationship between experience and improved performance; and
- The "selective referral" theory, which assumes that patients and physicians gravitate to the best physicians and hospitals because of their reputations for providing better care.

It is important to note that research also has found that once a certain threshold of volume of care is reached, the effect of better care at higher volumes weakens. This has been found in studies of cardiac surgery and organ transplantation. In addition, studies also have found that hospital and physician volume, combined, produces the best surgical results.

A study of 48,139 patients in New York State during 1986 examined the combined effect of hospital and physician volume (Hannan et al. 1989). The study found that in-patient mortality (patient deaths) for coronary artery bypass grafts, resection of abdominal aortic aneurysms, partial gastrectomies, colectomies, and total cholecystectomies was significantly lower when those procedures were performed by high-volume providers. The study found that the relationship between hospital volume and lower mortality was more significant for total cholecystectomies, but that physician volume was only marginally related to outcomes. For the four other procedures, physician volume was found to be more significant than hospital volume. The authors commented that:

"It is possible that the individual surgeon's experience is more critical for complicated, risky procedures and that the surgical team, hospital equipment, and hospital monitoring procedures are more important for less risky procedures."

Studies that have examined physicians' surgical volumes for heart procedures have prompted the American College of Cardiology and the American Heart Association to publish joint guidelines for coronary artery bypass graft surgery and cardiac catheterization. The coronary artery bypass graft guidelines, published in the *Journal of the American College of Cardiology* (March 1, 1991) recommend that: ·

"In general, a yearly minimum of 100 to 150 open heart operations, the majority of which are coronary artery bypass operations, should be performed by each surgeon caring for patients with ischemic heart disease."

For cardiac catheterization, joint American College of Cardiology and American Heart Association guidelines published in the *Journal of the American College of Cardiology* (November 1, 1991) recommend that for surgeons:

"Maintenance of proficiency should include an anticipated adult caseload of approximately 150 cases a year. This should be obtained within two years."

Although research found that high volume may be related to better quality of care for some medical procedures, those findings should not be the only criteria used in selecting a physician or hospital. The federal Office of Technology Assessment urges persons in need of medical treatment not to just "go by the numbers" in choosing a hospital or physician. New physicians continuously enter practice, new procedures are constantly being developed, and hospitals often offer new services. Furthermore, past volume levels may differ from current levels, and current levels may not predict future levels.

Research that has examined the relationship between hospital patient volume and patient outcomes is discussed in Chapter 3.

Other determinants of quality medical care

A major RAND study found large differences in the mortality rates of patients who were judged to have received good care versus those who were judged to have received poor care (Kahn et al. 1990). The substantial differences in quality of care that were identified were attributed to the skills of physicians and nurses.

The study collected detailed information from the medical records of over 14,000 patients in 297 hospitals during two time periods in the 1980s. The study used patient care "process scores" to measure whether patients received good or poor medical care. Physician and nurse cognitive scores were developed that measured the quality of data in the medical record. Technical diagnostic scores were developed to measure the use of diagnostic tests such as laboratory tests, blood gas tests, and electrocardiograms. In addition, technical therapeutic scores were developed to measure treatments and therapies such as medication, surgery, and physical therapy.

Four medical conditions were examined: congestive heart failure, acute myocardial infarction, pneumonia, and cerebrovascular accident (stroke). Seventeen percent of patients that received the best care died within 30 days of admission, while 23.6 percent of the patients that received the poorest care died within 30 days of admission. The authors noted, however, that not all patients who received poor care had poor outcomes.

Of all of the process scores, it was the quality of the therapy provided that had the most significant effect on quality. For example, patients with congestive heart failure who received the best therapeutic care had a mortality rate of 11 percent, while those who received the poorest care had a mortality rate of 21 percent, a two-fold difference.

RESEARCHING MEDICAL PROBLEMS

We live in an age of astounding advances in information technology. Both health care professionals and the public now have easy access to state-of-the-art medical information, including access to the most comprehensive medical data bases in the world. Agencies and organizations that make this medical information easily available include: the RAND Corporation; the National Cancer Institute and other National Institutes of Health; and the federal Agency for Health Care Policy and Research. In addition, there are other easily accessible sources of information on the diagnosis and treatment of medical problems such as the National Library of Medicine's MEDLINE system.

Unnecessary and inappropriate medical care occurs with some regularity, with experts estimating that about 20 percent of medical treatment is unnecessary. Nationally developed treatment guidelines can be consulted to obtain expert opinion when there are conflicting opinions between physicians, when there is uncertainty, or when there is a serious medical problem. However, medical practitioners may not always be aware of the latest research on the diagnosis and treatment of medical problems. In addition, according to Dr. Brook at RAND, "The number of machines, procedures, and drugs now exceeds the ability of most physicians to remember their proper use, complication rate, or efficacy," (Brook 1993). Practice guidelines often are readily available to both health care professionals and patients.

The National Cancer Institute

The National Cancer Institute (NCI) acts as an international clearinghouse for information about cancer. NCI serves both the scientific community and the public and offers a wide range of information, from technical and scientific data for physicians and researchers to booklets for patients. All NCI information is readily available to the public (non-physicians have access to the same information as physicians), and most services and publications are free.

The easiest way to obtain information from the NCI is to contact the Cancer Information Service, which provides information to patients, their families, health professionals and the public. The NCI's free Cancer Information Service can be reached by calling:

NCI Cancer Information Service
(800) 4-CANCER or (800) 422-6237

Callers from Florida are connected to the NCI Sylvester Comprehensive Cancer Center at Jackson Memorial Medical Center in Miami. The Sylvester Comprehensive Cancer Center is affiliated with the University of Miami School of Medicine. Both English and Spanish speaking cancer information specialists are available to assist callers from 9 a.m. to 10 p.m. Monday through Friday. All calls are confidential. The information specialists are trained to help both health care professionals and the public obtain appropriate information.

The Cancer Information Service makes available information on the latest cancer treatments, clinical trials, and physicians and facilities in Florida that are affiliated with the NCI. Information and publications available from the NCI's Cancer Information Service includes:
- Physician and patient statements on over 80 types of cancer, information on clinical trials, directories of physicians who treat cancer, and information on physicians and organizations engaged in cancer research;
- A series of general publications on cancer. Publications focus on cancer prevention, early detection, cancer treatment, advanced cancer, and living with cancer;
- "What You Need to Know About Cancer," NIH Publication No. 90-1566. This is a general information booklet for patients with cancer. There are 25 other publications in this series, each covering a different type of cancer, and including information about symptoms, diagnosis, treatment, and rehabilitation.
- "Scientific Information Services of the National Cancer Institute," NIH Publication No. 91-2683. This publication is written for physicians, other health care professionals, and researchers. Persons conducting research will find this publication to be a necessity. It describes all of the information services that are available from the National Cancer Institute, including information on how to order technical journals and monthly *Cancergrams*; and
- "Research Report" publications. This series includes detailed reports that discuss current research on the cause and prevention, symptoms, detection and diagnosis, and treatment of 17 different types of cancer.

For a complete list of NCI publications, write to:

The National Cancer Institute
Office of Cancer Communications
Building 31, Room 10A24
9000 Rockville Pike
Bethesda, Maryland 20892
(301) 496-5583

Physician Data Query system

The Physician Data Query (PDQ) system is updated monthly and contains cancer reports on over 80 different types of cancer. There are two types of PDQ cancer reports: *physician* information statements that describe the cancer, staging (the extent the cancer has spread), and treatment options; and *patient* information statements that include the same information that is in the physician information statements but in less technical language.

The PDQ system has three different information systems:

- The PDQ Cancer Information File contains the patient and physician statements discussed earlier, information on managing side effects, guidelines for early detection, and general information on clinical trials.
- The PDQ Protocol File contains detailed information on active and closed clinical trials and summaries of standard therapy protocols. Data on more than 1,300 active clinical trials include study objectives, patient eligibility and participating physicians. There are also summaries of the findings of more than 5,000 clinical trials.
- The PDQ Directory contains two separate directories: a physician directory and an organization directory. The physician directory has more than 15,000 physicians with their affiliations, medical specialities, and board certification. Being included in the physician directory does not mean that NCI endorses the physician. The organization directory lists hospitals and clinics that have cancer care programs and clinical trial groups.

All PDQ information is available free to both physicians and the public. Information from the PDQ system can be obtained by:

- calling (800) 4-Cancer and asking the cancer information specialist for PDQ information;
- using NCI's CancerFax; or
- using a computer terminal that is connected to the National Library of Medicine.

PDQ and CancerFax are registered trademarks.

CancerFax

The NCI has included the PDQ information discussed in the previous section in their CancerFax system. This information is obtained using a fax machine. CancerFax is available 24 hours a day, seven days a week and can be used by anyone. Because the NCI does not charge for the use of CancerFax, the telephone call is the only cost. CancerFax contains:

- Patient and physician statements on over 80 different types of cancer;
- Breast cancer prevention information;
- Information on the PDQ system; and
- Information on NCI publications.

Using CancerFax is a two-step process. First, call (301) 402-5874. Follow the instructions from the voice prompt to obtain a list of code numbers. Next, using a fax machine, call CancerFax back. Enter the code number that you received in your initial call for the information you want. Patient statements average four pages, while physician statements average seven. Some physician statements are much longer, however. The breast cancer statement is 30 pages.

American Cancer Society

The American Cancer Society (ACS) provides free information on cancer prevention, detection, treatment, rehabilitation, and support programs and facilities that provide mammography.

Mammography facility reports are available for seven ACS regions in Florida. Each regional report includes comparative information for each hospital, diagnostic center, clinic, or other facility in the region that provides mammography. These detailed reports include, for each facility, information on accreditation, the certification of personnel, the volume of mammographies performed each week, if breast ultrasounds are available, and cost information. To obtain regional mammography reports or other information from ACS, call (800) 227-2345.

Clinical practice guidelines

In recent years there has been an increased emphasis by medical researchers on developing clinical practice guidelines that embody state-of-the-art medical knowledge. Clinical practice guidelines, also known as practice parameters, are developed to help health care professionals and patients make appropriate medical decisions and to reduce unnecessary medical practices. Clinical practice guidelines are not, however, "cook book" medicine. Because there is uncertainty in medical decision making, clinical practice guidelines usually contain latitude for medical judgement.

Because practice guidelines are revised to reflect advances in medical science, when consulting them, it is important to know if they are current. When guidelines become obsolete, they are withdrawn or revised.

A Canadian study that examined the effect of the publication and dissemination of a National Institute of Health consensus statement on cesarean sections found there was "only a slight change from the previous upward trend" in c-section rates as a result of the release of the consensus statement (Lomas et al. 1989). The study concluded that, "Guidelines for practice may predispose physicians to consider changing their behavior, but unless there are other incentives or the removal of disincentives, guidelines may be unlikely to effect rapid change in actual practice." Another Canadian study, discussed earlier, found that c-sections could be sharply reduced when hospital "opinion leaders" were educated using techniques developed by the pharmaceutical industry (Lomas 1991).

AHCPR clinical practice guidelines

The federal Agency for Health Care Policy and Research (AHCPR) sponsors numerous medical effectiveness research projects to identify health care practices that are effective, appropriate, and of high quality. AHCPR supports two basic types of research: patient outcomes research to determine treatments that work best and research to develop clinical practice guidelines. AHCPR defines clinical practice guidelines as "recommendations designed to help health providers make better medical care decisions and reduce the use of ineffective or inappropriate services." The AHCPR clinical practice guidelines are developed by panels of health care experts who review scientific literature and arrive at a consensus of opinion.

According to AHCPR, each guideline "reflects the state of knowledge, current at the time of publication, on effective and appropriate care." The former director of AHCPR, J. Jarrett Clinton, M.D., states that AHCPR believes that if the guidelines are followed, "physicians will see an increase in patient satisfaction, more predictable outcomes, and better use of health care resources," (Clinton 1992). There are three AHCPR publications for each clinical practice guideline:

—*Clinical Practice Guideline* booklets, which contain a comprehensive discussion of each guideline for physicians and other health care practitioners;

—*Quick Reference Guides for Clinicians*, which are used in conjunction with the Clinical Practice Guideline; and

—consumer-oriented *Patient Guides.*

Guides either available from or under development by AHCPR include:

- *Acute Pain Management: Operative or Medical Procedures and Trauma*
- *Urinary Incontinence in Adults*
- *Pressure Ulcers in Adults: Prediction and Prevention*
- *Management of Functional Impairment Due to Cataract in the Adult*
- *Diagnosis and Treatment of Benign Prostatic Hyperplasia*
- *Depression in Primary Care Settings*
- *Management of Functional Impairment Due to Cataract in the Adult*
- *Provision of Comprehensive Care in Sickle Cell Disease*
- *HIV Positive Asymptomatic Patients: Evaluation and Early Intervention*
- *Management of Cancer-Related Pain*
- *Otitis Media in Children*
- *Diagnosis and Treatment of Heart Failure Secondary to Coronary Vascular Disease*
- *Post-Stroke Rehabilitation*
- *Treatment of Stage Two and Greater Pressure Ulcers*
- *Low Back Problems*
- *Screening for Alzheimer's and Related Dementias*
- *Quality Determinants of Mammography*

These publications are available at no charge from AHCPR. They also may be accessed by the National Library of Medicine's MEDLARS on-line computer system. All AHCPR publications are available to both physicians and non-physicians. To obtain clinical practice guideline publications from AHCPR, contact:

AHCPR Publications Clearinghouse
P.O. Box 8547
Silver Spring, Maryland 20907-8547
(800) 358-9295 or (301) 495-3453

RAND-AMA clinical practice guidelines

The RAND Corporation has one of the most prestigious medical effectiveness research programs in the nation. As of March 1993, RAND had developed seven clinical guidelines in conjunction with the American Medical Association (AMA) and 12 academic medical centers. Each includes a review of the literature and ratings of appropriateness and necessity. The seven clinical practice guidelines cover:

- percutaneous transluminal coronary angioplasty;
- coronary artery bypass graft surgery;
- coronary angiography;
- abdominal aortic aneurysm surgery;

- carotid endarterectomy;
- hysterectomy; and
- prenatal care.

A Canadian study discusses clinical decision making regarding carotid bruits and indications for surgery. This research was published by Sauve et al., "Does This Patient Have a Clinically Important Carotid Bruit?," *Journal of the American Medical Association*, Vol. 270, No. 15, December 15, 1993, pp. 2843–45.

AHCPR also has sponsored research to develop criteria that would indicate when a hysterectomy is necessary. "Indications for Hysterectomy" by Karen J Carlson, David H. Nichols, and Isaac Schiff was published in the March 25, 1993 issue of the *New England Journal of Medicine*, Vol. 328, No. 12, pp. 856–860.

RAND monographs are included in the bibliography of RAND publications entitled "Health-Related Research." Prices range from $7.50 to $20, plus shipping and handling. Ordering instructions can be obtained by contacting:

The RAND Corporation
Publications Department
PO Box 2138
Santa Monica, CA 90407-2138
(310) 393-0411, Ext. 6686

Selected RAND Abstracts contains subject and author indexes, citations, and abstracts. Five university libraries in Florida have subscriptions for RAND publications: the University of Miami Library, in Coral Gables; the University of Florida Library, in Gainesville; the Florida International University Library, in Miami; the Florida State University Library, in Tallahassee; and the University of South Florida Library, in Tampa.

National Institutes of Health medical consensus statements

The National Cancer Institute, the National Institute of Mental Health, and the other institutes that comprise the National Institutes of Health (NIH) convene conferences on various medical topics. According to the NIH, the conferences are convened to "evaluate available scientific information and to resolve safety and efficacy issues related to biomedical technology." The product of these conferences is a "consensus statement" that reflects the opinion of distinguished national experts.

Panels of national experts draft the consensus statements based on a review of the literature and discussions with researchers. The consensus statements are intended to, "advance understanding of the technology or issue in question and to be useful to health professionals and the public." The conferences are held at the National Institutes of Health campus in Bethesda, Maryland.

Although the NIH consensus statements are written primarily for physicians and the scientific community they contain a great deal of readily understandable information regarding the diagnosis and treatment of medical problems. The most important findings and conclusions are summarized in the conclusions and recommendations section at the end of each consensus statement.

Some of the consensus statements that are available from the NIH's Office of Medical Applications of Research:

Cancer

—*Adjuvant Chemotherapy for Breast Cancer* (1985)
—*Management of Clinically Localized Prostate Cancer* (1987)
—*Oral Complications of Cancer Therapies: Diagnosis, Prevention, and Treatment* (1989)
—*Adjuvant Therapy for Patients with Colon and Rectum Cancer* (1990)
—*Sunlight, Ultraviolet Radiation, and the Skin* (1989)
—*Treatment of Early-State Breast Cancer* (1990)
—*Diagnosis and Treatment of Early Melanoma* (1992)

As discussed earlier, treatment guidelines (physician and patient statements) on over 80 types of cancer, information on clinical trials, directories of physicians who treat cancer, and physicians and organizations active in cancer research can be obtained by contacting the National Cancer Institute at (800) 4-CANCER or by using the CancerFax system. NCI information, including physician treatment guidelines, is available to patients.

Mental health

—*Drugs and Insomnia: The Use of Medications to Promote Sleep* (1983)
—*Mood Disorders: Pharmacologic Prevention of Recurrences* (1984)
—*Electroconvulsive Therapy* (1985)
—*Differential Diagnosis of Dementing Diseases* (1987)
—*Treatment of Destructive Behaviors in Persons with Developmental Disabilities* (1989)
—*Treatment of Panic Disorder* (1991)
—*Diagnosis and Treatment of Depression in Late Life* (1991)

Women and children

—*Estrogen Use and Postmenopausal Women* (1979)
—*Febrile Seizures* (1980)
—*Cesarean Childbirth* (1980)
—*The Diagnosis and Treatment of Reye's Syndrome* (1981)
—*Defined Diets and Childhood Hyperactivity* (1982)
—*Diagnostic Ultrasound Imaging in Pregnancy* (1984)
—*Infantile Apnea and Home Monitoring* (1986)
—*Early Identification of Hearing Impairment in Infants and Young Children* (1993)
—*Effect of Antenatal Corticosteroids on Perinatal Outcomes* (1994)

The elderly

—*Osteoporosis* (1984)
—*Geriatric Assessment Methods for Clinical Decision Making* (1987)
—*Urinary Incontinence* (1988)
—*Noise and Hearing Loss* (1990)
—*Treatment of Sleep Disorders of Older Persons* (1990)

Dentistry

—*Removal of Third Molars* (1979)
—*Dental Sealants in the Prevention of Tooth Decay* (1983)
—*Anesthesia and Sedation in the Dental Office* (1985)
—*Dental Implants* (1988)

Other medical problems

—*Pain, Discomfort, and Humanitarian Care* (1979)
—*Computed Tomographic Scanning of the Brain* (1981)
—*Total Hip Joint Replacement* (1982)
—*Treatment of Hypertriglyceridemia* (1983)
—*Analgesic-Associated Kidney Disease* (1984)
—*Lowering Blood Cholesterol to Prevent Heart Disease* (1984)
—*Travelers' Diarrhea* (1985)
—*Health Implications of Obesity* (1985)
—*Health Implications of Smokeless Tobacco Use* (1986)
—*Prevention of Venous Thrombosis and Pulmonary Embolism* (1986)
—*Integrated Approach to the Management of Pain* (1986)
—*The Utility of Therapeutic Plasmapheresis for Neurological Disorders* (1986)
—*Platelet Transfusion Therapy* (1986)
—*Diet and Exercise in Noninsulin-Dependent Diabetes Mellitus* (1986)
—*Neurofibromatosis* (1987)
—*Magnetic Resonance Imaging* (1987)
—*Prevention and Treatment of Kidney Stones* (1988)
—*Cochlear Implants* (1988)
—*Therapeutic Endoscopy and Bleeding Ulcers* (1989)
—*Surgery for Epilepsy* (1990)
—*Diagnosis and Management of Asymptomatic Primary Hyperthyroidism* (1990)
—*Gastrointestinal Surgery for Severe Obesity* (1991)
—*Acoustic Neuroma* (1991)
—*Triglyceride, High Density Lipoprotein, and Coronary Heart Disease* (1992)
—*Gallstones and Laparoscopic Cholecystectomy* (1992)
—*Impotence* (1992)
—*Morbidity and Mortality of Dialysis* (1993)

Consensus statements are available at no cost from the National Institutes of Health:

The Office of Medical Applications of Research
National Institutes of Health
Building 1, Room 260
Bethesda, Maryland 20892
(301) 496-1143

Medical specialty society practice guidelines

The American College of Cardiology and the American Heart Association have developed guidelines for diagnostic and surgical procedures of the heart. The guidelines are published in the *Journal of the American College of Cardiology*. Medical school libraries and certain other libraries subscribe to this journal. Libraries that do not have subscriptions, such as local public libraries, often can obtain copies of these articles through inter-library loan programs. These guidelines, written for health care professionals and hospitals, include:

"Guidelines and Indications for Coronary Artery Bypass Graft Surgery." *Journal of the American College of Cardiology*, Vol. 17, No. 3, March 1, 1991, pages 543–89.

"ACC/AHA Guidelines for Cardiac Catheterization and Cardiac Catheterization Laboratories." *Journal of the American College of Cardiology*, Vol. 18, No. 5, November 1, 1991, pages 1149–82.

"ACC/AHA Guidelines for Percutaneous Transluminal Coronary Angioplasty." *Journal of the American College of Cardiology*, Vol. 12, No. 2, August 1988, pages 529–45. (A revised guideline was expected to be published late in 1993).

"Guidelines for Coronary Angiography." *Journal of the American College of Cardiology*, Vol. 10, No. 4. October 1987, pages 935–50.

"Guidelines for the Early Management of Patients with Acute Myocardial Infarction." *Journal of the American College of Cardiology*, Vol. 16, No. 2, August 1990, pages 249–92.

"Guidelines for Implantation of Cardiac Pacemakers and Antiarrhythmia Devices." *Journal of the American College of Cardiology*, Vol. 18. No. 1. July 1991, pages 1–13.

"ACC/AHA Guidelines for Electrocardiography." *Journal of the American College of Cardiology*, Vol. 19. No. 3, March 1, 1992, pages 473–81.

"Guidelines for Clinical Intracardiac Electrophysiologic Studies." *Journal of the American College of Cardiology*, Vol. 14, No. 7, December 1989, pages 1827–42.

"ACC/AHA Guidelines for the Clinical Application of Echocardiography." *Journal of the American College of Cardiology*, Vol. 16, No. 7, December 1990, pages 150528.

"Guidelines for the Management of Congestive Heart Failure." (Under development, expected publication in 1994.)

It is important to note that guidelines are sometimes revised to account for advances in medical science. The American College of Cardiology can be contacted to learn if a guideline has been updated or if a guideline on a new topic has been published:

American College of Cardiology
Special Projects
9111 Old Georgetown Road
Bethesda, Maryland 20814

Several medical specialty societies publish catalogs that include policy statements, educational material, and practice guidelines for medical problems. The medical specialty societies listed below can be contacted to obtain ordering information:

American Academy of Pediatrics
Publications Department
PO Box 927
Elk Grove Village, Il 60009-0927
(800) 433-9016

American College of Physicians
Customer Service
(800) 523-1546

American Academy of Family Physicians
Order Department
(800) 944-0000

American Academy of Obstetricians
and Gynecologists
Resource Center
(202) 863-2518

AMA *Directory of Practice Parameters*

The American Medical Association (AMA) publishes *Directory of Practice Parameters: Titles, Sources, and Updates*. This directory includes about 1,500 practice guidelines and standards. (Full text practice parameters are available on CD-ROM, *Practice Parameters on CD-ROM*, 1994). Some of the libraries that subscribe to MEDLINE may have the AMA directory and the CD-ROM full text product. Libraries affiliated with hospitals, medical schools, and nursing programs in universities and community colleges also may have these publications. In 1994 the cost of the directory was $99 for members and $149 for non-members. The CD-ROM version was $995 for a single-user version. For information on how to order AMA practice guideline products, contact:

Ordering Department
The American Medical Association
P.O. Box 109050
Chicago, Il 60610-9050
(800) 621-8335

MEDLINE and the National Library of Medicine

The National Library of Medicine's MEDLARS (Medical Literature Analysis and Retrieval System) computer system is designed for physicians, health care professionals, and the scientific community. MEDLARS has over 34 separate computer data bases and is the most comprehensive medical data base in existence.

- MEDLINE contains more than seven million bibliographic citations from more than 3,600 international biomedical journals covering medicine, nursing, dentistry, veterinary medicine, and the preclinical sciences.
- CANCERLIT contains more than 800,000 citations and abstracts from medical journals and other sources on cancer research.
- PDQ contains cancer treatment information, clinical trial information, and information on physicians and cancer treatment facilities.

The Evidence-Based Medicine Working Group, a prestigious group of physicians and medical researchers in Canada and the U.S., has begun to publish a series of articles to help physicians use medical research to make the best treatment decisions. The group is chaired by Gordon H. Guyatt, M.D., of McMaster University in Hamilton, Ontario. These new publications will replace the *Readers' Guides* that were published by McMaster University in 1981, which have been translated into seven foreign languages and are heavily referenced in clinical literature.

The new series, *Users' Guides to the Medical Literature*, is published in the *Journal of the American Medical Association (JAMA)*. As this book went to press, two articles had been published in *JAMA*, with additional articles slated to be published throughout 1994. The first article, "How to Get Started," (Nov. 3, 1993) includes a discussion on how to use MEDLINE to identify articles that can be consulted to help solve clinical problems. The second (Dec. 1, 1993) gives advice on how to determine if an article has valid results.

MEDLINE can be used to locate the articles in this series by searching for *Users' Guides to the Medical Literature*. Article reprint requests should be directed to:

Gordon H. Guyatt, M.D., Chairman
The Evidence-Based Medicine Working Group
McMaster University Health Sciences Centre
1200 Main Street West, Room 2C12
Hamilton, Ontario
Canada L8N 3Z5

MEDLINE can be used to identify articles that discuss specific medical problems, conditions, and treatment options (see Lindberg et al. 1993). MEDLINE may be searched by using subject headings or by using key words. MEDLINE includes Medical Subject Headings (MeSH) and Publication Type (PT) codes that can be used to narrow searches to include only those articles that meet specific criteria. According to the Evidence-Based Medicine Working Group, using "META-ANALYSIS" for a PT code is more likely to identify a methodologically sound article than using "REVIEW." In addition, "PRACTICE GUIDELINE" has been added as a search term. The key words "breast cancer" and "chemotherapy" will identify all journal articles that discuss chemotherapy as a treatment for breast cancer. The abstract (summary) of the articles that meet the search specifications then can be retrieved from MEDLINE.

Some Florida libraries charge for MEDLINE search time. According to the National Library of Medicine, a typical search takes about 10 to 15 minutes of computer time and the typical charge is about $35 an hour. Therefore, the average charge is about $6 to $9. Some libraries use a CD-ROM (compact disk) version of MEDLINE, for which there usually is not a charge. The CD-ROM version is very easy to use and very fast. Persons with minimal computer skills should have little difficulty using it. Libraries in Florida with MEDLARS include hospital medical libraries, academic libraries, and National Library of Medicine Resource Libraries.

Physicians and others with home computers also can subscribe to the MEDLARS system and use MEDLINE through a modem. For information on subscribing to MEDLARS, contact:

MEDLARS Management Section
National Library of Medicine
Building 38A, Room 4N421
8600 Rockville Pike
Bethesda, Maryland 20894
(800) 638-8480

Three National Network libraries in Florida are designated as "Resource Libraries": the University of Florida in Gainesville; the University of South Florida in Tampa; and the University of Miami. All of these libraries make MEDLARS services available to the public, participate in an on-line inter-library document loan program, and have staff who are trained in using the MEDLARS data bases.

Libraries With Public Access to MEDLINE
Member Library of National Network of Libraries of Medicine

Bradenton
Manatee Memorial Hospital
Wentzel Medical Library
206 2nd Street, E.
Bradenton, FL 34208
(813) 746-5111

Fort Lauderdale
Holy Cross Hospital
Medical Staff Library
4725 N. Federal Highway
Fort Lauderdale, FL 33308
(305) 771-8000

Gainesville
University of Florida
Health Sciences Library
Gainesville, FL 32610-0206
(904) 392-4018

Jacksonville
University of Florida Health Science Center
Borland Library
PO Box 44226
Jacksonville, FL 32231-4226
(904) 549-3240

Melbourne
Holmes Regional Medical Center
Medical Library
1350 South Hickory Street
Melbourne, FL 32901
(407) 727-7000

Miami
Baptist Hospital
Health Sciences Library
8900 N. Kendall Drive
Miami, FL 33176
(305) 596-6506

University of Miami School of Medicine
Louis Calder Memorial Library
PO Box 016950
Miami, FL 33101
(305) 547-6749

Orlando
Florida Hospital
Medical Library
601 E. Rollins Street
Orlando, FL 32803-1248
(407) 897-1860

Florida Hospital/East Orlando
Health Sciences Library
7727 Lake Underhill Drive
Orlando, FL 32822
(407) 277-8110

Sarasota
Sarasota Memorial Hospital
Medical Library
1700 S. Tamiami Trail
Sarasota, FL 34239-3555
(813) 953-1730

Tallahassee
Florida A & M University
Schools of Nursing/Allied Health
Sciences Library
Florida A & M University
Tallahassee, FL 32307
(904) 599-3900

Florida State University
Paul Dirac Science Library
Tallahassee, Florida 32306-2047
(904) 644-5534

Tampa
Shriners Hospital for Crippled Children
Professional Library
12502 North Pine Drive
Tampa, FL 33612-9499
(813) 972-2250

Tampa General Hospital
Medical Library
PO Box 1289, Davis Islands
Tampa, FL 33601
(813) 251-7328

University Community Hospital
Medical Library
3100 E. Fletcher Avenue
Tampa, FL 33613-4688

University of South Florida
Health Sciences Center Library
12901 Bruce B. Downs Blvd.
Tampa, FL 33612-4799
(813) 974-2123

If you do not see a convenient library listed, non-network libraries that may have MEDLINE and make it available to the public include libraries in universities and community colleges with nursing programs. When contacting libraries to inquire if they have MEDLINE, ask for "reference."

There are other libraries with MEDLINE in Florida that do not make this service available to the public. Most of these are hospital medical libraries. However, it may be possible to use MEDLINE in these facilities through a physician who has hospital staff privileges.

Special medical data bases

The Online Journal of Clinical Trials makes available articles that have been accepted for publication in scientific journals but have not yet appeared in print. Subscribers thus have access to new studies weeks or even months before publication. The Online Journal of Clinical Trials is a joint project of the American Association for the Advancement of Science and the Online Computer Library Center. The system can be accessed by using an IBM compatible personal computer and modem. For information contact:

Director of Publications
Online Journal of Clinical Trials
AAAS
1333 H Street, N.W.
Washington, D.C. 20005

The Reproductive Toxicology Center makes available REPROTOX, a computer data base that contains information on the effects of more than 4,000 chemical and physical agents on reproduction. The data base can be accessed by a personal computer and modem.

According to the Reproductive Toxicology Center, "Advances in synthetic chemistry have led to an increasingly complex chemical environment that includes drugs, food additives, pesticides, and radiation, as well as water and air pollutants. It is estimated that persons of childbearing age are routinely exposed to thousands of agents." The center "promotes understanding about the effects of the chemical and physical environment on human fertility, pregnancy, and development." To obtain more information contact:

Reproductive Toxicology Center
Columbia Hospital for Women Medical Center
2440 M Street, N.W., Suite 217
Washington, D.C. 20037-1404
(202) 293-5137

AHCPR *Health Technology Assessment Reports*

The Agency for Health Care Policy and Research (AHCPR) also sponsors research that evaluates the safety and effectiveness of new medical diagnostic and treatment technologies. To evaluate each medical technology, the AHCPR conducts a literature review and obtains advice from national experts, including medical speciality societies. The results are then analyzed and an assessment report is prepared as part of the "Health Technology Assessment Reports" series.

Since 1981, when the *Health Technology Assessment Report* series began, more than 140 reports have been released. Selected topics include:
  • *Extracorporeal Shock Wave Lithotripsy Procedures for the Treatment of Kidney Stones* (1985), PB86-121811/AS

- *Percutaneous Ultrasound Procedures for the Treatment of Kidney Stones* (1985), PB86-121829/AS
- *Transurethral Ureteroscopic Lithotripsy Procedures for the Treatment of Kidney Stones* (1987), PB88-2050113
- *Continuous Positive Airway Pressure for the Treatment of Obstructive Sleep Apnea in Adults* (1986), PB87-190374/AS
- *Patient Selection Criteria for Percutaneous Transluminal Coronary Angioplasty* (1985), PB86-133808/AS
- *Magnetic Resonance Imaging* (1985), PB86-132131/AS
- *Apheresis in the Treatment of Guillain-Barre Syndrome* (1985), PB86-151024/AS
- *Endoscopic Electrocoagulation in the Treatment of Upper Gastrointestinal Bleeding* (1986), PB88-157797/AS
- *Cardiac Rehabilitation Services* (1987), PB90-101346
- *Chemical Aversion Therapy for the Treatment of Alcoholism* (1987), PB89-156681
- *Endoscopic Laser Photocoagulation in the Treatment of Upper Gastrointestinal Bleeding* (1987), PB90-101338.
- *Reassessment of Autologous Bone Marrow Transplantation* (1988), PB90-101098
- *Assessment of Liver Transplantation* (1990), PB90-101304
- *Diagnosis and Treatment of Impotence* (1990), PB90-101411
- *Extracranial-Intracranial Bypass to Reduce the Risk of Ischemic Stroke* (1990), PHS91-3473.
- *Cardiac Catheterization in a Freestanding Setting* (1989), PB90-101213
- *Assessment of Liver Transplantation* (1990), PB90-101304

All *Health Technology Assessment Reports* are free. To obtain a list of the reports or to order a report, contact:

AHCPR Publications Clearinghouse
P.O. Box 8547
Silver Spring, Maryland 20907-8547
(800) 358-9295 or (301) 495-3453

InfoTrac Health Reference Center database

Some public libraries have the InfoTrac Health Reference Center computer system, an easy-to-use medical information system. It is an excellent source of general health care information on alcohol and drug abuse, nutrition guidelines, disease and treatment information, AIDS, cancer and heart conditions, pregnancy and childbirth, sports medicine and training, and other topics. The system includes articles from the popular media, abstracts and articles from many professional journals such as the Journal of the American Medical Association, definitions of medical terms and problems, and other health information. The data base is updated monthly and contains articles from more than 160 publications.

In 1992, about a dozen Florida libraries subscribed to the InfoTrac system. According to Infotrac, these usually were the main public libraries in the larger Florida cities. To learn the location of the nearest library that has the InfoTrac Health Reference Center, telephone:

Basic Products Group
Information Access Company
(800) 227-8431

National Institute on Aging

The National Institute on Aging sponsors research and publishes extensively on aging and health care problems. Information is available for free to both health care professionals and the public. Of particular interest is the research bulletin series. In addition, the National Institute on Aging published an excellent 240-page "Resource Directory for Older People" which is also available for free. For a list of their publications, or to request a publication, contact:

National Institute on Aging
Information Center
PO Box 8057
Gaithersburg, MD 20898-8057
(800) 222-2225

Institutes of the National Institutes of Health

Twelve institutes comprise the National Institutes of Health. The National Institute also houses three national centers. All can be contacted to obtain research articles, bibliographies, and other information. They are:
—National Institute on Aging
—National Institute of Allergy and Infectious Diseases
—National Institute of Arthritis and Musculoskeletal and Skin Diseases
—National Cancer Institute
—National Institutes of Child Health and Human Development
—National Institute on Deafness and Other Communications Disorders
—National Institute of Diabetes and Digestive and Kidney Diseases
—National Institutes of Dental Research
—National Institute of Environmental Health Sciences
—National Eye Institute
—National Institutes of General Medical Sciences
—National Heart, Lung, and Blood Institute
—National Institutes of Mental Health
—National Institutes of Neurological Disorders and Stroke
—National Center for Human Genome Research
—National Center for Nursing Research
—National Center for Research Resources

All of the National Institute of Health institutes and centers share the same address:

Public Health Service
Building 31
9000 Rockville Pike
Bethesda, Maryland 20892

STATE AND NATIONAL SOURCES OF INFORMATION FOR PERSONS WITH SPECIFIC HEALTH PROBLEMS

AIDS
AIDS Clinical Trials
U.S. Public Health Service
(800) 874-2572

National AIDS Clearinghouse
U.S. Public Health Service
(800) 458-5231

Florida AIDS Hotline
(800) FLA-AIDS

Florida AIDS Hotline (Spanish)
(800) 545-SIDA

Florida AIDS Hotline (Creole)
(800) AIDS-101

National AIDS Hotline
(800) 342-AIDS

Alcohol and drug abuse
National Clearinghouse for Alcohol
and Drug Information
(800) 729-6686

Families Anonymous
PO Box 528
Van Nuys, CA 91408

Allergies
(also see Asthma)

American Academy of Allergy and
  Immunology
(800) 822-2762

Alzheimer's Disease
Alzheimer's Association
(800) 272-3900

Anxiety disorders
Anxiety Disorders Association of
  America
6000 Executive Boulevard, Suite 200
Rockville, Maryland 20852-4004

Arthritis
Arthritis Foundation
(800) 283-7800

National Arthritis and Musculoskeletal
  and Skin Diseases Information
  Clearinghouse
(301) 495-4484

Asthma
Asthma and Allergy Foundation
(800) 7-ASTHMA

Balance Disorders
Vestibular Disease Association
P.O. Box 4467
Portland, Oregon 97208-4467
(800) 837-8428

Blood pressure
National High Blood Pressure Association
(301) 951-3260

Burns
Phoenix Society
(215) 946-4788

Cancer
AMC Cancer Information
(800) 525-3777

American Cancer Society Cancer
  Response Line
(800) ACS-2345

National Cancer Institute
Cancer Information Service
(800) 4-CANCER

(see discussion in Chapter One)
Y-Me Breast Cancer Support Program
(800) 221-2141

Cerebral Palsy
United Cerebral Palsy Association
(800) USA-1UCP

Cleft Palate
American Cleft Palate Association
(800) 24-CLEFT

Cystic Fibrosis
Cystic Fibrosis Foundation Association
(800) 344-4823 or (301) 881-9130

Diabetes
American Diabetes Association
(800) ADA-DISC

National Diabetes Information
  Clearinghouse
(301) 468-2162 or 496-7433

Juvenile Diabetes Foundation
International Hotline
(800) 223-1138

Digestive diseases
National Digestive Disease Education and
Information Clearinghouse
(301) 496-9707

National Foundation for Ileitis and Colitis
(212) 685-3440

United Ostomy Association
(213) 413-5510

Disabling conditions
(also see Hearing and speech)

Canine Companions for Independence
(800) 767-BARK

IBM National Support Center for Persons
with Disabilities
(800) IBM-2133 Voice/TTD

Job Accommodation Network
(800) 526-7234

Library of Congress National Library
Services for the Blind and Physically
Handicapped
(800) 424-8567

National Center for Youth with Disabilities
(800) 333-NCYD

National Easter Seals Society
(800) 221-6827

National Handicapped Sports and
Recreational Association
(301) 217-0960 or
(202) 393-7505

National Head Injury Foundation Family
Helpline
(800) 444-6443

National Information Center for Children
and Youth with Handicaps
(800) 999-5599

National Information System for Health
Related Services—Chronically Ill and
Developmentally Disabled Children Up
to Age 21
(800) 922-9234

National Rehabilitation Information Center
(800) 34-NARIC

Domestic violence
Domestic Violence Hotline
(800) 333-SAFE

Down Syndrome
National Down Syndrome Congress
(800) 232-6372

National Down Syndrome Society
(800) 221-4602

Elderly
American Association of Retired Persons
Health Advocacy Services
(202) 434-2277

National Institute on Aging
(800) 222-2225

Emphysema
Emphysema Anonymous
(813) 334-4226

Epilepsy
Epilepsy Foundation of America
Landover, Maryland
(301) 459-3700

Epilepsy Information Hotline
Epilepsy Foundation of America
(800) 332-1000

Eyes
National Eye Care Project Helpline
(800) 222-3937

Food addiction
National Food Addiction Hotline
(800) 872-0088

General health
National Health
Information Center
(800) 336-4797
(703) 522-2590 (in Virginia)

National Heart, Lung, and Blood
Institute Education Programs
Information Center
(301) 951-3260

Headache
National Headache Foundation
(800) 843-2256

Hearing and speech

American Speech-Language Hearing
  Association
(800) 638-8255

Better Hearing Institute Helpline
(800) 424-8576

Deafness Research Foundation
(800) 535-3323

Dial A Hearing Screening Test
(800) 222-EARS

Ear Foundation
(800) 545-4327

Hearing Helpline
(800) 327-9355

National Hearing Aid Helpline
(800) 521-5247

National Information Center on Deafness
(202) 651-5109

Tele-Consumer Hotline
(800) 332-1124

Heart problems

American Heart Association
(800) AHA-USA1

Impotence

Impotence Information Center
(800) 843-4315

Recovery of Male Potency
(800) 835-7667

Kidney disease
(see Urological Disorders)

Lead poisoning

National Lead Information Center
(800) 532-3394

Learning disorders
(also see Handicapping Conditions)

The Orton Dyslexia Society
(800) ABCD-123

Liver diseases

American Liver Foundation
(800) 223-0179

Lung diseases

Asthma Information Line
(800) 822-ASMA

National Jewish Center's
Lung Line
(800) 222-5864

Lung Line
National Asthma Center
(800) 222-5864

Lupus

American Lupus Society
(800) 331-1802

Lupus Foundation of America
(800) 558-0121
(212) 685-4118 (New York)

Terri Gotthelf Lupus Research
  Institute
(800) 82-LUPUS

Mental health
(see Chapter 7)

Multiple Sclerosis

National Multiple Sclerosis Society
(800) 624-8236 (recording)
(800) 227-3166 (staff member)

Nutrition

American Dietetic Association
Consumer Nutrition Hot Line
(800) 366-1655

Lifeline Foundation
(enteral or parenteral feeding)
(617) 784-3250

Orthopaedic problems

American Academy of Orthopaedic
  Surgeons
Orthopaedic Research Education
  Foundation
(708) 698-9980

Osteoporosis

National Osteoporosis Foundation
(202) 223-2226

Pain

American Chronic Pain Association
Monroeville, Pennsylvania
(412) 856-9676

National Chronic Pain Outreach
  Association
Bethesda, Maryland
(301) 652-4998

Paralysis and spinal cord injury
(also see Handicapping Conditions)

American Paralysis Association
(800) 225-0292

APA Spinal Cord Injury Hotline
(800) 526-3456

National Rehabilitation Information
Clearinghouse
(800) 34-NARIC

National Spinal Cord Injury Association
(800) 962-9629

National Stroke Association
(800) 367-1990

Parkinson's Disease
American Parkinson Disease Association
(800) 223-2732 or (212) 732-9550

National Parkinson Foundation
(305) 547-6666 (in Florida)
(800) 327-4545 (national)

Parkinson's Education Program
(800) 344-7872

Poisoning
Poison Control Center
(800) 282-3171

Pregnancy
American College of Obstetricians and
Gynecologists
409 12th Street, S.W.
Washington, D.C. 20024

ASPO/Lamaze
(800) 368-4404

International Childbirth Education
Association
(800) 624-4934

LaLeche League International
(800) 525-3243

National Abortion Federation
1-800-772-9100

Pregnancy Counseling Services
(800) 368-3336

Healthy Baby Hotline
(800) 451-BABY

Psoriasis
National Psoriasis Foundation
(503) 297-1545

Rare disorders
American Leprosy Missions
(800) 543-3131

Amyotrophic Lateral Sclerosis
Association
(800) 782-4747

Amyotrophic Lateral Sclerosis Society
(213) 990-2151

National ALS Foundation
(212) 679-4016

Ankylosing Spondylitis Association
(800) 777-8189

Batten Disease Support
(800) 448-4570

Centers for Disease Control
Rare Disease Hotline
(800) 456-3505

Cooley's Anemia Foundation
(800) 221-3571

Cornelia de Lange Syndrome Foundation
(800) 223-8355

Crohn's and Colitis Foundation
(800) 343-3637

Histiocytosis-X Association of America
(800) 548-2758

Huntington's Disease Foundation of
America
(212) 757-0443

Huntington's Disease Society of America
(800) 345-4372

Iron Overload Disease Association
433 Westwind Drive
North Palm Beach, FL 33408
National Lymphedema Network
(800) 541-3259

Meniere's Network
(800) 545-4327

Muscular Dystrophy Association
(212) 986-3240

Myasthenia Gravis Foundation
(800) 541-5454
(212) 889-8157 (New York)

American Narcolepsy Association
(800) 222-6085

National Neurofibromatosis Foundation
(800) 323-7938

National Organization for Rare Disorders
(800) 999-6673
(203) 746-6518 (in Connecticut)
(212) 686-1057 (in New York)

National Information Center for Orphan
   Drugs and Rare Diseases
(800) 456-3505

National Reye's Syndrome Foundation
(800) 233-7393

National Retinitis Pigmentosa Foundation
(800) 638-2300

Sarcoidosis Family Aid and Research
   Foundation
(800) 225-6872

Scleroderma Foundation
(800) 722-HOPE

Sturge-Weber Disease Foundation
800) 627-5482

Tourette Syndrome Association
(800) 237-0717

National Tuberous Sclerosis Assn.
(800) 225-6872

Sexuality
Sex Information and Education Council of
   the United States
(212) 673-3850

National STD Hotline
(800) 227-8922

American Assoc. of Sex Educators
   Counselors, & Therapists
435 N. Michigan Ave, Suite 1717
Chicago, Ill. 60611-4067

Sickle Cell Disease
National Association for Sickle Cell
   Disease
(800) 421-8453

Spina Bifida
Spina Bifida Information and Referral
(800) 621-3141

Stress
American Institute of Stress
124 Park Avenue
Yonkers, New York 10703

Stroke
Courage Stroke Network
(800) 553-6321

American Heart Association
(800) AHA-USA1

Sudden Infant Death Syndrome
American SIDS Institute
(800) 232-SIDS

National SIDS Foundation
(800) 221-SIDS

Urological disorders
American Kidney Fund
(800) 638-8299

National Kidney Foundation
(800) 622-9010
(212) 889-2210

Simon Foundation
(800) 23-SIMON

Vision
American Council of the Blind
(800) 424-8666

American Foundation for the Blind
(800) 232-5463

Guide Dog Foundation for the Blind
(800) 548-4337

The Lighthouse National Center
(800) 334-5497

National Association for Parents of the
   Visually Impaired
(800) 562-6265

National Center for Sight
(800) 221-3004

National Eye Care
Eye exams for low-income elderly
(800) 222-EYES

National Eye Research Foundation
(800) 621-2258

Women
(also see Pregnancy)

Endometriosis Association
(800) 992-ENDO

PMS Access
(800) 222-4767

National Institute of Health
Office of Research on Women's Health
(301) 402-1770

Women's Health Initiative
(information on post-menopausal women
and hormone replacement therapy)
(301) 402-2900

Women, Infants and Children Information Line
(nutrition program for pregnant or
breastfeeding women with
low-incomes)
(800) 342-3556

CHAPTER 2
Choosing a physician

As medical science advances, choosing a physician becomes an increasingly difficult decision. To receive high quality health care for serious medical problems, it is important for a physician to stay current with state-of-the-art information on diagnosis and treatment and to be affiliated with the best health care facilities.

Although the selection of a physician is a very important decision, studies have not identified good "predictors" that identify physicians with superior skills. Some health care writers state that a physician's reputation may well be the most important indication, particularly for surgical or other specialty care.

Research has found that surgical expertise is related to how frequently a procedure is performed. As discussed in Chapter 3, joint American College of Cardiology and American Heart Association guidelines call for physicians and hospitals to meet certain surgical volume thresholds to maintain proficiency. In addition, it is reasonable to assume that, in general, physicians who are affiliated with medical schools and teaching hospitals, and physicians who participate in clinical trials, may have more current medical knowledge and expertise than other physicians.

The choice of a primary care physician—a family practitioner, obstetrician, pediatrician, or specialist in internal medicine—is an important decision not only to ensure that appropriate care is received for routine problems, but also to help ensure that one is referred to the best specialists. The emphasis the primary care practitioner places on good health habits also can be important. Finally, although medical skills obviously are critically important, it also is important for physicians, particularly primary care physicians, to have good communication skills.

An article published in the *Journal of the American Medical Association* argues that a good physician-patient relationship is time-consuming, and that physicians should "persuade" rather than "impose" a course of treatment. The article concluded that,

> *"The essence of doctoring is a fabric of knowledge, understanding, teaching, and action, in which the caring physician integrates the patient's medical condition and health-related values, makes a recommendation on the appropriate course of action, and tries to persuade the patient of the worthiness of this approach and the values it realizes,"* (Emanuel and Emanuel 1992).

STUDIES ON PHYSICIANS AND QUALITY OF CARE

According to a 1988 federal Office of Technology Assessment (OTA) study on the quality of medical care, physicians who perform high volumes of certain procedures may be more successful in maintaining or improving their skills. Nurses and other hospital staff who care for high volumes of certain types of patients also may become more skilled and proficient.

A study sponsored by the National Center for Health Research examined the relationship between the volume of patients treated by physicians and hospital quality of care (Kelly and Hellinger 1987). The study examined more than 11,000 non-surgical patients who were treated for acute myocardial infarction (AMI) in 146 hospitals during 1977. The study found that the *hospital* volume of treating AMI patients was not a factor in patient survival. Rather, the study found AMI patients were more likely to survive if their *physicians* treated high volumes of AMI patients. In addition, AMI patients treated in teaching facilities affiliated with a medical school were found to have higher survival rates than AMI patients treated in hospitals not affiliated with medical schools. The study found that the outcomes of nonsurgical heart patients "do not depend on operating room staff and are less dependent on complex medical equipment."

The *Medical Outcomes Study* analyzed the use of medical services by more than 20,000 adults seen by some 300 physicians in private practice in HMOs during 1986 (Greenfield et al. 1992 and Rosenblatt 1992). The physicians (family practitioners, general internists, endocrinologists, and cardiologists) were located in Boston, Chicago and Los Angeles. This is the first large scale study that has examined the interrelationship between the specialties of physician, the practice setting (physician office or HMO), the use of medical resources, and patient outcomes. Patient outcome findings had not been published as this book was went to press. The study took into account the severity of patients' illnesses and examined the care that they received. Key findings include:

- Private practice physicians, paid on a fee-for-service basis, hospitalized patients at a rate 41 percent higher than physicians employed by HMOs.
- Although HMO patients had 8 percent more office visits than private practice patients, private practice patients took 12 percent more prescription drugs than HMO patients.
- A future *Medical Outcomes Study* report will examine whether the additional medical services that were provided by the non-HMO physicians result in better patient outcomes.

The *Medical Outcomes Study* also has reported findings on how satisfied patients were in the care they received in private practice and HMO settings (Rubin et al. 1993). Although solo practice and fee for service settings were rated the highest, and group and prepaid/HMO settings the lowest, the differences in ratings were not great. The study found that 65 percent of patients seen by solo physicians paid under the fee for service system rated their care "excellent" in contrast to 59 percent in solo prepaid settings. Fifty percent of patients seen by multispecialty groups paid under fee for service arrangement, 46 percent in multispecialty group prepaid settings, and 49 percent in HMOs rated their care excellent. According to the authors, some of the differences in ratings may be attributed to the fact that solo practices had "lower proportions of new visits and greater continuity of care." HMOs saw larger proportions of new patients who had not established a relationship with a physician.

QUALIFICATIONS AND PROFESSIONAL EXPERTISE

Some physicians either are members of medical speciality boards or are eligible for membership. The former are referred to as "board-certified," while the latter are referred to as "board-eligible." There are two large nationally recognized medical speciality boards, the American Board of Medical Specialities and the Advisory Board for Osteopathic Specialists. To be a certified member, a physician must meet certain requirements such as completing a certain amount of training and passing an examination.

Although it is reasonable to assume that certification by a medical speciality board would be a good indicator of professional skills, research does not always support this view. The 1988 OTA study reviewed 13 studies published between 1976 and 1986 that examined board certification as an indicator of the quality of medical care. The report stated that although board certification helps to identify physicians who meet a standard set of qualifications and who pass a certification examination, board certification does not reflect the amount of experience, or measure proficiency, in the speciality. The report concluded that board certification was not a good predictor to identify physicians who provide high quality care. However, OTA cautioned that methodological problems in the design of these studies (such as small samples and a lack of data on how ill patients were) may have limited the accuracy of their findings. Some more recent studies have, however, found that hospitalized patients treated by board-certified physicians have better outcomes.

The criteria below, some of which were drawn from articles and books, may be useful in choosing either a primary care physician or a specialist. However, it is important to note that there is no evidence in the medical research literature regarding the effectiveness or validity of any of these criteria, with the exception of board certification.

- The opinions of nurses, particularly nurses who work in hospitals, and other health care professionals can be useful in selecting a physician. If a physician has admitting privileges at the best hospital or hospitals in your community, this may be an indication of professional excellence.
- A physician who teaches and who also maintains a private practice may have more current medical knowledge and expertise than a physician who does not teach. Likewise, physicians who participate in clinical trials or other scientific studies may have more specialized knowledge and expertise than others.
- Physicians who are members of Alpha Omega Alpha (AOA) had exceptionally high grades in medical school. Membership in the AOA is an academic honor extended to the best medical school students. In 1990, the AOA had more than 100 chapters and 50,000 members nationally. There are about 725,000 physicians in the U.S.; AOA membership includes about 7 percent of them.
- If complex surgery is needed, such as open heart surgery, the frequency with which the surgeon performs the procedure could be important. Many studies have shown a relationship between good outcomes and high volume for certain surgical procedures. For example, joint guidelines published by the American College of Cardiology and the American Heart Association recommend that, "in general, a yearly minimum of 100 to 150 open heart operations, the majority of which are coronary artery bypass operations, should be performed by each surgeon caring for patients with ischemic heart disease." Those preparing to undergo a new or complex surgical procedure should ask how often the surgeon has performed the procedure, what training the surgeon has received, and how successful the surgeon has been.
- The American Board of Medical Specialists, which can be reached by telephone at (800) 776-2378, provides information on whether a physician is certified by one of its 23 boards. These include boards of family practice, internal medicine, surgery, plastic surgery, thoracic surgery, and radiology.
- The initials F.A.C.P. after the name of a physician with a specialty in internal medicine indicates that he or she is a fellow in the American College of Physicians. Membership criteria include a requirement that the physician has made significant contributions to medical research or teaching, or has demonstrated clinical excellence. The FACP can be reached by telephone at (800) 523-1546.

- The National Cancer Institute (NCI) maintains a computer directory of physicians who are registered with them. The NCI can be reached at (800) 4-CANCER. Upon request a cancer information specialist will look in both the PDQ Protocol File and in the PDQ Physician Directory to determine whether a physician participates in active clinical trials or specializes in cancer treatment.
- If a physician has a degree in osteopathic medicine, the American Osteopathic Association (AOA) can be contacted to learn whether he or she is certified by the Advisory Board of Osteopathic Specialists in one of 18 medical specialities. The AOA certification office can be reached by telephone at (800) 621-1773.
- The Florida Department of Business and Professional Regulation can be contacted at (800) 342-7940 to learn whether "probable cause" has been found in pending complaints against a physician or whether disciplinary action has been taken in closed cases.

OTHER CONSIDERATIONS

In addition to medical expertise, there are other factors that can be considered in selecting a physician:
- Is the physician attentive and a good listener?
- Does the physician take the time to adequately explain his or her diagnostic and treatment decisions?
- Are complete answers provided to patients' questions? Bringing a written list of questions may help patients avoid forgetting to ask a pertinent question.
- Does the physician emphasize preventive care? Are good health habits such as diet and exercise discussed?
- Is a thorough medical history taken, including information on the medical problems of family members?
- Does the physician accept Medicare assignment? Physicians who accept assignment bill Medicare directly and accept the Medicare charge limit as payment in full. A list of Florida physicians who accept Medicare assignment can be obtained by calling Medicare Part B Customer Service at (800) 333-7586.
- Does the physician use economical laboratory, radiology, and treatment facilities? A recent state-sponsored study found that, because of overutilization costs were much higher when Florida physicians referred patients to diagnostic imaging centers, clinical laboratories, radiation therapy centers, and physical therapy or rehabilitation centers in which they held a financial interest.

Those who do not have health insurance and are paying the bill themselves should ask what price the physician will charge in relation to what he or she is paid by Medicare and private insurance companies for the same service. Sometimes persons without health insurance are charged higher fees than persons with insurance.

SECOND OPINIONS

Second opinions are an accepted medical practice, particularly for surgery. Second opinions are particularly important for severe problems, rare problems, or problems that are difficult to diagnose. The U.S. Department of Health and Human Services recommends that in the Medicare program patients should consider getting a second opinion when surgery is recommended for a non-emergency condition, such as tonsillitis, gall bladder procedures, hysterectomies, hernia repairs and cataract operations. When getting a second opinion, it is important to request that medical records be sent to the second physician to avoid repeating medical tests. The agency suggests that the following questions be posed to the physician:

- What is the problem?
- Have all the necessary tests been performed to confirm the diagnosis?
- What are the benefits and risks of proposed surgery?
- How long will the recovery period be and what is involved?
- How much experience has the surgeon had with this type of operation?
- What percentage of operations performed by the physician have been successful?
- What will happen if the surgery isn't done?
- Are there other ways to treat the condition?

The Medicare program has a hotline that provides the names of specialists who will provide second opinions. The Second Surgical Opinion Hotline can be reached at (800) 638-6833.

CHAPTER 3
Florida hospitals

There are substantial differences among Florida hospitals in the services they provide. Some hospitals treat a wide range of medical and surgical problems, while others specialize in the care of certain types of patients or certain medical problems. Hospitals vary in the numbers and specialties of physicians on their staffs, in the proportion of elderly persons they treat, in their number of hospital beds, in the use of beds by patients (occupancy), and in the severity and complexity of the illnesses and injuries they treat.

The services provided by acute care hospitals are discussed in this chapter. A handful of hospitals are not discussed—state mental and tuberculosis hospitals, prison hospitals, and hospitals on military bases. Chapter 7 discusses psychiatric hospitals and hospitals that treat persons for alcohol or drug problems. Chapter 8 discusses Veterans Administration hospitals.

SELECTING A HOSPITAL

Most often patients go to a particular hospital on the advice of their physician. Patients who choose a hospital themselves are in the minority. The findings of a national survey in 1989 on hospital patient satisfaction, however, found that patients who choose their hospital are more satisfied than those who go to a hospital on the advice of their physician. The survey found that only 26 percent of hospital selections were made by patients, while physicians made 58 percent of the selections. The remaining 16 percent were joint decisions, decisions made by health maintenance organizations (HMOs) or insurance companies, or emergency admissions.

As this book went to press, information regarding the quality of care provided by individual Florida hospitals was not available. Over the next few years, however, hospital-specific information regarding the quality of care provided by individual hospitals likely will become available to the public through accreditation organizations and state and federal agencies. The development of hospital quality of care measures is a very active area of research. Until that information becomes publicly available, however, the only data that sheds light on hospital quality is from national studies—and these studies have examined groups of hospitals, rather than individual ones.

The quality of care provided by hospitals is known to vary substantially. For example, a RAND study of 16,758 Medicare patients in 297 hospitals located in Florida and four other states found that patients who were cared for in hospitals with the lowest "process of care" scores (a measurement of quality of care) were 25 percent more likely to die within 30 days following their hospitalization than patients that received care in hospitals with higher scores (see Brook 1993). The study examined patients with one of four medical problems: congestive heart failure, heart attack, pneumonia, or stroke. Other studies have found differences in patient mortality rates among hospitals for open heart surgery and other surgical procedures. Researchers have found, however, that when different medical problems or procedures are studied in individual hospitals, the hospital often does not have either uniformly good or uniformly poor quality of care (Chassin 1993).

Many studies have examined whether patient volume and other hospital characteristics influence the quality of care that patients receive. Although many of these studies were conducted with very sophisticated research designs, and have yielded important perspectives on hospital care, their findings apply to groups of hospitals, rather than to individual hospitals.

Research studies that examine hospital quality often have found that for certain types of surgery, patient outcomes are often better in hospitals that perform a high volume of similar surgical procedures. Other recent research studies have found that patient outcomes are better in teaching hospitals, large urban hospitals, financially strong hospitals, and hospitals that care for large numbers of patients with specific medical illnesses or surgical problems. Research findings related to hospital volume for organ transplantation, open heart surgery, and cardiac catheterization are discussed later in this chapter.

The federal Office of Technology Assessment (OTA) (1988) cautions that one should not just "go by the numbers" regarding hospital or physician volume, but should consider other factors.

Many physicians have admitting privileges at more than one hospital. Almost all hospitals have a "physician referral" department to help persons who are interested in being admitted to a specific hospital but who do not have a physician to admit them. Hospitals often list their physician referral line in the telephone directory along with their other departments.

Hospital accreditation

The 1988 OTA study entitled, *The Quality of Medical Care, Information for Consumers*, reviewed research that examined the relationship between hospital quality and accreditation. Although OTA found that research studies have not determined that accredited hospitals or hospitals recognized by the National Cancer Institute (NCI), the American College of Surgeons, or other organizations, provide better care than other hospitals, the study stated, "It seems worthwhile for consumers to seek hospitals that have been judged by independent experts to have the appropriate resources to provide care, either overall or for specific conditions."

There are two organizations that accredit general hospitals, the Joint Commission for Accreditation of Healthcare Organizations (JCAHO) and the American Osteopathic Association (AOA). In addition, the Commission on Accreditation of Rehabilitation Facilities accredits hospitals that provide rehabilitative care. Hospitals accredited by these organizations also are included in this chapter but the JCAHO list of acute care general hospitals was limited to those hospitals that received the highest accreditation rating.

To improve the credibility and validity of accreditation, JCAHO will begin to use a new system to measure hospital performance in 1994. This new system will use patient outcomes and performance standards to accredit hospitals. Initially, only hospitals that volunteer to participate in the program will be included. By 1996, the new system is expected to include all hospitals. This program, the Indicator Monitoring System, will include obstetrics and anesthesia indicators during 1994. In 1995, trauma, oncology and cardiovascular care indicators will be added, and indicators that measure medication use and infection control will be included in 1996. According to JCAHO, these performance indicators will provide "relevant, reliable and valid" data for individual hospitals.

Hospital characteristics and quality of care

The 1988 OTA study reviewed 26 research studies that examined 15 different procedures and diagnoses provided by hospitals and physicians. OTA found that there was "rather substantial evidence that worse outcomes occur at lower volumes for most of the procedures and diagnoses that have been studied." Key findings in the OTA report are:

- "The evidence for hospitals overwhelmingly showed worse outcomes at lower volumes for coronary artery bypass surgery (CABG), intestinal operations, total hip replacement, cardiac catheterization, abdominal aortic aneurysm, and biliary tract surgery."
- The majority of studies that examined hysterectomies, prostatectomy operations, newborn diseases, appendectomies, hernia operations, acute myocardial infraction, and vascular surgery also found that worse outcomes occur at lower volumes.
- The majority of studies that examined stomach operations and fractures of the femur failed to find a relationship between volume and outcome.
- Research studies of cardiac surgery and organ transplantation have found that when a threshold is reached, the effect of better care at higher volumes weakens.
- Studies of cardiac surgery have found that a high combination of hospital and individual physician volume often produces the best surgical results.

Several studies have examined the relationship between the characteristics of hospitals and patient outcomes. Hospital characteristics have included size, location, medical staffing, medical school affiliation, numbers of patients, and financial viability. Because this research is very complex, researchers frequently qualify their research findings by stating that their findings are "a first step" in identifying types of hospitals that provide good care or that their findings are "suggestive."

A national study (Kelly and Hellinger 1986) sponsored by the Public Health Service examined patient mortality in 160 hospitals in 1977. This study included a disproportionate number of hospitals that were large, urban, affiliated with medical schools, and private non-profit. The study found that:

- Patients with intestinal cancer who were treated in hospitals that were members of the Council of Teaching Hospitals (COTH) were almost 4 percent less likely to die than patients treated in hospitals that were not affiliated with medical schools.
- Patients with abdominal aneurysms who were treated in COTH hospitals were found to be 5 percent less likely to die. The study also found a relationship between low mortality and a high volume for surgery patients with peptic ulcers.

A national study involving 3,100 general hospitals in 1986 was published in the *New England Journal of Medicine* (Hartz et al. 1989). The hospitals in the study were disproportionately urban and the patients studied were adults. The study took into account how severely ill the patients were. The study found that the training of the medical staff was the hospital characteristic "most closely associated" with patient survival and that "teaching hospitals may provide better care than other hospitals." In addition, the study concluded that because high occupancy may be related to a hospital's economic health "greater financial stability may be associated with an improved quality of care." According to the Hartz study,

> *"The characteristics most strongly associated with a lower mortality rate were a higher percentage of physicians who were board-certified specialists*

and a higher occupancy rate. Lower adjusted mortality rates were also associated with higher payroll expenses per hospital bed, teaching hospitals, private not-for-profit hospitals, hospitals with a greater percentage of nurses who were R.N.s, a higher level of technological sophistication, and larger hospitals."

Other researchers also have found financial viability to be related to better quality of care. A study, which used *Harvard Medical Practice Study* data from the state of New York, determined that hospitals most likely to have patients suffer medical injuries as a result of negligent care were those with the lowest operating costs (Burstin et al. 1993). The study also found that negligent care was "more pronounced among hospitals with fairly entrenched financial difficulties." The authors noted that because financially distressed hospitals often care for the poor, "efforts to improve the quality of care in these institutions may be warranted."

A National Cancer Society study of 5,766 breast cancer patients in 99 geographically dispersed hospitals in Illinois during 1988 also suggests that the financial condition and the size of the hospital may be factors that affect quality of care, with large financially strong hospitals providing better care than others (Hand et al. 1991).

A recent national study, sponsored by the federal Agency for Health Care Policy and Research (AHCPR) examined mortality rates for 974,000 acute myocardial infarction (AMI) patients in 426 hospitals, including 146,000 patients in 62 hospitals who received coronary artery bypass graft (CABG) surgery, 130,000 patients in 337 hospitals who received hip replacements, 56,000 neonatal patients in 222 hospitals with respiratory distress syndrome, and 37,000 patients in 330 hospitals who received inguinal hernia repair surgery (Farley and Ozminkowski 1992). The study was conducted during the seven-year period between 1981 and 1987 and found that:

- "Increasing volume in a hospital leads to significantly lower adjusted mortality rates for . . . AMI, hernia repairs, and respiratory distress syndrome in neonates;"
- Nursing intensity was a factor in reducing mortality rates for AMI. The study reported that "greater nursing intensity, measured by registered nurses per patient day, [had] a sizable positive effect;"
- There also was a significant positive relationship between high volume and good outcomes for CABG. "This correlation appears to be due to referral patterns in which hospitals that improve their outcomes attract larger numbers of patients," the study said; and
- Substantial effects of volume on outcomes were not found for hip replacements.

A RAND study included over 14,000 patients who were age 65 and older in 297 hospitals in 30 geographic areas of Florida and four other states in different regions (Keeler et al. 1992). The hospitals were selected to represent hospitals nationally with regard to city size, percentage of Medicare patients, hospital size, teaching intensity, patient mortality for the five diseases studied, and type of ownership.

The hospitals were studied during two time periods, from 1981 to 1982 and again from 1985 to 1986. Half of the patients were hospitalized in the first time period and half during the second time period. The study examined patients with one of five diagnoses: congestive heart failure, acute myocardial infarction, pneumonia, stroke, and hip fracture. The study found that:

- "Quality of care varies from state to state, but teaching, larger, and more urban hospitals have better quality in general than nonteaching, small, and rural hospitals;"

- There was a four percentage point difference in the estimated expected increase in mortality for the patients studied between the hospital group with the lowest quality (rural hospitals) and the hospital group with the highest quality (major teaching hospitals); and
- "Quality of care was strongly related to teaching. More teaching [was] associated with better quality."

Two recent studies (Turner and Ball 1992; Stone et al. 1992) examined the relationship between hospital experience in treating AIDS patients and patient mortality. Both studies found that patient mortality was lower in hospitals with greater experience in treating AIDS patients. Turner and Ball examined 10,538 adult patients with AIDS in 258 hospitals nationwide during 1986 and 1987. Stone et al. examined 806 patients with AIDS who received care at 40 hospitals in Massachusetts during 1987.

The Stone study found substantial differences in patient mortality between low- and high-experience hospitals. At high-experience hospitals inpatient mortality was 9.8 percent. Low-experience hospitals had an inpatient mortality rate of 19 percent. The authors commented that the better patient outcomes at high-experience hospitals did not appear to be related to cost, to the length of the hospital stay, or to more use of the intensive care unit. According to the authors, "It is certainly plausible that hospitals that are more familiar with the disease will develop more effective diagnostic and therapeutic strategies and thereby achieve better results."

An editorial accompanying the Stone article in the *Journal of the American Medical Association* gave three possible explanations of why hospitals with less experience in treating persons with AIDS were found to have poorer outcomes than hospitals with more experience (Shapiro and Greenfield 1992).

> *"First, failure of early recognition of complications may have led to rapid, fatal progression before appropriate therapy could be introduced. Second, less experienced physicians might not have known the appropriate dosing of medications . . . or when to switch to another medication when the patient was not improving. Third, less experienced providers might not have been aware of newer modalities."*

Individual hospital mortality data

The use of hospital mortality data to identify hospitals that provide good (or bad) care is highly controversial (see Park et al. 1990 and Green and Wintfeld 1993). Many factors can influence patient mortality. Hospitals that provide excellent care to very ill patients may have higher mortality rates than hospitals which do not care for severely ill patients. Hospitals that care for large numbers of the elderly may have higher mortality rates than hospitals that have lower proportions of the elderly. It is important that hospital mortality rates be adjusted for these and other factors.

There is no consensus in the research literature regarding the validity of using routinely collected mortality data to identify individual hospitals that provide either excellent or poor care. Some researchers argue that two or more years of mortality data that takes into account the health risk and health status of patients might be used as a quality measure for individual hospitals. A recently published multi-year study of California patients who underwent coronary artery bypass graft surgery found that routinely collected risk-adjusted mortality data could consistently identify hospitals that provided better care to high risk patients (Luft and Romano 1993). Other studies, which have used clinical data obtained from individual patient records (rather than routinely reported administrative data), have reported findings that suggest that quality of care differences between hospitals can be identified (Keeler et al. 1992 and Chassin 1993).

TEACHING AND RESEARCH HOSPITALS

As of January 1992, there were 24 hospitals in Florida that had programs accredited by the Accreditation Council for Graduate Medical Education. The 24 hospitals include six statutory teaching and research hospitals and 18 other teaching hospitals. To be designated as a statutory teaching hospital, the hospital must have seven or more residency programs and 100 or more residents. The six statutory teaching hospitals are affiliated with medical schools and they are the backbone of hospital-based academic medicine in Florida. All act as regional referral centers.

Compared with other hospitals, teaching hospitals provide the greatest range of advanced diagnostic and therapeutic medical services, such as neonatal intensive care, organ transplantation, open heart surgery, and intensive care for burn patients. Several research studies have found that patients who are treated in teaching hospitals affiliated with medical schools have better outcomes that other hospitals.

A study of Florida's teaching hospitals published in March 1988 found that Medicare patients have the longest stays in the statutory teaching hospitals, averaging almost 10 days. In the other teaching hospitals, the average stay for Medicare patients was 9.2 days and in non-teaching hospitals the average stay was 8.4 days.

**Teaching hospitals with programs
accredited by the Accreditation Council
for Graduate Medical Education
1992**

City	Hospital	Number of residency programs
Statutory teaching hospitals		
Gainesville	Shands Hospital	45
Jacksonville	University Hospital	15
Miami	Jackson Memorial	44
Miami Beach	Mount Sinai Medical Center	13
Orlando	Orlando Regional	8
Tampa	Tampa General/H. Lee Moffitt	36
Other teaching hospitals		
Daytona Beach	Halifax Medical Center	1
Fort Lauderdale	North Beach Hospital	1
Gainesville	Alachua General Hospital	1
Jacksonville	Nemours Children's Clinic	2
Jacksonville	St. Vincent's Medical Center	1
Miami	Doctor's Hospital	2
Miami	Miami Children's Hospital	3
Miami	South Shore Hospital	1
Miami	Ann Bates Leach Eye Hospital	1
Miami Beach	Miami Beach Community	1
Orlando	Florida Hospital	2
Orlando	Florida Elks Children's Hospital	1
Pensacola	Sacred Heart Hospital	2
St. Petersburg	All Children's Hospital	5

St. Petersburg	Bayfront Medical Center	3
Tallahassee	Tallahassee Memorial Regional MC	1
Tampa	U of South Fla Psychiatry Center	2
Tampa	Shriners Hosp for Crippled Children	1

Source: American Medical Association, Directory of Graduate Medical Education Programs 1992–1993

OSTEOPATHIC HOSPITALS

There are two types of physicians, medical doctors (M.D.s) and doctors of osteopathy (D.O.s). Both M.D.s and D.O.s practice traditional methods of medicine.

Osteopathic medicine emphasizes a "whole person" approach to medical care and osteopathic physicians use generally accepted medicines, surgical methods, and diagnostic techniques. According to the American Osteopathic Association (AOA), "Osteopathic medicine is a system of medical care with a philosophy that combines the needs of the patient with current medical science, an emphasis on the interrelationship between structure and function, and an appreciation of the body's ability to heal itself."

With its focus on musculoskeletal structure, manipulative therapy, prevention, and wellness, the AOA says, "The osteopathic physician acts as a teacher to help patients take more responsibility for their own well-being and change unhealthy patterns. Sports medicine is also a natural outgrowth of osteopathic medicine because of its focus on the musculoskeletal system, osteopathic manipulative treatment, diet, exercise and fitness."

In 1992, there were 15 osteopathic medical colleges in the United States, including one in Miami, the Southeastern University of the Health Sciences. Ten of the 15 osteopathic medical colleges were founded between 1969 and 1981.

All 50 states license osteopathic physicians for the practice of medicine and surgery. Florida has approximately 1,800 osteopathic physicians. In March 1993, 11 hospitals were accredited by the AOA. Chapter 11 includes information on accreditation organizations.

Osteopathic hospitals accredited
by the American Osteopathic Association
March 1993

County	Hospital	City
Broward	Universal Medical Center	Plantation
Dade	Westchester General	Miami
Hillsborough	Centurion Hospital	Tampa
Lee	Gulf Coast Hospital	Ft. Myers
Orange	Florida Hospital East Orlando	Orlando
Palm Beach	Humana, Palm Beaches	Palm Beach
Palm Beach	Wellington Regional	W. Palm Beach
Pinellas	Metropolitan General	Pinellas Park
Pinellas	Sun Coast Hospital	Largo
Pinellas	University General Hospital	Seminole
Volusia	Peninsula Medical Center	Ormond Beach

Source: American Osteopathic Association (September, 1992).

To check on the accreditation status of an osteopathic hospital, contact:

American Osteopathic Association
(800) 621-1773

HOSPITAL COMMUNITY BENEFITS STANDARDS PROGRAM

Two Florida hospitals participate in the Hospital Community Benefits Standards program. JCAHO or AOA-accredited hospitals are eligible to participate. The program is supported by the W.K. Kellogg Foundation. Participating hospitals are required to develop a systematic program, consisting of various activities and projects designed to give more explicit shape and identity to what they are doing to fulfill their community commitment. Standards call for hospital-sponsored projects that are designed to improve the health status of persons in the community, address the health problems of minorities and the poor, and contain community health care cost increases.

In June 1992, the Florida participants were Lee Memorial Hospital in Fort Myers and Tampa General Hospital in Tampa. Program information can be obtained by contacting:

Hospital Community Benefit Standards Program
New York University
113 University Place, 9th Floor
New York, New York 10003
(212) 998-7494

EMERGENCY ROOMS AND TRAUMA CENTERS

About one-fourth of all adults use a hospital emergency room over a two-year period. The percentage of children using emergency rooms is higher, at 46 percent. Hospital emergency rooms are the appropriate medical facility to visit when immediate attention is needed for a serious medical problem, but they are expensive because they are staffed and equipped to care for persons with serious medical problems that need prompt attention.

Patients with minor health care problems can receive the care they need at "walk-in" physician care centers. For minor problems, both the wait for treatment and the cost of care is likely to be much less at a physician care center than at a hospital emergency room.

Although most hospitals have emergency rooms, emergency medical capabilities vary. Large hospitals generally are staffed and equipped to treat more serious medical conditions than small hospitals. The smaller the hospital, the more likely it is that a patient with a life-threatening medical problem will be stabilized and transferred to another hospital that has the needed equipment and specialists. Not surprisingly, a national study found that emergency room costs increase as the size of the hospital increases.

Hospitals with the most sophisticated emergency rooms are designated as trauma centers. Trauma centers are staffed and equipped to treat the most serious injuries, such as head and spinal cord injuries, and victims of severe accidents. In Florida, there are state standards that divide trauma centers into three groups: Level I Trauma Centers, Level II Trauma Centers, and Pediatric trauma referral centers. Level I facilities provide emergency care to patients with the most complex medical conditions. Only the very large hospitals, which have diversified physician specialist staffs, are able to meet the criteria designated as Level I trauma centers. In fact, all four Level I trauma centers are statutory teaching hospitals. Some trauma centers also are designated as pediatric trauma centers.

Trauma centers		
1993		
Hospital	*City*	*Type*
University Hospital	Jacksonville	Level I & Pediatric
Jackson Memorial	Miami	Level I & Pediatric
Orlando Regional MC	Orlando	Level I & Pediatric
Tampa General	Tampa	Level I & Pediatric
Broward General MC	Ft. Lauderdale	Level II & Pediatric
N. Broward Med Center	Ft. Lauderdale	Level II & Pediatric
Memorial Hospital	Hollywood	Level II & Pediatric
Plantation General	Plantation	Pediatric
Miami Children's	Miami	Pediatric
Delray Community	Delray Beach	Level II
Halifax Medical Center	Daytona Beach	Level II
Lee Memorial	Ft. Myers	Level II
Delray Community	Palm Beach	Level II
St. Mary's Hospital	Palm Beach	Level II
Baptist Hospital	Pensacola	Level II
Sacred Heart	Pensacola	Level II
West Fla Regional MC	Pensacola	Level II
Bayfront Medical Center	St. Petersburg	Level II
St. Joseph's Hospital	Tampa	Level II

Source: Emergency Medical Services Office, 1993.

COMPREHENSIVE REHABILITATION

Thirty-six Florida's hospitals were licensed in 1992 to provide comprehensive rehabilitation services. Comprehensive rehabilitation services include restoring lost bodily functions, treating persons with congenital abnormalities, and treating persons with specific diseases or medical conditions. Patients include those who have suffered strokes, head and spinal cord injuries, amputations, hip fractures, or who have arthritis or other medical problems that restrict limb movement.

Treatment is provided by an interdisciplinary staff skilled in medical and rehabilitation nursing, speech and occupational therapy, and social services. Many hospitals that do not provide comprehensive rehabilitative services provide speech, occupational, or rehabilitative therapy to persons with less severe medical problems.

Hospitals that provide		
comprehensive rehabilitative services		
Calendar year 1991		
County	*Name of Hospital*	*Patient Days*
Alachua	Upreach Pavilion	10,137
Brevard	Sea Pines Rehabilitation Hospital	24,430
Broward	Holy Cross Hospital	9,981
Broward	Memorial Hospital Hollywood	7,838
Broward	N. Broward Med Center (Licensed 1991)	1,850

Broward	St. John's Rehabilitation Hospital	2,377
Broward	Sunrise Hospital	37,657
Collier	Naples Community Hospital	7,839
Dade	AMI Parkway Regional Medical Center	3,933
Dade	Baptist Hospital of Miami	11,397
Dade	Bon Secours Hospital	14,105
Dade	Jackson Memorial Hospital	16,699
Dade	Mt. Sinai Medical Center	13,296
Dade	South Miami Hospital	7,197
Dade	West Gables Rehabilitation Hospital	9,842
Duval	Memorial Regional Rehab Center	23,819
Escambia	HCA West Florida Regional MC	14,147
Hillsborough	Tampa General Hospital	18,428
Indian River	Treasure Coast Rehabilitation	16,571
Lake	Leesburg Regional (Licensed 1991)	648
Lee	Lee Memorial Hospital	13,748
Leon	Capital Rehabilitation Hospital	14,507
Manatee	HCA L.W. Blake Memorial Hospital	6,939
Orange	Florida Hospital, Orlando	15,124
Orange	Humana Hospital, Lucerne	5,525
Orange	Orlando Regional MC Sand Lake	4,600
Palm Beach	Pinecrest Hospital	21,522
Palm Beach	St. Mary's Hospital	4,385
Pinellas	Bayfront Medical Center	7,729
Pinellas	Healthsouth Rehabilitation Center	12,408
Pinellas	Sun Coast Hospital (Licensed 1991)	274
Pasco	Riverside Hospital	6,023
Polk	Winter Haven Hospital	5,122
Sarasota	Rehabilitation Institute	20,747
Sarasota	Sarasota Memorial Hospital	7,559
Volusia	Peninsula Med Center (Licensed 1991)	4,307

Source: *Florida Hospital Bed Utilization*, January 1, 1991 to December 31, 1991, Volume II, Agency for Health Care Administration (1992). This publication, which contains data reported by hospitals, may be obtained from the state Agency for Health Care Administration or reviewed in a State of Florida depository library.

The Commission on Accreditation of Rehabilitation Facilities (CARF) was established in 1966 as a private, not-for-profit organization. CARF accredits rehabilitation and other facilities that meet its national standards. According to CARF, one of the purposes of the Commission is to "Develop and maintain current, state-of-the-art standards which can be used by organizations to measure their level of performance, to promote consumer-responsiveness, and to strengthen their programs." Information on accreditation organizations is included in Chapter 11.

Commission on Accreditation
of Rehabilitation Facilities
Accredited facilities
as of December 4, 1992

Bradenton	Mediplex Rehabilitation	CIR:N
Bradenton	HCA L.W. Blake Hospital	CIR:H
Coral Gables	HEALTHSOUTH Sports Medicine & Rehab.	OMR
Daytona	Easter Seal Society of Volusia/Flagler	OMR
Daytona	Florida C.O.R.F.	OMR
Delray Beach	Pinecrest Rehabilitation Hosp	CIR:H, OMR
Ft. Lauderdale	Holy Cross Hospital	CIR:H
Ft. Lauderdale	Sunrise Rehabilitation Hosp	CIR:H, OMR
Ft. Myers	Lee Memorial Hospital	CIR:H
Gainesville	UpReach Pavilion	CIR:H
Hialeah	Palmetto Outpatient Rehab Center	OMR
Hollywood	Memorial Hospital	CIR:H
Jacksonville	Medical Rehab. Center, Jacksonville	OMR
Jacksonville	Memorial Regional Rehab. Center	CIR:H
Largo	HEALTHSOUTH Rehab. Hospital	CIR:H, OMR
Melbourne	Easter Seal Center	OMR
Melbourne	Sea Pines Rehab. Hospital	CIR:H, OMR
Miami	Baptist Hospital of Miami	CIR:H, OMR
Miami	Bon Secours Hospital	CIR:H
Miami	CMS WorkAble of South Miami	OMR
Miami	Easter Seal Society of Dade County	OMR
Miami	HEALTHSOUTH Reg. Rehab. Center	CIR:N, OMR
Miami	Jackson Memorial Hospital	CIR:H
Miami	South Miami Hospital	CIR:H
Miami	West Gables Rehab. Hospital	CIR:H
Miami Beach	Lehrman Back Center	OMR
Miami Beach	Mt. Sinai Medical Center	CIR:H
Miami Beach	Parkway Reg. Medical Center	CIR:H, OMR
Naples	Naples Community Hospital	CIR:H
Naples	Naples Rehabilitation Center	OMR
Ocala	HEALTHSOUTH Sports Med.& Rehab. Cntr	OMR
Orange Park	Northeast Florida Rehab. Inc.	OMR
Orlando	Sand Lake Hospital	OMR
Orlando	Florida Hospital Rehab. Center	CIR:H
Orlando	Humana Hospital - Lucerne	CIR:H
Orlando	Comprehensive Med. Rehab. Center	OMR
Ormond Beach	Peninsula Medical Center	CIR:H
Palm Beach	Rehab. Cntr for Children & Adults	OMR
Panama City	Gulf Coast Rehabilitative Services	OMR
Pensacola	HCA West Fla Regional Medical Cntr	CIR:H
Pinellas Park	Easter Seal Rehabilitation Center	OMR
Pompano Beach	North Broward Medical Center	CIR:H
St. Petersburg	Bayfront Medical Center	CIR:H
Sarasota	Rehab. Institute of Sarasota	CIR:H, OMR

Sarasota	Sarasota Memorial Hospital	CIR:H
Tallahassee	Capital Rehabilitation Hospital	CIR:H
Tamarac	Neurological Rehabilitation Center	OMR
Tampa	Tampa General Hosp Rehab. Center	CIR:H
Vero Beach	Treasure Coast Rehab. Hospital	CIR:H, OMR
Winter Haven	Mid-Florida Rehabilitation Center	CIR:H

CIR:H Comprehensive inpatient rehabilitation: hospital
CIR:N Comprehensive inpatient rehabilitation: skilled nursing home
OMR: Outpatient medical rehabilitation

Source: Commission on Accreditation of Rehabilitation Facilities.

To obtain a current list of CARF-accredited facilities, contact:

Commission on Accreditation of Rehabilitation Facilities
101 N. Wilmot Road, Suite 500
Tucson, Arizona 85711
(602) 748-1212

JCAHO accredits hospitals that provide rehabilitation services. The chart below lists those speciality hospitals that were accredited as of February 1993. The service codes indicate which services the facility was accredited for on the date the facility was examined.

Joint Commission on Accreditation of
Healthcare Organizations
Accredited rehabilitation hospitals
February 1993

Hospital	City	Service codes
Pinecrest Rehabilitation Hosp	Delray Beach	E Q BB CC DD EE FF GG
Sunrise Rehabilitation Hosp	Ft Lauderdale	E L O Q R S W AA BB CC DD EE FF
Memorial Regional Rehab Cntr	Jacksonville	Not Avail.
Healthsouth Rehab. Hospital	Largo	E L Q BB CC DD EE FF
Sea Pines Rehab Hospital	Melbourne	E BB CC DD EE
West Gables Rehab. Hosp	Miami	E Q BB CC DD EE FF
Healthsouth Reg Rehab. Cntr	Miami	E S BB CC
Bon Secours/Villa Maria	North Miami	Not Avail.
Rehabilitation Inst Of Sarasota	Sarasota	E BB CC DD EE FF
Capital Rehabilitation Hospital	Tallahassee	A B E L Q BB CC DD EE FF
Treasure Coast Rehab Hospital	Vero Beach	Not Avail.

JCAHO accreditation service codes:

A	Medical/Surgical, Acute Care	S	Ultrasound
B	Pediatric, Acute Care	BB	Physical Therapy
E	Physical Medicine and Rehab	CC	Occupational Therapy
L	Electrocardiography	DD	Recreational Therapy
Q	Diagnostic X-Ray	EE	Respiratory Therapy
R	Magnetic Resonance Imaging	FF	Speech Pathology
W	X-Ray Radiation Therapy	GG	Psychiatric Educational Srvcs

Source: JCAHO (February 22, 1993).

JCAHO may be contacted to learn whether a hospital currently is accredited and makes available an accreditation history of hospitals from the mid-1970s. Chapter 11 includes information on how to contact the JCAHO.

OBSTETRICAL CARE

Hospitals vary in their capability of providing medically advanced care to newborns with medical complications. Hospitals that provide advanced care to newborns have neonatal intensive care units.

There are three levels of patient care in hospitals for newborns: Level I, Level II, and Level III. Hospitals with Level I newborn nurseries provide routine delivery and infant care to women who have a normal delivery and normal baby. Level I hospitals are primarily small hospitals. High-risk patients and newborns with complex medical problems are transferred either to hospitals with Level II or Level III services, depending upon the severity of the medical problem.

Hospitals with Level II services provide care to complicated obstetrical cases (high-risk patients) and to newborns with certain medical problems. Level II care frequently is referred to as "intermediate care." The most technologically advanced obstetrical and neonatal care is provided by hospitals with Level III intensive care services. These hospitals act as regional centers for the treatment of newborns with severe medical problems. Level III units are staffed by physicians and obstetrical nurses who have advanced specialist training in the care of newborns with severe medical problems.

According to a 1988 study by the federal Office of Technology Assessment (OTA), "The evidence strongly suggests that the likelihood of survival among very low birthweight babies (babies weighing less than 1,500 grams at birth) is highest if the baby is born in a hospital designated a Level III neonatal facility." The OTA study also stated that four studies had found that worse outcomes occurred in hospitals that had low patient volume.

Very large hospitals, including the statutory teaching hospitals and children's specialty hospitals, usually provide Level III care. In addition, the 192-bed St. Joseph's Women's Hospital in Tampa, a specialty hospital that is devoted exclusively to women, provides Level III care.

Hospitals with
Level III neonatal intensive care units
Calendar year 1991

County	Hospital	Total patient days
Alachua	Shands Teaching Hospital*	7,158
Broward	Broward General Medical Center*	7,194
Broward	HCA Plantation General	3,969
Broward	Memorial Hospital Hollywood*	3,815
Dade	Jackson Memorial Hospital*	17,911
Dade	Miami Children's	5,039
Dade	North Shore Medical Center	638
Duval	University Medical Center*	9,644
Escambia	Sacred Heart*	5,911

County	Hospital	Total patient days
Hillsborough	Brandon Hospital	1,759
Hillsborough	St. Joseph's Women's Hospital—Tampa	2,886
Hillsborough	Tampa General*	6,755
Lee	Lee Memorial	2,748
Leon	Tallahassee Memorial	4,667
Orange	Orlando Regional/Arnold Palmer*	14,913
Orange	Florida Hospital—Orlando	3,112
Palm Beach	Good Samaritan	1,678
Palm Beach	St. Mary's Hospital*	2,459
Pinellas	All Children's Hospital*	6,231
Sarasota	Sarasota Memorial	684

*Regional Perinatal Intensive Care Center (RPICC) as of March 1993. These centers are required to meet certain requirements regarding physician and nurse staffing and equipment.

Source: *Florida Hospital Bed Utilization*, January 1, 1991 to December 31, 1991, Volume II, Agency for Health Care Administration (1992). This publication, which contains data reported by hospitals, may be obtained from the Agency for Health Care Administration or reviewed in a State of Florida depository library.

Hospitals with
Level II neonatal intensive care units
Calendar year 1991

County	Hospital	Total patient days
Alachua	Alachua General Hospital	1,504
Alachua	Shands Hospital*	4,295
Brevard	J.E. Holmes Regional Medical Center	4,258
Broward	Broward General Medical Center*	6,634
Broward	Coral Springs Medical Center	3,245
Broward	HCA Northwest Regional	775
Broward	Holy Cross Hospital	1,768
Broward	Memorial Hospital—Hollywood*	2,445
Broward	Plantation General	2,311
Clay	Orange Park Medical Center	350
Dade	Baptist Hospital	3,852
Dade	Hialeah Hospital	1,815
Dade	Jackson Memorial Hospital*	26,635
Dade	Mercy Hospital	463
Dade	Miami Children's	2,548
Dade	Mt. Sinai Medical Center	2,662
Dade	North Shore Medical Center	2,270
Dade	South Miami Hospital	4,744
Duval	Baptist Medical Center	9,699
Duval	Memorial Med Cntr of Jacksonville	3,527
Duval	St. Vincent's Medical Center	2,180
Escambia	Sacred Heart Hospital*	7,222
Hillsborough	Brandon Hospital	1,856
Hillsborough	St. Joseph's Women's Hospital—Tampa	4,102
Hillsborough	Tampa General Hospital*	5,630

Lee	Lee Memorial Hospital	4,218
Leon	Tallahassee Memorial	4,556
Manatee	Manatee Memorial	2,284
Martin	Martin Memorial	395
Orange	Florida Hospital Orlando	2,975
Orange	Orlando Regional/Arnold Palmer*	4,217
Orange	Winter Park Memorial Hospital	604
Palm Beach	AMI Palm Beach Gardens	425
Palm Beach	Bethesda Memorial	3,781
Palm Beach	Good Samaritan Hospital	1,577
Palm Beach	St. Mary's Hospital*	5,937
Palm Beach	West Boca Medical Center	2,843
Pinellas	All Children's Hospital*	8,656
Pinellas	Bayfront Medical Center*	3,843
Pinellas	Mease Hospital Dunedin	1,130
Pinellas	Morton F. Plant Hospital	1,322
Polk	Lakeland Regional Medical Center	4,720
Polk	Winter Haven Hospital	2,395
Sarasota	Sarasota Memorial Hospital	2,538
Volusia	Halifax Memorial Hospital	2,783

*RPICC as of March 1993. These centers are required to meet certain requirements regarding physician and nurse staffing and equipment.

Source: *Florida Hospital Bed Utilization*, January 1, 1991 to December 31, 1991, Volume II, Agency for Health Care Administration (1992). This publication, which contains data reported by hospitals, may be obtained from the Agency for Health Care Administration or reviewed in a State of Florida depository library.

Hospitals that provide Level I obstetrical services*
1992

County	Name of Hospital
Alachua	North Florida Regional Medical Center
Bay	Bay Medical Center
Bay	HCA Gulf Coast Community
Brevard	Cape Canaveral Hospital
Brevard	Holmes Regional
Brevard	Jess Parish Memorial
Brevard	Wuesthoff Memorial
Broward	Coral Springs Medical Center
Broward	Doctor's General Plantation
Broward	Imperial Point Medical Center
Broward	Pembroke Pines Hospital
Broward	Westside Regional Medical Center
Charlotte	Bon Secours & St. Joseph Hospital
Citrus	Citrus Memorial
Citrus	Seven Rivers Community
Collier	Naples Community Hospital
Dade	AMI Palmetto General

Dade	Healthsouth Doctors Hospital
Dade	Miami Beach Community Hospital
Dade	Parkway Regional Medical Center
Dade	SMH Homestead Hospital
Desoto	Desoto Memorial
Duval	Methodist Hospital
Duval	Riverside Hospital
Escambia	Baptist Hospital
Escambia	HCA West Florida Regional Medical Center
Escambia	University Hospital and Clinic
Hernando	Brooksville Regional
Highlands	Walker Memorial
Hillsborough	St. Joseph's Hospital
Hillsborough	South Florida Baptist Hospital
Hillsborough	University Community
Indian River	Indian River Memorial Hospital
Indian River	Sebastian Hospital
Jackson	Jackson Hospital
Lake	Lake Medical Center
Lake	Waterman Medical Center
Leon	Tallahassee Community
Manatee	HCA L.W. Blake Hospital
Manatee	Manatee Memorial
Marion	Munroe Regional Medical Center
Monroe	DePoo Health Systems
Nassau	Nassau General
Okaloosa	Ft. Walton Beach Hospital
Okeechobee	HCA Raulerson Memorial
Orange	Princeton Hospital
Orange	Lucerne Medical Center
Orange	West Orange Memorial Hospital
Orange	Winter Park Memorial
Osceola	Osceola Regional Hospital
Palm Beach	AMI Palm Beach Gardens
Palm Beach	Everglades Memorial
Palm Beach	West Boca Medical Center
Pasco	Dade City Hospital
Pasco	East Pasco Medical Center
Pasco	HCA New Port Richey Hospital
Pasco	Riverside Hospital
Pinellas	Mease Hospital
Pinellas	St. Anthony's Hospital
Pinellas	St. Petersburg General Hospital
Pinellas	Sun Coast Hospital
Pinellas	Women's Medical Center
Polk	Bartow Memorial
Polk	Lake Wales Hospital
Polk	Polk General Hospital
Polk	Winter Haven Hospital
Putnam	HCA Putnam Community
St. Lucie	Lawnwood Regional Medical Center

St. Johns ....Flagler Hospital
Santa Rosa ....HCA Santa Rosa Medical Center
Sarasota ....Venice Hospital
Seminole.............................Central Florida Regional
Volusia ....Halifax Medical Center
Volusia ....West Volusia Memorial

*Level II and Level III hospitals, shown in previous tables, also have Level I services.

Source: Agency for Health Care Administration (1993) and (1994).

Hospital cesarean sections

Cesarean section is the most common hospital surgical procedure, both in Florida and nationally. Nationally, c-section rates (the percentage of all deliveries that are done by cesarean section) have increased more than four fold between 1970, when the rate was only 5.5 percent, and 1991, when the rate was 23.5 percent. Over the past several years, Florida's c-section rate has been above the national average and was 25.1 percent in 1992. C-section rates, however, have been declining slightly over the past several years, both nationally and in Florida. Florida's rate was 27.3 percent in 1988, 26.7 percent in 1989, 26.5 percent in 1990, and 25.2 percent in 1991. In 1992, hospital c-section rates ranged from a low of 12.8 percent to a high of 44.2 percent across Florida hospitals.

An article in the *Journal of the American Medical Association* examined c-section rates in selected countries (Notzon 1990). The article reported that in 1985 the United States had a rate of 23 percent. Canada had a rate of 19 percent, while Denmark and Italy had rates of 13 percent, Sweden and Norway had a rate of 12 percent, Switzerland had a rate of 11 percent, and New Zealand, England, and the Netherlands had rates of 10 percent. The World Health Organization states, "There is no justification in any specific geographic region to have more than 10–15 percent cesarean section births."

A 1990 Florida Health Care Cost Containment Board study stated that the reasons for the increase in c-section rates over the past 20 years are unclear. However, the report stated that the following factors were the most frequently mentioned explanations for the increase in c-section rates:

- The threat of malpractice lawsuits;
- Obstetrical policy on repeat cesarean sections;
- Obstetrical training and the belief in the superior outcome from c-sections;
- Economic incentives to perform high-cost c-sections (in 1991, the average charge in Florida hospitals for c-section deliveries was $6,446);
- The relative ease of the procedure to physicians; and
- An increase in the average age of motherhood.

In an editorial in the *Journal of the American Medical Association* two physicians from Northwestern University Medical School wrote,

> *"In our current litigious environment where patients expect a perfect obstetric outcome and physicians using available knowledge are eager to try new technologies to improve that outcome, is it surprising that we have seen an escalation of cesarean delivery rates to a level that now appears unreasonable? (Jonas and Dooley 1989)."*

A study examined the incidence of cesarean delivery for 60,490 women who delivered at 31 New York hospitals during 1984 (Localio et al. 1993). The study found that women were more likely to have c-sections in hospitals where physicians paid high malpractice insurance premiums. The study took into account clinical risk, the socio-economic status of patients, and the characteristics of physicians and hospitals. The study stated that, "The malpractice risk effect might be operating at the group or hospital level more than at the individual physician level. A claim against a physician affects the peer group as a whole."

If a study were conducted in Florida that used the Localio methodology, the findings likely would be similar. This is because Dade and Broward counties have the highest premium costs for obstetrical malpractice insurance. These two counties also have, on average, the highest c-section rates in the state. Conversely, areas in Florida with the lowest c-section rates have the lowest rates of malpractice insurance. It is important to note that Florida's malpractice insurance climate for obstetricians is perhaps the worst in the United States. Annual premiums for malpractice insurance in excess of $100,000 for obstetricians are very common in Southern Florida and in other urban areas. Because of high cost, some obstetricians, particularly in South Florida, do not carry medical liability insurance but rather maintain sufficient assets to comply with Florida law.

In 1988, the American Academy of Pediatrics and the American College of Obstetricians and Gynecologists published a revised edition of *Guidelines for Perinatal Care* which stated, "Recent data show that 50-80 percent of patients who attempt to deliver vaginally after a cesarean birth have successful vaginal births. Unless there are contraindications to vaginal delivery, women with one previous cesarean delivery should be counseled to undergo labor in their current pregnancy."

An article published in the *Journal of the American Medical Association* examined the association of nonclinical factors on repeat cesarean sections (Stafford 1991). According to the study, repeat c-sections comprise 36 percent of all c-sections, and nationally only 12.6 percent of women who previously have had c-sections give birth vaginally. Stafford examined the records of 45,425 women who gave birth in hospitals in California during 1986 who had previous c-sections. The study found the highest repeat c-section rates were for women with private health insurance, women who delivered in proprietary hospitals, and women who gave birth in hospitals with lower numbers of births.

An earlier study by the same author examined strategies for controlling c-section rates. It found that "...formal programs aimed at modifying practices within individual hospitals appear to be the most successful" (Stafford 1990). These internal hospital programs require second opinions before a c-section is performed and a detailed review of all c-sections after they are performed by the hospital's obstetricians. A more recent study found that c-section rates could be sharply reduced by using educational techniques used by the pharmaceutical industry (Lomas et al. 1991).

A program in a Chicago hospital was designed to reduce c-section rates (Myers and Gleicher 1988). Physicians volunteered to participate in the program and were required to obtain a second opinion before performing a c-section. All c-sections underwent peer review and objective criteria for the four most common indicators for c-sections were developed. The study found that as a result of the program:

- The hospital's c-section rate fell from 17.5 percent of 1,697 deliveries to 11.5 percent of 2,301 deliveries during the first two years of the program.
- Deliveries that were operative vaginal deliveries fell from 10.4 percent to 4.3 percent during the same period.

The authors concluded that, "...an initiative within an obstetrics department can reduce cesarean-section rates substantially without adverse effects on the outcome for mother or infant."

Appendix B contains reported c-section rates for all Florida hospitals. In examining hospital c-section rates, it is important to bear in mind that the physicians on the hospital's medical staff perform c-sections, not the hospital. The hospital's average c-section rate is the average of all physicians on staff who deliver; individual physicians may either have higher or lower rates.

OPEN HEART SURGERY

Open heart surgery is one of the most sophisticated surgical procedures, requiring highly skilled cardiac surgeons and specially trained anesthesiologists, perfusionists, and nurses. The expertise of these specially trained cardiac surgical teams is maintained by performing a sufficiently high volume of surgeries. The literature is particularly convincing with regard to finding that better patient outcomes generally occur when patients are treated by surgeons who perform cardiac surgery frequently and in hospitals where large numbers of cardiac patients undergo surgery.

It is important to note that research studies also have found that when a threshold is reached, the effect of volume on better care weakens. This has been found in studies of cardiac surgery and organ transplantation. A study of coronary artery bypass graft (CABG) surgery in teaching hospitals in Pennsylvania stated that, "All studies have found the effect (of volume on patient mortality) to be weaker at higher volume levels, and most authors have noted a threshold of about 200 to 250 CABG procedures per year (Williams et al. 1991).

CABG surgery is the most common open heart procedure and has a high rate of success. According to a task force report by the American College of Cardiology and the American Heart Association (Kirklin et al. 1991), "In general, about 96.5 percent of heterogeneous groups of patients survive at least 1 month after the operation, and 95 percent, 88 percent, 75 percent and 60 percent, respectively, survive 1, 5, 10 or 15 or more years after the operation."

In addition to CABG, open heart surgery also is performed to correct congenital heart defects, to repair damage from cardiac diseases, to replace heart valves, to repair aneurysms, and to treat other cardiac problems. Some patients may benefit from alternative nonsurgical methods of treating heart disease. These alternative methods include percutaneous transluminal coronary angioplasty (PCTA), streptokinase, and the use of intravascular stents. Other procedures, including laser-heated thermal probes, hot balloons and catheter-tip turbines, are under study.

Many research studies have found that hospitals with the lowest mortality rates for CABG have the highest volume. Joint guidelines published by the American College of Cardiology and the American Heart Association recommend that (Kirklin et al. 1991):

- "At least 200 to 300 open heart operations, the majority of them coronary artery bypass operations, should be performed annually by hospitals caring for patients with ischemic heart disease."
- "At least 100 to 150 open heart operations, the majority of which are coronary artery bypass operations, should be performed annually by each surgeon caring for patients with ischemic heart disease. The cardiac surgeon should, in most instances, be certified by the American Board of Thoracic Surgery or an equivalent certifying body in another country."
- "Hospital CABG programs should have at least two qualified cardiac surgeons and both surgeons should practice only in a single institution."

A study of hospital mortality in New York for cardiac surgery patients during 1989 found that patient mortality was the lowest when both surgeon and hospital volume was high (Kirklin et al. 1991 and Hennan et al. 1991). Conversely, patient mortality was found to be highest when both surgeon and hospital volume was low. The study, which examined the outcomes of 12,448 patients, also found that the volume (number of operations) of surgeons was a better predictor of patient mortality than hospital volume.

Risk-adjusted hospital mortality rates by annual hospital and surgeon patient volume
Coronary artery bypass grafts
State Of New York, 1989

Surgeon Volume	Hospital Volume 28–199	Hospital Volume 200–699	Hospital Volume 700+
60 or less	13.3%	9.7%	5.0%
60-99	4.7%	4.9%	4.6%
100-179	5.5%	4.2%	3.9%
180 or more	6.1%	3.1%	2.7%

Note: Data are risk-adjusted hospital mortality rates for 12,448 patients in the state of New York in 1989 and include coronary bypass operations and other cardiac surgery cases. The statewide mortality rate was 3.7 percent. Patient data were obtained for 126 surgeons.

Source: Reprinted with permission from (Kirklin et al.) *Journal of the American College of Cardiology* (March 1, 1991); and Medical Care (Hannan et al. 1991), J.B. Lippincott publishing company; and John W. Kirklin, M.D., chairman ACC/AHA Task Force on Assessment of Diagnostic and Therapeutic Cardiovascular Procedures (1993).

A study of 18,986 CABG surgery patients in 77 California hospitals (Showstack et al. 1987) found that there were fewer deaths in hospitals that performed more than 200 cardiac bypass operations annually and that patients spent fewer days in these hospitals. The Showstack study, published by the *Journal of the American Medical Association*, found that 5.2 percent of the patients died in hospitals that performed 20 to 100 operations annually. The study found that, in general, as the volume of surgery increased, the patient death rate declined. For hospitals with between 101 and 200 operations, the death rate was 3.9 percent. The rate was 4.1 percent for hospitals performing between 201 and 350 procedures, and the rate was 3.1 percent for hospitals performing more than 350 operations.

Showstack also found that patient outcomes were, in general, better in high-volume hospitals. Hospitals that performed between 20 and 100 operations annually had a poor outcome rate of 21.7 percent. The rate was 15.5 percent for hospitals performing between 101 and 201 operations. Hospitals performing between 201 and 350 procedures had a rate of 11.8 percent, and hospitals performing more than 350 operations had a rate of 12 percent. Poor outcomes were defined as deaths in the hospital combined with postoperative lengths of stay beyond 15 days.

A 1987 National Center for Health Services Research study (Kelly and Hellinger 1987) found that patients with atherosclerosis who undergo a CABG operation or a cardiac catheterization procedure are more likely to survive in hospitals with high volumes of these procedures. The study found that the presence of a coronary care unit (CCU) in the hospital lowered patient deaths by 3.2 percent. The study cited other research which found that patient deaths within 30 days of a bypass operation have declined over the past ten years from between 6 percent and 7 percent to fewer than 3 percent.

Kelly and Hellinger also found that for persons with acute myocardial infarction (AMI), who did not undergo surgery, the hospital volume of treating AMI patients was not a factor in patient survival. The study found AMI patients were more likely to survive if their physicians treated high volumes of AMI patients. In addition, patients who were treated by physicians who were board-certified in family practice or internal medicine were more likely to survive compared to patients who were treated by physicians who were not board certified. AMI patients treated in teaching facilities affiliated with a medical school were found to have higher survival rates than AMI patients treated in hospitals not affiliated with medical schools. The study found that the outcomes of nonsurgical heart patients ". . . do not depend on operating room staff and are less dependent on complex medical equipment."

Two studies published in the August 14, 1991 issue of the *Journal of the American Medical Association* examined CABG surgery in-hospital mortality. One study (Williams, Nash, and Goldfarb 1991) examined 4,613 patients over a 30-month period in five major teaching hospitals in Philadelphia who underwent coronary artery catheterization and CABG surgery during the same admission. The authors found that: there were threefold differences in the mortality rates of individual surgeons; patient mortality rates were not associated with the number of procedures performed by surgeons; and the intensity of hospital services was not related to patient mortality.

The other JAMA study examined 3,055 CABG patients during a 22-month period between 1987 and 1989 in five regional medical centers in New England (O'Connor et al. 1991). The study was undertaken to determine if patient severity of illness (case mix) was associated with in-hospital mortality. The study included data from all of the 18 surgeons who performed cardiothoracic surgery in Maine, New Hampshire, and Vermont. The study found the crude in-hospital mortality rate averaged 4.3 percent, and varied between 3.1 percent and 6.3 percent. Mortality rates for individual surgeons varied from 1.9 percent to 9.2 percent. The study concluded that, "The observed differences in in-hospital mortality rates among institutions and among surgeons in northern New England are not solely the result of differences in [how severely ill the patients were] and may reflect differences in currently unknown aspects of patient care. Understanding this variation requires a detailed understanding of the processes of care."

Some patients may undergo surgery for uncertain or inappropriate reasons. A RAND Corporation study of 386 random bypass surgery patients in three hospitals in an unidentified western state (Winslow et al. 1988) found that 56 percent of the patients received bypass surgery for appropriate reasons, 30 percent were uncertain, and 14 percent were performed for inappropriate reasons. However, a more recent study of 1,338 patients who underwent isolated coronary artery bypass graft surgery in the State of New York in 1990 had very different findings. The New York study, also conducted by RAND, found almost 91 percent were appropriate, 7 percent uncertain, and only 2.4 percent were inappropriate (Leape et al. 1993; also see Chassin 1993). The authors noted that since the time the earlier study was undertaken, "The practice of coronary revascularization has changed remarkably. Bypass surgery has become safer and medical therapy has improved. Most importantly, PTCA has emerged as an alternative method of revascularization. For all of these reasons it is appropriate to reassess whether there is still substantial overuse of coronary artery bypass surgery." The authors noted that the research findings "may not be generalizable to the country as a whole." The "exemplary outcomes" reported by the study were attributed, in part, to the regulatory environment in New York that included oversight by the Cardiac Advisory Committee in New York's Department of Health.

Appendix C contains adult and pediatric open heart surgery utilization data for Florida hospitals.

ANGIOPLASTY AND CARDIAC CATHETERIZATION

Cardiac catheterization is performed in "laboratories" either to diagnose heart and circulatory problems, or as a therapy to treat coronary artery disease. As with CABG surgery, research studies have found that cardiac catheterization volume may be a factor in patient outcomes. Cardiac catheterization involves passing a radiopaque catheter into the heart. The catheter either obtains pressure measurements, samples blood, injects radiographic contrast material or other substances, conducts electrophysiologic studies, or obtains material for endomyocardial biopsies. Another test is a right ventriculogram, which involves taking an x-ray of the right ventricle of the heart.

As a diagnostic procedure, coronary angiography is the standard test for diagnosing coronary artery disease. Coronary angiography is performed during cardiac catheterization. A RAND Corporation study of 1,335 patients who underwent coronary angiography in New York during 1990 found that 76 percent of the angiographies were appropriate, 20 percent uncertain, and 4 percent inappropriate (Bernstein et al. 1993). Half of the patients who underwent the procedure had either unstable angina (28 percent) or chronic stable angina (22 percent). No inappropriate use of coronary angiography was found for unstable angina, and only 3 percent of the patients with chronic stable angina were found to have received coronary angiography inappropriately. Other types of patients had high inappropriate rates: chest pain of unknown origin, 40 percent; asymptomatic patients, 27 percent; and patients who underwent the procedure following a myocardial infarction, 13 percent. However, these patients represented relatively small percentages of those who underwent the procedure. Patients with chest pain of unknown origin comprised 3 percent of all patients, asymptomatic patients 4 percent, and patients who received the procedure after a myocardial infarction comprised 7 percent.

As a therapeutic treatment, cardiac catheterization has replaced the need for open heart surgery for some patients. Percutaneous transluminal coronary angioplasty (PTCA) is the most common therapeutic procedure. PTCA is used to clear coronary arteries that have been narrowed by plaque deposits. A balloon-tipped catheter is inserted into the artery; the balloon is then inflated and deflated to break up the plaque.

A RAND Corporation study of 1306 patients who underwent PTCA in New York State during 1990 determined that 58 percent of the patients underwent PTCA for appropriate reasons. Thirty-eight percent of the patients were found to have undergone the procedure for uncertain reasons, and 4 percent were found to be inappropriate (Hilborne et al. 1993). The authors stated that there were several explanations for the high "uncertain" rate. Most important is a shortage of outcomes data which is needed to make a definitive judgment on appropriateness. In addition, some researchers question the long-term benefit of PTCA. Finally, PTCA medical practice is undergoing rapid change because of new catheter designs and the use of alternative procedures such as coronary atherectomy and coronary stenting.

Catheter catherectomy is a recent therapeutic technique that uses diamond tips, rather than expanding and contracting balloons, to destroy plaque. Another procedure is balloon valvuloplasty, which is performed to relieve valve stenosis. Valve stenosis is a complication of rheumatic fever and comprises about 10 percent of all heart disease.

Other new technologies to remove plaque from the peripheral arteries include mechanical atherectomy and various types of intravascular stents. Like many areas of medicine, new cardiac procedures are being developed at a fast pace as new knowledge is acquired and technology advances. An experimental cardiac diagnostic technique uses nuclear magnetic resonance imaging. This diagnostic technique does not expose patients to ionizing radiation.

According to the guidelines of an American College of Cardiology and American Heart Association task force on cardiac catheterization (Pepine et al. 1991):

- Cardiac catheterization laboratories for adults should maintain a minimum caseload of at least 300 a year.
- Pediatric laboratories should maintain a minimum caseload of at least 150 children per year. "It is particularly important that infants and all patients with complex congenital heart disease be catheterized only in centers with active pediatric cardiac surgical programs."
- Physician guidelines call for 150 adult cases per year and 50 to 100 pediatric cases per year. In addition, "A laboratory physician should be a fully accredited member of the hospital staff and, ideally, be specialty certified or at least board qualified with the intention of taking boards at the earliest possible date."
- "In view of the lack of appropriately controlled safety and the need for data for hospital-based, mobile, or free-standing laboratories operating without on-site (accessible by gurney) cardiac surgery facilities . . . further development of these services cannot be endorsed at this time."
- Cardiac catheterization programs that are not located in hospitals that also have in-house cardiovascular surgery (open heart surgery) programs "will offer limited services" and "must" have formal arrangements with a hospital that does perform cardiovascular surgery.
- PTCA, balloon valvuloplasty, transseptal puncture, transthoracic left ventricular puncture, and myocardial biopsy, should not be performed in a hospital without an in-house surgical program.
- "Laboratories without surgery available on site will see less variety in the condition of patients undergoing evaluation. They must exercise particular caution to not accept unstable, acutely ill, or other high-risk patients."
- "Patients at high risk for catheterization-associated complications should be referred to centers where on-site surgery is available for stabilization and diagnostic catheterization procedures."

The study conducted by Kelly and Hellinger (1987) discussed in the open heart surgery section found that patients who undergo a cardiac catheterization procedure are more likely to survive in hospitals that perform a high volume of these procedures. However, a relationship between surgeon volume and patient outcomes was not found.

According to Kelly and Hellinger, "The dominant effect of the volume of similar surgical cases treated by hospitals may reflect the importance of a learning-by-doing effect for operative and postoperative staff, the reliance on complex medical equipment during surgical procedures, or other characteristics of high volume hospitals. The most appropriate entity for measuring the effect of experience on treating surgical patients may be the experience of the operating room staff in performing similar types of procedures."

Appendix D contains Florida hospital adult and pediatric cardiac catheterization utilization data.

ORGAN TRANSPLANTATION

Organ transplantation is one of the most sophisticated of all surgical operations. Advances in surgical techniques and in the development of immunosuppressive drugs have increased the feasibility and success of organ transplants.

In September 1992, the federal government began releasing patient survival rates for hospitals with organ transplant programs (Public Health Service 1992). According to the initial study, 92.9 percent of patients who received a kidney transplant were alive one year after surgery. The one year survival rate for patients receiving a pancreas transplant was 88.7 percent, 82.1 percent for heart, 74.4 percent for liver, 53.9 percent for lung, and 53.3 percent for heart/lung. These data are averages for all 531 transplant programs in the country for patients who received transplants from Oct. 1, 1987 through Dec. 31, 1989. A second, more sophisticated, study was expected to be released in late 1993.

The study found that transplant programs that frequently performed procedures had consistently high patient survival rates. Low volume programs were found to have "widely variable" results. However, the report stated that, "Differences between programs performing few transplants may not be statistically significant since the numbers of transplants performed at these programs are so small."

A study of heart transplantation published in the *New England Journal of Medicine* (Laffel et al. 1992) examined 1,123 patients who received heart transplants in 56 hospitals from 1984 to 1986. The study was designed to determine the relationship between experience and patient mortality. The study found that the "previous training of cardiologists was strongly related to [lower] mortality." Although the study found that there was a positive relationship between surgical experience and better outcomes for patients, a relationship between total volume of transplants and patient mortality was not found.

The United Network for Organ Sharing has published a guide that lists questions patients might ask the transplant staff when visiting a transplant hospital. These questions include:

- What is the hospital's experience in transplanting this particular organ?
- What are the organ and patient survival rates at this hospital?
- Is there a special nursing unit for transplant patients?
- Will I be asked to participate in research studies?

Patients and physicians may obtain at no charge hospital survival rates for up to 10 transplant programs, a user's guide that explains how to interpret the survival rates, a patient guide to use in selecting a transplant hospital, and general information about organ donation, including donor cards, by contacting:

United Network for Organ Sharing
1100 Boulders Parkway, Suite 500
Richmond, Virginia 23225
(800) 243-6667

In August 1992, ten Florida hospitals performing organ transplants were members of the United Network for Organ Sharing (UNOS).

UNOS member hospitals with transplant programs
August 1992

County	Hospital	Organs
Alachua	Shands Hospital	Heart
	Shands Hospital	Liver
	Shands Hospital	Kidney
Dade	Jackson Memorial	Heart
	Jackson Memorial	Lung
	Jackson Memorial	Heart/Lung
	Jackson Memorial	Liver
	Jackson Memorial	Kidney
	Jackson Memorial	Pancreas
	Miami Children's Hospital	Heart

Duval	Methodist Medical Center	Kidney
Hillsborough	St. Joseph's Hospital	Heart
Hillsborough	Tampa General	Heart
	Tampa General	Liver
	Tampa General	Kidney
Lee	SW Florida Regional MC	Kidney
Leon	Tallahassee Memorial	Heart
Orange	Florida Hospital	Kidney
Pinellas	All Children's	Kidney

Source: U.S. Department of Health and Human Services, 1992.

Becoming an organ donor

Despite recent medical advances in organ transplantation, there are far too few donors. It has been estimated that only one in four persons in need of a transplant receives it. Each year approximately 2,000 persons die waiting for a transplant because organs are not available. In August 1992, almost 28,000 persons were on waiting lists nationally to receive an organ.

In Florida, it is a simple matter to become a potential donor. The Department of Highway Safety and Motor Vehicles has a form for potential donors to complete. Donors' driver's licenses are stamped, indicating that the driver is a potential donor.

Another way to become a potential donor is to sign and carry an organ donor card. The United Network for Organ Sharing (UNOS) offers a guide on organ donation. To obtain the free guide, which contains an organ donor card, contact UNOS.

Be sure to notify, and discuss your desire to be an organ donor with, your next of kin. According to UNOS, "Although this can be a difficult decision, many families find that when faced with such a tragedy, donating organs for transplantation provides great consolation and comfort."

The Public Health Service also publishes information on organ transplantation and organ donation. To obtain a copy of *Questions and Answers About Organ Transplantation* and other information contact:

Public Health Service
HRSA, Bureau of Health Resources Development
Division of Organ Transplantation
5600 Fishers Lane
Parklawn Building, Room 11a-22
Rockville, Maryland 20857
(301) 443-7577

EYE, HEART, AND HAND SURGERY

Although there is only one specialty eye surgery hospital in Florida, the Ann Bates Leach Eye Hospital in Miami, most large hospitals have physicians that perform ophthalmological surgery. The Ann Bates Leach Eye Hospital is affiliated with the Bascom Palmer Eye Institute, which has a residency program with the University of

Miami medical school.

The Miami Heart Institute, with 258 beds, is located in Miami Beach. This is the only specialty hospital in Florida dedicated solely to the treatment of patients with heart conditions. The Miami Heart Institute performs open heart surgery and cardiac catheterization but does not have a heart transplant program.

Although not technically a specialty hospital, the 27-bed Ramadan Hospital and Hand Surgery Center specializes in hand surgery. Ramadan is located in Lake Butler in Union County, a short drive from Gainesville.

CHILDREN'S HOSPITALS

There are seven hospitals in Florida that specialize in the treatment of children. All of the children's hospitals are nonprofit and two are supported by fraternal organizations. The Shriners Hospital for Crippled Children specializes in the care of handicapped children. The Wolfson Children's Hospital is affiliated with Baptist Hospital in Jacksonville. Most children's hospitals are affiliated with medical schools and have residency programs.

Florida children's hospitals		
County	*Hospital*	*Number Beds*
Dade	Miami Children's Hospital	208
Duval	Wolfson Children's (Baptist Hospital)	90
Escambia	Sacred Heart Children's Hospital	50
Hillsborough	Shriners Hospital for Crippled Children	60
Lake	Florida Elks Children's Hospital	100
Orange	Orlando RMC/Palmer Children & Womens	255
Pinellas	All Children's Hospital	113

Source: Agency for Health Care Administration.

The St. Jude Children's Research Hospital in Memphis, Tennessee, is a nationally recognized children's specialty hospital. Information regarding admissions, treatments and services offered by St. Jude can be obtained by contacting:

St. Jude Children's Research Hospital
P.O. Box 1818
Memphis, TN 38101-9903

CANCER TREATMENT

Two national organizations, the National Cancer Institute and the Commission on Cancer of the American College of Surgeons have programs that recognize hospital cancer treatment programs.

National Cancer Institute-affiliated hospitals

There are two categories of hospitals that are affiliated with the National Cancer Institute (NCI): comprehensive cancer centers and clinical cancer centers. Florida has one NCI-approved comprehensive cancer hospital, the Sylvester Comprehensive Cancer Center at the University of Miami and Jackson Memorial Hospital. Nationally, there are 42 NCI-supported treatment centers.

Florida has four hospitals that participate in the NCI Community Clinical Oncology

Program (CCOP). CCOP hospitals participate in NCI sponsored research studies that include clinical trials. Obtaining treatment at an NCI-affiliated hospital has several advantages because NCI hospitals conduct clinical trials in addition to providing traditional cancer treatments. Clinical trials have the potential to help patients with cancers that cannot be successfully treated by traditional means. Clinical trials also may provide new information to help others.

Hospitals with cancer programs
approved by the National Cancer Institute
1992

City	Name of Hospital	Type
Miami	Sylvester Comp Cancer Center (Jackson Memorial Hospital)	Comprehensive
Miami Beach	Mt. Sinai Medical Center	CCOP
Orlando	Orlando Regional Medical Center	CCOP
Pensacola	Sacred Heart Children's Hospital	CCOP
St. Petersburg	All Children's Hospital	CCOP

Source: National Cancer Institute, 1992.

To be eligible for NCI clinical trials, it is important to contact the NCI when cancer is first diagnosed and before non-NCI treatment begins. Clinical trial programs enroll patients who have not received prior treatment. This is necessary to obtain unbiased scientific data regarding the effects of experimental treatments. The same clinical trial program may be offered at several NCI community clinical oncology program sites. Depending upon the clinical trial, community hospitals in Florida may participate as NCI community clinical oncology program sites. Participation in clinical trial programs is free.

The main NCI center in Bethesda, Maryland, conducts specialized experimental cancer investigations. The NCI pays for all costs, including hospitalization, lodging, food, and travel for patients who are treated in specialized programs.

Information regarding the specialized cancer treatments offered at all 42 national NCI centers, can be obtained by calling the NCI. These free information services include information on treatment, information on NCI affiliated physicians, numerous publications on cancer, cancer literature searches, and other services, including a "quit smoking" hotline.

National Cancer Institute
(800) 4-CANCER

American College of Surgeons cancer programs

The Commission on Cancer of the American College of Surgeons approves cancer programs at hospitals. Forty-eight non-military hospitals in Florida have approved programs. The Naval Hospital in Jacksonville also has an approved program.

Approval by the American College of Surgeons (ACS) is not based on success in treating cancer patients. According to ACS, the program is, "Intended to measure process rather than outcome." The ACS places emphasis on the education of health care professionals in, "new knowledge based on clinical research." The basic criteria that are used to approve programs "stress the importance of multidisciplinary cancer conferences and accurate recording of diagnostic and treatment data in a cancer registry for meaningful patient-care evaluation."

Hospitals with cancer programs
approved by the American College of Surgeons
1992

City	Name of Hospital	Type
Boca Raton	Boca Raton Community Hospital	CHCP
Boynton Beach	Bethesda Memorial Hospital	CHCP
Bradenton	Manatee Memorial Hospital	CHCP
Cape Coral	Cape Coral Hospital	CHCP
Clearwater	Morton Plant Hospital	COMP
Daytona Beach	Halifax Medical Center	COMP
Dunedin	Mease Health Care	COMP
Ft. Lauderdale	Broward General Medical Center	CHCP
Ft. Myers	Lee Memorial Hospital	CHCP
Ft. Myers	S.W. Florida Regional Med. Cntr.	CHCP
Gainesville	Shands Hospital	THCP
Jacksonville	Wolfson Children's	SHCP
Jacksonville	St. Vincent's Medical Center	CHCP
Jacksonville	University Medical Center	THCP
Jupiter	Jupiter Hospital	CHCP
Lake Worth	JFK Medical Center	CHCP
Lakeland	Lakeland Regional Medical Center	CHCP
Largo	HCA Largo Medical Center	CHCP
Largo	Sun Coast Hospital	CHCP
Melbourne	Holmes Regional Medical Center	COMP
Miami	Baptist Hospital of Miami	COMP
Miami	Cedars Medical Center	COMP
Miami	Jackson Memorial Hospital	THCP
Miami	Mercy Hospital	CHCP
Miami	North Shore Medical Center	COMP
Miami	South Miami Hospital	CHCP
Miami Beach	Mt. Sinai Medical Center	THCP
Naples	Naples Community Hospital	CHCP
Ocala	Marion Community Hospital	COMP
Ocala	Munroe Regional Medical Center	COMP
Orlando	Florida Regional Medical Center	COMP
Orlando	Orlando Regional Medical Center	THCP
Pensacola	Baptist Hospital	COMP
Pensacola	Sacred Heart Hospital	CHCP
Pensacola	West Florida Regional Med. Cntr.	COMP
Rockledge	Wuesthoff Hospital	CHCP
Sarasota	Sarasota Memorial Hospital	CHCP
St. Petersburg	Bayfront Medical Center	CHCP
St. Petersburg	St. Anthony's Hospital	CHCP
Stuart	Martin Memorial Hospital	CHCP
Tallahassee	Tallahassee Memorial	COMP
Tampa	H. Lee Moffitt Cancer Center	THCP
Tampa	St. Joseph's Hospital	COMP
Tampa	Tampa General Hospital	THCP

Tampa	University Community Hospital	COMP
Titusville	Parrish Medical Center	CHCP
Venice	Venice Hospital	CHCP
Vero Beach	Indian River Memorial Hospital	CHCP

THCP = Teaching Hospital Cancer Program
COMP = Community Hospital Comprehensive Cancer Program
CHCP = Community Hospital Cancer Program
SHCP = Special Hospital Cancer Program

Source: American College of Surgeons, 1992.

Lists of ACS approved programs and other information can be obtained from:

**Cancer Department
American College of Surgeons
55 East Erie Street
Chicago, IL 60611
(312) 664-4050, Ext. 209**

BURN TREATMENT

Although most general hospitals provide care to patients who have suffered burns, the treatment of severely burned persons is specialized. Only four hospitals in Florida provide care to severely burned persons. These hospitals are Shands Teaching Hospital, Tampa General Hospital, Orlando Regional Medical Center, and Jackson Memorial Hospital. The burn units at Jackson Memorial and Tampa General are much larger than those at Shands or Orlando Regional. Very severely burned patients may be flown to the Brooke Army Hospital at Fort Sam Houston, Texas, which has a nationally recognized program for burn victims.

The table below shows Florida's hospitals with burn units for severely burned patients.

Florida hospitals with burn units
February 1993

County	Hospital	Staffed beds
Alachua	Shands Teaching Hospital	6
Dade	Jackson Memorial Hospital	28
Hillsborough	Tampa General Hospital	18
Orange	Orlando Regional Medical Center	6

Source: Agency for Health Care Administration, 1993.

Long-term acute care

Three hospitals, Vencor Hospital in Fort Lauderdale, Vencor Hospital in Coral Gables, and Vencor Hospital in Tampa, specialize in providing long-term acute care services to medically-complex and catastrophically ill patients with neurological disorders, central nervous system disorders, and cardio-pulmonary disorders. In addition, these hospitals also specialize in child and adult pulmonary patients who are ventilator-dependent, require assisted or partial ventilator support, or need supplemental oxygen and bronchial hygiene.

Seven hospitals have long-term care programs accredited by the Joint Commission on Accreditation of Healthcare Organizations. These seven hospitals are listed in the "JCAHO Accredited Long-Term Facilities" section of Chapter Four.

SPECIAL DIAGNOSTIC AND THERAPEUTIC EQUIPMENT

Technologically advanced equipment has greatly increased the ability of physicians to diagnose and successfully treat a variety of medical conditions. High-tech equipment for the treatment of diseases includes lithotripters and various megavoltage radiation therapy devices. Technologically advanced diagnostic equipment includes computerized tomographic (CT) scanners (commonly called "cat" scanners), magnetic resonance imaging (MRI) systems, and digital vascular imaging (DVI) systems. All of this equipment is standard in technologically advanced general hospitals.

CT scanners are the "oldest" technologically-sophisticated diagnostic device, introduced in the 1970s. The early CT scanners scanned the cranium; today's machines scan the entire body. A CT scanner, like an x-ray machine, uses radiation to produce images. However, unlike an x-ray machine which takes a single image, CT scanners take multiple images from many different angles. CT scanners also take images in much finer detail than x-ray machines. CT scanners have become a standard piece of diagnostic equipment in hospitals. Even some small rural hospitals have contracts with firms that provide mobile CT scanners.

Extracorporeal shockwave lithotripters use ultrasonic sound waves to dissolve certain types of kidney stones. Patients are immersed in water for 30 to 60 minutes while being exposed to highly focused ultrasonic sound waves. Lithotripters represent a major breakthrough in technology because they replace invasive surgery. Prior to mid-1986, Shands Teaching Hospital in Gainesville was the only hospital in Florida with an extracorporeal shockwave lithotripter. Lithotripters now are standard equipment in large hospitals. Hospitals without them usually are visited by mobile units.

Magnetic resonance imaging (MRI) systems use radio waves, rather than radiation, to produce diagnostic images. MRI systems produce three-dimensional images that are particularly useful in the diagnosis of cancer, multiple sclerosis, cerebrovascular diseases, heart disease, and complications resulting from pregnancy. In addition, MRI scans are useful for spinal or brain surgery. New refinements in MRI technology are continually being made and still greater improvements are expected in the future.

Digital vascular imaging (DVI) equipment is primarily used for the diagnosis of vascular diseases. DVI systems use a computer to display several x-ray images simultaneously. The information is then stored on video discs.

JCAHO-ACCREDITED HOSPITALS

The Joint Commission on Accreditation of Healthcare Organizations (JCAHO) accredits hospitals that comply with certain standards. These standards prescribe minimum essential levels of performance and are designed to promote quality health care. The JCAHO has four categories of hospital accreditation:
- Accreditation with commendation. Fewer than 10 percent of hospitals receive this distinction. As of April 1993, only 16 Florida acute care hospitals had received this designation;
- Accreditation (80 percent to 85 percent of hospitals are in this category);
- Conditional accreditation (about 5 percent of hospitals); and

- Denied accreditation (only a small percentage of hospitals are denied accreditation, possibly because hospitals that cannot meet JCAHO accreditation standards likely do not apply for accreditation).

Readers should consult the "Accreditation Organizations" section of Chapter 11 for additional information on accredited facilities. Persons interested in obtaining current information regarding the accreditation status of a hospital can contact the JCAHO. JCAHO information is available to anyone.

Acute care hospitals
accredited with commendation by JCAHO
April 1993

Hospital	*City*
Aventura Medical Center	Aventura
Bethesda Memorial Hospital	Boynton Beach
Hca L.W. Blake Hospital	Bradenton
Brandon Hospital	Brandon
Dade City Hospital	Dade City
Destin Hospital	Destin
Vencor Hospital	Ft Lauderdale
Ft Walton Beach Med Center	Ft Walton Beach
Memorial Hospital Of Hollywood	Hollywood
Bayonet Point/Hudson Med Cntr	Hudson
Osceola Regional Hospital	Kissimmee
Plantation General Hospital	Plantation
Pompano Beach Medical Center	Pompano Beach
St Petersburg General Hospital	St Petersburg
University Pavilion Hospital	Tamarac
Helen Ellis Memorial Hospital	Tarpon Springs

Source: JCAHO, April 1993.

ACUTE CARE HOSPITALS

Listed below are the names, addresses, and telephone numbers of Florida acute care general hospitals, rehabilitation hospitals, and other specialty hospitals. Psychiatric and substance abuse specialty hospitals are listed at the end of Chapter 7.

Alachua County
Alachua General Hospital
801 S.W. 2nd Ave
Gainesville 32602
(904) 372-4321

HCA North Florida Regional Medical
    Center
State Road 26 At I-75
Gainesville 32602
(904) 333-4100

Shands Teaching Hospital
1600 S.W. Archer Road
Gainesville 32610
(904) 395-0400

Upreach Pavilion
8900 N.W. 39th Ave
Gainesville 32602
(904) 338-0091

Baker County
Ed Fraser Memorial Hospital
159 North 3rd St
Macclenny 32063
(904) 259-3151

Bay County
Bay Medical Center
615 North Bonita Ave
Panama City 32401
(904) 769-1511

HCA Gulf Coast Community Hospital
449 West 23rd St
Panama City 32405
(904) 769-8341

Bradford County
Bradford County Hospital
922 East Call St
Starke 32091
(904) 964-6000

Brevard County
Cape Canaveral Hospital
701 W. Cocoa Beach Causeway
Cocoa Beach 32931
(407) 799-7171

J.E. Holmes Regional Medical Center
1350 South Hickory St
Melbourne 32901
(407) 727-7000

Jess Parrish Memorial Hospital
951 North Washington Ave
Titusville 32796
(407) 268-6100

Sea Pines Rehabilitation Hospital
101 Florida Ave
Melbourne 32901
(407) 984-4600

Wuesthoff Memorial Hospital
110 Longwood Ave
Rockledge 32955
(407) 636-2211

Broward County
AMI North Ridge Hospital
5757 North Dixie Highway
Fort Lauderdale 33334
(305) 776-6000

Broward General Medical Center
1600 South Andrews Ave
Fort Lauderdale 33316
(305) 355-4400

Coral Springs Medical Center
3000 Coral Hills Drive
Coral Springs 33065
(305) 344-3000

Doctors Hospital of Hollywood
1859 Van Buren St
Hollywood 33020-5145
(305) 920-9000

Florida Medical Center Hospital—Fort
  Lauderdale
5000 West Oakland Park Blvd
Fort Lauderdale 33313
 (305) 735-6000

HCA N.W. Regional Hospital
5801 Colonial Drive
Margate 33063
(305) 974-0400

Hollywood Medical Center
3600 Washington St
Hollywood 33021
(305) 966-4500

Holy Cross Hospital
4725 North Federal Highway
Fort Lauderdale 33308
(305) 771-8000

Imperial Point Medical Center
6401 North Federal Highway
Fort Lauderdale 33308
(305) 776-8500

Manor Oaks
2121 East Commercial Blvd
Fort Lauderdale 33308
(305) 771-8400

Memorial Hospital-Hollywood
3501 Johnson St
Hollywood 33021
(305) 987-2000

Memorial Hospital West
703 N. Flamingo Road
Pembroke Pines 33028
(305) 436-5000

North Beach Hospital
2835 North Ocean Blvd
Fort Lauderdale 33308
(305) 568-1000

North Broward Medical Center
201 Sample Road
Pompano Beach 33064
(305) 941-8300

Pembroke Pines Hospital
2301 University Drive
Pembroke Pines 33024
(305) 962-9650

Plantation General Hospital
410 N.W. 42nd Ave
Plantation 33317
(305) 587-5010

Pompano Beach Medical Center
600 S.W. 3rd St
Pompano Beach 33060
(305) 782-2000

Saint John's Rehabilitation Hospital
3075 N.W. 35th Ave
Lauderdale Lakes 33311
(305) 739-6233

Sunrise Rehabilitation Hospital
4399 Nob Hill Road
Sunrise 33321
(305) 749-0300

Universal Medical Center
6701 West Sunrise Blvd
Plantation 33313
(305) 581-7800

University Hospital
7201 North University Drive
Tamarac 33321
(305) 721-2200

Vencor Hospital
1516 East Las Olas Blvd
Fort Lauderdale 33301
(305) 764-8900

Westside Regional Medical Center
8201 West Broward Blvd
Plantation 33324
(305) 473-6600

Calhoun County
Calhoun General Hospital
424 Burns Ave
Blountstown 32424
(904) 674-5411

Charlotte County
Fawcett Memorial Hospital
21298 Olean Blvd
Port Charlotte 33952
(813) 629-1181

Medical Center Hospital
809 East Marion Ave
Punta Gorda 33950
(813) 639-3131

Saint Joseph's Hospital of Port Charlotte
2500 Harbor Blvd
Port Charlotte 33952
(813) 625-4122

Citrus County
Citrus Memorial Hospital
502 Highland Blvd
Inverness 32652
(904) 344-6582

Seven Rivers Community Hospital
6201 North Suncoast Blvd
Crystal River 32629
(904) 795-6560

Clay County
Humana Hospital—Orange Park
2001 Kingsley Ave
Orange Park 32073
(904) 272-8500

Collier County
Naples Community Hospital
350 Seventh St North
Naples 33939
(813) 263-5114

Columbia County
Lake City Medical Center
1701 West Duval St
Lake City 32055
(904) 752-2922

Lake Shore Hospital
560 East Franklin St
Lake City 32055
(904) 755-3200

Dade County
Anne Bates Leach Eye Hospital
900 N.W. 17th St
Miami 33136
(305) 326-6000

Aventure Hospital
20900 Biscayne Blvd
Miami 33180
(305) 932-0250

Baptist Hospital of Miami
8900 North Kendall Drive
Miami 33176
(305) 596-1960

Bon Secours Hospital
1050 N.E. 125th St
North Miami 33161
(305) 891-8850

Cedars Medical Center
1400 N.W. 12th Ave
Miami 33181
(305) 325-4515

Coral Gables Hospital
3100 Douglas Road
Coral Gables 33134
(305) 445-8461

Deering Hospital
9333 S.W. 152nd St
Miami 33157
(305) 371-2000

Douglas Gardens Hospital
5200 N.E. 2nd Ave
Miami 33137
(305) 751-8626

Golden Glades Regional Medical Center
17300 NW 7th Avenue
Miami 33169
(305) 654-3000

Healthsouth Doctors Hospital
5000 University Drive
Coral Gables 33146-2094
(305) 666-2111

Hialeah Hospital
651 East 25th St
Hialeah 33013
(305) 693-6100

Jackson Memorial Hospital
1611 N.W. 12th Ave
Miami 33136
(305) 549-6754

Kendall Regional Medical Center
11750 Bird Road
Miami 33175
(305) 223-3000

Larkin General Hospital
7031 S.W. 62nd Ave
South Miami 33143
(305) 666-6500

Mercy Hospital - Miami
3663 South Miami Ave
Miami 33133-4237
(305) 285-2121

Miami Beach Community Hospital
250 West 63rd St
Miami Beach 33141
(305) 868-5000

Miami Children's Hospital
6125 S.W. 31st St
Miami 33155
(305) 666-6511

Miami Heart Institute
4701 North Meridian Ave
Miami Beach 33140
(305) 672-1111

Mount Sinai Medical Center
4300 Alton Road
Miami Beach 33140
(305) 674-2222

North Shore Medical Center
1100 N.W. 95th Street
Miami 33150
(305) 835-6000

Palm Springs General Hospital
1475 West 49th St
Hialeah 33012
(305) 558-2500

Palmetto General Hospital
2001 West 68th St
Hialeah 33016
(305) 823-5000

Pan American Hospital
5959 N.W. 7th St
Miami 33126
(305) 264-1000

Parkway Regional Medical Center
160 N.W. 170th St
North Miami Beach 33169
(305) 651-1100

SMH Hospital
160 N.W. Thirteenth St
Homestead 33030
(305) 248-3232

South Miami Hospital
7400 S.W. 62nd Ave
South Miami 33143
(305) 661-4611

South Shore Hospital and Medical Center
630 Alton Road
Miami Beach 33139
(305) 672-2100

University of Miami Hospital and Clinics
1475 N.W. 12th Ave
Miami 33136
(305) 547-6418

Vencor Hospital
5190 S.W. 8th St
Coral Gables 33134
(305) 445-1364

Victoria Hospital
955 N.W. 3rd St
Miami 33128
(305) 545-8050

West Gables Rehabilitation Hospital
2525 SW 75th Avenue
Miami 33155
(305) 262-6800

Westchester General Hospital
2500 S.W. 75th Avenue
Miami 33155
(305) 264-5252

Desoto County
Desoto Memorial Hospital
900 North Robert Ave
Arcadia 33821
(813) 494-3535

Duval County
Baptist Medical Center
800 Prudential Drive
Jacksonville 32207
(904) 393-2000

Baptist Medical Center The Beaches
1350 13th Ave South
Jacksonville Beach 32250
(904) 247-2900

Jacksonville Medical Center
4901 Richard St
Jacksonville 32207
(904) 737-3120

Memorial Regional Rehabilitation Center
3625 University Blvd S.
Jacksonville 32216
(904) 399-6111

Methodist Medical Center
580 West Eighth St
Jacksonville 32209
(904) 798-8000

Riverside Hospital
2033 Riverside Ave
Jacksonville 32204
(904) 387-7000

Saint Luke's Hospital
4201 Belford Road
Jacksonville 32216-5898
(904) 296-3700

Saint Vincent's Medical Center
1800 Barrs St
Jacksonville 32203
(904) 387-7300

University Hospital of Jacksonville
655 West Eighth St
Jacksonville 32209
(904) 350-6899

Escambia County
Baptist Hospital
1000 West Moreno St
Pensacola 32501
(904) 434-4804

Sacred Heart Hospital of Pensacola
5151 North Ninth Ave
Pensacola 32504
(904) 474-7000

West Fla Regional Medical Center
8383 North Davis Highway
Pensacola 32514
(904) 478-4460

Flagler County
Memorial Hospital—Flagler
Moody Boulevard, SR 1
Bunnell 32010
(904) 437-2211

Franklin County
Emerald Coast Hospital
Washington Square
Apalachicola 32320
(904) 653-8853

Gadsden County
Gadsden Memorial Hospital
Highway 90 East
Quincy 32351
(904) 875-1100

Gulf County
Gulf Pines Hospital
102 Twentieth St
Port Saint Joe 32456
(904) 227-1121

Hamilton County
Hamilton County Memorial Hospital
506 N.W. 4th St
Jasper 32052
(904) 792-2101

Hardee County
Hardee Memorial Hospital
533 West Carlton St
Wauchula 33873
(813) 773-3101

Hendry County
Hendry General Hospital
524 West Sagamore St
Clewiston 33440
(813) 983-9121

Hernando County
Brooksville Regional Hospital
55 Ponce DeLeon Boulevard
Brooksville 34605
(904) 796-5111

HCA Oak Hill Hospital
11375 Cortez Blvd.
Spring Hill 33526
(904) 597-3023

Spring Hill Regional Hospital
10461 Quality Drive
Spring Hill 34609
(904) 796-1450

Highlands County
Highlands Regional Medical Center
3600 South Highlands Ave
Sebring 33870
(813) 385-6101

Walker Memorial Hospital
2501 U.S. 27 North
Avon Park 33825-1200
(813) 453-7511

Hillsborough County
AMI Town & Country Hospital
6001 Webb Road
Tampa 33615
(813) 885-6666

Brandon Hospital
119 Oakfield Drive
Brandon 33511
(813) 681-5551

Centro Asturiano Hospital
1302 21st Ave
Tampa 33605
(813) 248-1680

Centurion Hospital of Carrollwood
7171 North Dale Mabry
Tampa 33614
(813) 935-1191

Doctors' Hospital of Tampa
4801 North Howard Ave
Tampa 33603
(813) 879-1550

H. Lee Moffit Cancer Center & Research
  Institute
12901 North 30th St
Tampa 33612
(813) 972-4673

Memorial Hospital of Tampa
2901 Swann Ave
Tampa 33609
(813) 873-6400

Shriners' Hospital for Crippled Children
12501 North 30th St
Tampa 33612
(813) 972-2250

South Bay Hospital
4016 State Road 674
Sun City Center 33570
(813) 634-3301

South Florida Baptist Hospital
301 North Alexander
Plant City 33566
(813) 757-1200

St. Joseph's Hospital
3001 Dr. Martin Luther King
Tampa 33677-4227
(813) 870-4000

St. Joseph's Women's Hospital—Tampa
3030 West Buffalo Ave
Tampa 33607
(813) 879-4730

Tampa General Hospital
Davis Islands
Tampa 33601
(813) 251-7000

University Community Hospital
3100 E. Fletcher Avenue
Tampa 33613
(813) 971-6000

Vencor Hospital—Tampa
4555 South Manhattan Ave
Tampa 33611
(813) 839-6341

Holmes County
Doctors Memorial Hospital
401 East Byrd Ave
Bonifay 32425
(904) 547-4271

Indian River County
Indian River Memorial Hospital
1000 36th St
Vero Beach 32960
(407) 567-4311

Sebastian Hospital
13695 U.S. Highway 1
Sebastian 32958
(407) 589-3186

Treasure Coast Rehabilitation Hospital
1600 37th St
Vero Beach 32960
(407) 778-2100

Jackson County
Campbellton-Graceville Hospital
1305 College Drive
Graceville 32440
(904) 263-4431

Jackson Hospital
800 Hospital Drive
Marianna 32446
(904) 526-2200

Lake County
Florida Elks Children's Hospital
633 Umatilla Blvd
Umatilla 32784
(904) 669-2171

Leesburg Regional Medical Center
600 East Dixie Ave
Leesburg 32748
(904) 365-4505

South Lake Mem Hospital
847 Eighth St
Clermont 32711
(904) 394-4071

Waterman Medical Center
201 North Eustis St.
Eustis 32726
(904) 589-3333

Lee County
Cape Coral Hospital
636 Del Prado Blvd
Cape Coral 33904
(813) 574-2323

East Pointe Hospital
1500 Lee Blvd
Lehigh Acres 33936
(813) 369-2101

Gulf Coast Hospital
13681 Doctors Way
Fort Myers 33912
(813) 768-5000

Lee Memorial Hospital
9981 Healthpark Circle
Fort Myers 33901
(813) 433-7799

S.W. Florida Regional Medical Center
3785 Evans Ave
Fort Myers 33901
(813) 939-8583

The Glade Center
10140 Deer Farm Road
Fort Myers 33906
(813) 275-8081

Leon County
Capital Rehabilitation Hospital
1675 Riggins Road
Tallahassee 32308-5315
(904) 656-4800

Tallahassee Community Hospital
2626 Capital Medical Blvd
Tallahassee 32308
(904) 656-5000

Tallahassee Memorial Regional Medical
    Center
Magnolia Dr & Miccousukee Rd
Tallahassee 32308
(904) 681-1155

Levy County
Nature Coast Regional Hospital
125 South West Seventh St
Williston 32696
(904) 528-2801

Madison County
Madison County Memorial Hospital
201 East Marion St
Madison 32340
(904) 973-2271

Manatee County
HCA L.W. Blake Memorial Hospital
202 59th St West
Bradenton 33529
(813) 792-6611

Manatee Memorial Hospital
206 2nd St East
Bradenton 34208
(813) 746-5111

Marion County
Marion Community Hospital
1431 S.W. First St
Ocala 32678
(904) 732-2700

Munroe Regional Medical Center
131 S.W. 15th St
Ocala 32678
(904) 351-7200

Martin County
Martin Memorial Hospital
300 Hospital Drive
Stuart 33495
(407) 287-5200

Monroe County
Fishermans Hospital
3301 Overseas Highway
Marathon 33050
(305) 743-5533

Health System Depoo
5900 West Junior College Rd
Key West 33040
(305) 294-5531

Mariners Hospital
50 High Point Road
Tavernier 33070
(305) 852-9222

Nassau County
Nassau General Hospital
1700 East Lime St
Fernandina Beach 32034
(904) 261-3627

Okaloosa County
Destin Hospital
996 Airport Road
Destin 32541
(904) 654-7600

Ft Walton Beach Medical Center
1000 Mar-Walt Drive
Fort Walton Beach 32548
(904) 862-1111

HCA Twin Cities Hospital
Highway 85 N. & College Blvd
Niceville 32578
(904) 678-4131

North Okaloosa Medical Center
151 Redstone Ave. S.E.
Crestview 32536
(904) 682-9731

Okeechobee County
HCA Raulerson Hospital
1796 Highway 441 North
Okeechobee 33472
(813) 763-2151

Orange County
Florida Hospital—Altamonte Springs
601 E. Altamonte Drive
Altamonte Springs 32701
(407) 830-4321

Florida Hospital—Apopka
201 N. Park Ave
Apopka 32703
(407) 889-1000

Florida Hospital Center for Rehabilitation
    and Wellness
5165 Adanson Street
Orlando, FL 32804
(407) 897-1785

Florida Hospital—East Orlando
7727 Lake Underhill Road
Orlando, FL 32822
(407) 277-8110

Florida Hospital—Orlando
601 East Rollins Ave
Orlando 32803
(407) 896-6611

Lucerne Hospital
818 South Main Lane
Orlando 32801
(407) 649-6111

Orlando Regional Med. Center
1414 South Kuhl Ave
Orlando 32806
(407) 841-5111

Orlando Regional Med. Center—Sand
  Lake
9400 Turkey Lake Road
Orlando 32819
(407) 351-8500

Princeton Hospital
1800 Mercy Drive
Orlando 32808
(407) 295-5151

West Orange Hospital
555 North Dillard St
Winter Garden 32787
(407) 656-1244

Winter Park Memorial Hospital
200 North Lakemont Ave
Winter Park 32792-3273
(407) 646-7495

Osceola County
Kissimmee Mem. Hospital
200 Hilda St
Kissimmee 34741
(407) 846-4343

Saint Cloud Hospital
2906 17th St
Saint Cloud 32769
(407) 892-2135

Osceola Regional Hospital
700 West Oak St
Kissimmee 32742
(407) 846-2266

Palm Beach County
AMI Palm Beach Gardens Medical Center
3360 Burns Road
Palm Beach Gardens 33410
(407) 622-1411

Bethesda Memorial Hospital
2815 South Seacrest Blvd
Boynton Beach 33435
(407) 737-7733

Boca Raton Community Hospital
800 Meadows Road
Boca Raton 33486
(407) 395-7100

Delray Community Hospital
5352 Linton Blvd
Delray Beach 33484
(407) 495-3100

Everglades Memorial Hospital
200 South Barfield Highway
Pahokee 33476
(407) 924-5201

Glades General Hospital
1201 South Main St
Belle Glade 33430
(407) 996-6571

Good Samaritan Hospital
Palm Beach Lakes Blvd
West Palm Beach 33402
(407) 655-5511

J.F. Kennedy Medical Center
4800 South Congress Ave
Atlantis 33462
(407) 965-7300

Jupiter Hospital
1210 S. Old Dixie Highway
Jupiter 33458
(407) 747-2234

Palm Beach Medical Center
2201 45th St
West Palm Beach 33407
(407) 842-6141

Palm Beach Regional Hospital
2829 Tenth Ave North
Lake Worth 33460
(407) 967-7800

Palms West Hospital
13001 State Road 80
Loxahatchee 33470
(407) 798-3300

Pinecrest Rehabilitation Hospital
5360 Linton Blvd
Delray Beach 33445
(407) 495-0400

Saint Mary's Hospital
901 45th St
West Palm Beach 33407
(407) 844-6300

Wellington Regional Medical Center
10101 Forest Hill Blvd
West Palm Beach 33414
(407) 798-8500

West Boca Medical Center
21644 St Road 7
Boca Raton 33428
(407) 488-8000

Pasco County
Dade City Hospital
1550 Fort King Road
Dade City 33525
(813) 567-6726

East Pasco Medical Center
7050 Gall Blvd
Zephyrhills 33541
(813) 788-0411

HCA Bayonet Point Hudson Medical
    Center
14000 Fivay Road
Hudson 34667
(813) 863-2411

HCA New Port Richey Hospital
5637 Marine Parkway
New Port Richey 34656
(813) 848-1733

Riverside Hospital of New Port Richey
6600 Madison Street
New Port Richey 34652
(813) 842-8468

Pinellas County
All Children's Hospital
801 Sixth St South
St Petersburg 33701
(813) 898-7451

Bayfront Medical Center
701 Sixth St South
St Petersburg 33701
(813) 893-6111

Clearwater Community Hospital
1521 East Druid Road
Clearwater 34616
(813) 447-4571

Edward White Hospital
2323 Ninth Ave North
St Petersburg 33733
(813) 323-1111

Gulf Coast Hospital
3030 Sixth St South
St Petersburg 33705
(813) 823-1122

HCA Medical Center Hospital-Largo
201 S.W. 14th St
Largo 34649
(813) 586-1411

Healthsouth Rehabilitation Center
901 N Clearwater/Largo Road
Largo 34640
(813) 586-2999

Helen Ellis Hospital
1395 South Pinellas Ave
Tarpon Springs 34689
(813) 942-5000

Northside Hospital
6000 49th St North
St Petersburg 33709
(813) 521-4411

Mease Hospital-Countryside
3231 McMullen Booth Road
Safety Harbor 34695
(813) 725-6111

Mease Hospital-Dunedin
833 Milwaukee Ave
Dunedin 34698
(813) 733-1111

Metropolitan General Hospital
7950 66th St North
Pinellas Park 34665
(813) 545-2580

Morton Plant Hospital
323 Jeffords Street
Clearwater 34616
(813) 462-7000

Palms of Pasadena Hospital
1501 Pasadena Ave South
St. Petersburg 33707
(813) 381-1000

St. Anthony's Hospital Care Center
1200 7th Ave North
St Petersburg 33705
(813) 825-1100

St. Petersburg General
6500 38th Ave North
St Petersburg 33710
(813) 384-1414

Sun Coast Hospital
2025 Indian Rocks Road
Largo 34649
(813) 581-9474

University General Hospital
10200 Seminole Blvd
Seminole 34648
(813) 397-5511

Women's Hospital & Medical Center
9675 Seminole Blvd.
Seminole 34642
(813) 393-4646

Polk County
Bartow Memorial Hospital
1239 East Main
Bartow 33830
(813) 533-8111

Heart of Florida Hospital
Tenth St At Wood Ave
Haines City 33844
(813) 422-4971

Lake Wales Hospital
410 South Eleventh St
Lake Wales 33859
(813) 676-1433

Lakeland Regional Medical Center
Lakeland Hills Blvd
Lakeland 33802
(813) 687-1100

Morrow Memorial Hospital
105 Arneson Avenue
Auburndale 33823
(813) 967-8511

Polk General Hospital
2010 East Georgia St
Bartow 33830
(813) 533-1111

Winter Haven Hospital
200 Avenue F, N.E.
Winter Haven 33881
(813) 293-1121

Putnam County
HCA Putnam Community Hospital
Highway 20 West
Palatka 32178
(904) 328-5711

Saint Johns County
Flagler Hospital
400 Health Park Blvd.
St Augustine 32086
(904) 825-4400

Flagler Hospital West
1933 U.S. Highway 1
St. Augustine 32086
(904) 829-5155

St. Lucie County
HCA Medical Center of Port St. Lucie
1800 S.E. Tiffany Ave
Port St. Lucie 34952
(407) 335-4000

Lawnwood Regional Medical Center
1700 South 23rd St
Fort Pierce 34950-0188
(407) 461-4000

Santa Rosa County
Gulf Breeze Hospital
1110 Gulf Breeze Parkway
Gulf Breeze 32561
(904) 934-2000

Jay Hospital
221 South Alabama St
Jay 32565
(904) 675-4532

Santa Rosa Medical Center
1450 Berry Hill Road
Milton 32570
(904) 623-9741

Sarasota County
Doctors Hospital of Sarasota
2750 Bahia Vista St
Sarasota 34239
(813) 366-1411

Englewood Community Hospital
700 Medical Blvd
Englewood 34223
(813) 475-6571

Rehabilitation Institute of Sarasota
3251 Proctor Road
Sarasota 33581
(813) 921-8600

Sarasota Memorial Hospital
1700 South Tamiami Trail
Sarasota 34239
(813) 953-1300

Venice Hospital
540 The Rialto
Venice 34285
(813) 485-7711

Seminole County
Central Florida Regional Hospital
1401 West Seminole Blvd
Sanford 32771
(407) 321-4500

South Seminole Community Hospital
555 West State Road 434
Longwood 32750
(407) 767-1200

Suwannee County
Suwannee Hospital
5th Street
Live Oak 32060
(904) 362-1413

Taylor County
Doctors Memorial Hospital
407 East Ash St
Perry 32347
(904) 584-0800

Union County
Ramadan Hand Institute
850 East Main St
Lake Butler 32054
(904) 496-2323

Volusia County
Daytona Beach Medical Center
400 North Clyde Morris
Daytona Beach 32020
(904) 239-5000

Fish Memorial Hospital—Deland
245 E. New York Avenue
Deland 32721
(904) 734-2323

Fish Memorial Hospital—New Smyrna
  Beach
401 Palmetto St
New Smyrna Beach 32069
(904) 427-3401

Halifax Medical Center
303 North Clyde Morris Blvd
Daytona Beach 32015
(904) 254-4000

Memorial Hospital—Ormond Beach
875 Sterthaus Ave
Ormond Beach 32074
(904) 676-6000

Peninsula Medical Center
264 South Atlantic Ave
Ormond Beach 32074
(904) 672-4161

West Volusia Memorial Hospital
701 W. Plymouth
Deland 32721
(904) 734-3320

Walton County
Walton Regional Hospital
21 College Avenue
Defuniak Springs 32433
(904) 892-5171

Washington County
N.W. Florida Community Hospital
300 Highway #280
Chipley 32428
(904) 638-1610

CHAPTER 4
Florida nursing homes

Nursing homes provide general, restorative, and rehabilitative nursing to persons who need skilled nursing and medical supervision 24 hours a day. A physician must prescribe admission to a nursing home, and all residents remain under the care of a physician once they are admitted. An individual plan of care, which includes medical and dietary requirements, is prepared by the physician for each resident and must be reviewed regularly by the facility's professional staff. Nursing homes care for two principal types of residents, those in need of short-term care, such as patients needing rehabilitative care, and those in need of long-term care. There are two types of nursing homes. Skilled nursing facilities provide 24-hour skilled nursing care to the very ill and incapacitated. Intermediate care facilities care for moderately ill and mildly incapacitated persons needing less intensive medical care.

Alternatives to the intensive—and expensive—care provided in nursing homes include adult congregate living facilities or ACLFs, continuing care facilities, or home care. Chapter 5 discusses retirement homes that provide health care services. Chapter 6 discusses home health care. Key factors that are used in making the nursing home decision include:

- Is 24-hour skilled nursing in a medically intensive environment needed?
- Has living at home and arranging for home health and other support services been considered? What is the family situation? Can members of household assist with care?
- Has living in an ACLF or continuing care facility been considered?
- Which option provides the greatest independence and promotes the highest quality of life for the person in need of care?
- What are the financial implications of each option?

CHARACTERISTICS OF NURSING HOME RESIDENTS

Although there are some residents in nursing homes who are able to move about without assistance, most are in wheelchairs or are unable to leave their beds. A small proportion of residents have been recently discharged from hospitals and require care for short periods of time. These residents include persons recovering from surgery, strokes, broken bones, heart attacks, and other medical problems. The majority of residents are long-term residents, principally the elderly and those with serious medical problems. The "Nursing Home Use after Age 65" section of Chapter 9 discusses research studies that have estimated the nursing home use by persons age 65 and older.

In Florida, approximately 16 percent of nursing home discharges are due to recovery from illnesses, and another 22 percent are due to requests by residents or family members. Most of the remaining discharges either are deaths in the nursing home, or transfers to hospitals where death often occurs. According to an article in the *New England Journal of Medicine* (Libow and Starer 1989):

- At any one time 5 percent of persons over 65 reside in nursing homes;
- Twenty-five percent of those over 65 will spend some time in a nursing home;
- Of The average stay in a nursing home is 2.9 years;
- The average resident is an 86-year-old female who has multiple concurrent illnesses; and
- The female to male ratio is 2.5:1.

In Florida, 2.1 percent of the population over age 65 lives in nursing homes. This is about half the national average. Approximately 44 percent of Florida's nursing home residents are 85 years of age or older, and 36 percent are between 75 and 84. The majority of nursing home residents (63 percent) are admitted directly from hospitals. About 20 percent, who generally are older residents, are admitted from home. The remaining 17 percent are admitted from other nursing homes or health care facilities.

A national study of nursing home patients conducted in 1985 determined that although the average length of stay was 14.6 months, 64 percent of residents were discharged in less than 6 months. Thirty percent left in less than six months and returned to live in the community (Liu, Manton and Liu 1990). This study found that residents who did not leave in less than six months stayed 31.9 additional months, for a total nursing home stay of 37.9 months.

Another national study of nursing home residents sponsored by the Public Health Service examined the functional status and mental health status of residents of nursing homes (Lair and Lefkowitz 1990). This research found that:
- 55 percent of women and 48 percent of men experienced urinary incontinence; and
- 61 percent of women and 53 percent of men had limitations in four or more activities of daily living, such as bathing, dressing, using the toilet, walking, and eating.
- Almost 52 percent of males and 46 percent of females had behavioral problems. Males were almost twice as likely to hurt another as women (16 percent versus 9 percent). For both sexes, 31 percent had problems getting upset and/or yelling, and 11 percent wandered.
- Almost 30 percent of all nursing home residents experienced psychotic symptoms, 43 percent had dementia, 64 percent had at least one symptom of depression and 68 percent had at least one psychiatric symptom, such as dullness, withdrawal, impatience, delusions, or hallucinations. At almost all ages, women were more likely to have multiple symptoms than men.

The prevalence of depression among newly admitted nursing home residents was examined in a study by research psychiatrists from the John Hopkins University School of Medicine (Rovner et al. 1991). This study examined 454 new nursing home admissions to eight Baltimore area nursing homes between February 1987 and March 1988 and followed these residents for one year. The communities the patients were from were mostly white and middle class. The study found that 12.6 percent of the residents had a major depressive disorder and 18.1 percent had depressive symptoms. Major depressive disorder, but not depressive symptoms, were found to increase the likelihood of death. The authors concluded that,

"Because depression is a prevalent and treatable condition associated with increased mortality, recognition and treatment in nursing homes is imperative."

SERVICES PROVIDED BY NURSING HOMES

Nursing homes care for all of the medical, physical, social, and psychological needs of residents. All nursing homes provide the following:

- **Medical services**—All residents are admitted to a nursing home on the orders of a physician, and remain under the care of a physician during their stay. Physicians develop resident care plans, determine dietary requirements, prescribe medications, and order restorative and rehabilitative procedures.
- **Nursing services**—All nursing homes provide 24-hour nursing care that includes administering medications, giving injections and performing catheterizations. Most provide restorative nursing, physical therapy, speech therapy, and occupational therapy. Nursing homes vary in the sophistication of nursing care that they provide. Only about a third of nursing homes accept paralyzed residents or provide tracheotomy care, and about 20 percent care for persons who have seizures.
- **Personal services**—Nursing home staff help residents with the activities of daily living, including getting out of bed, bathing, eating, dressing, and toileting.
- **Social and recreational services**—All nursing homes provide social and recreational activities for residents. Common activities include games, music, arts and crafts, and exercise programs.

Some nursing homes have special care units for residents with Alzheimer's and other forms of dementia. According to a September 1992 federal Office of Technology Assessment (OTA) report, at least half of all nursing home residents have dementia and the number of nursing homes with "special care units" is increasing rapidly. The OTA cautions that while some persons may receive excellent care in special care units, special care units "vary greatly." They differ with regard to patient care philosophies and goals, physical design features, staff-to-resident ratios, activity programs, and other characteristics. Although the OTA report cautions that it is not known "exactly what constitutes effective nursing home care" for those with dementia, families could better evaluate special care units if nursing homes provided the following information about special care units:

- What is special about the unit;
- How the unit differs from nonspecialized units in the nursing home;
- Whether there are behavior problems that cannot be handled; and
- Whether it is expected that individuals in the special care unit will be discharged before their death and, if so, for what reasons.

The Alzheimer's Association has a facility referral service that provides information on local ACLFs and nursing homes that have special units for Alzheimer's patients. The Alzheimer's Association may be contacted by calling:

Alzheimer's Association
(800) 272-3900

RESEARCH AND QUALITY OF CARE

A study was conducted in Rhode Island to examine the quality of care that nursing homes provided (Spector and Takada 1991). More than 2,600 nursing home residents in 80 nursing homes were included in the study. The study was sponsored by the National Center for Health Services Research. The study included residents of nursing homes that provided intermediate care. These residents were less likely to be deficient in activities of daily living (ADLs) than residents of skilled nursing facilities.

The study found that nursing homes that provided the best quality of care had staff who interacted more with residents, had a low turnover of registered nurses, had "sufficient" private pay patients, had few patients receiving care for skin breakdowns, and had high participation rates in organized activities. Key findings included the following:

- More staff or more resources are not always the answer for improving the quality of life and life expectancy of nursing home residents. Rather, sufficient staff relative to needs (staff-ADL interaction), continuity of leadership (low turnover of RNs), and factors related to the ability to attract a sufficient percentage of private-pay residents are important aspects of quality.
- Nursing homes that have a low proportion of residents receiving skin care and have low participation rates in organized activities after controlling for case mix (how ill the patients are), may increase the risk of negative outcomes.
- Urinary catheters should be used sparingly, because of the potential risk of increased functional decline and reduced likelihood of improvement.
- Underuse as well as overuse of psychoactive drugs may affect the likelihood of patients improving.

VISITING A NURSING HOME RESIDENT

An article in *Aging* magazine discussed ways to "brighten the day" of a nursing home resident (DHHS 1993). According to the article, a visit can mean much more than a gift. Recommended ways to cheer up a nursing home resident during a visit included: watching videocassettes of family events or looking through family photo albums, singing or listening to familiar music, or playing games or doing crafts together. Ideas for gifts include jogging suits or other "active" clothing, socks with grippers, handkerchiefs, and lotions and other personal skin care items in plastic bottles. For alert residents, gifts that encourage activity may be good choices. These might include bird feeders, window gardens, baskets of yarn, or subscriptions to favorite magazines. Those who are cognitively impaired may enjoy dolls, musical chimes, and mobiles.

SELECTING A NURSING HOME

Choosing a nursing home for long-term care is rarely a true choice option. This is because many nursing homes are filled to capacity, and because nursing homes often seek certain types of patients, particularly private pay and Medicare patients in need of skilled rehabilitation, I.V. care, ventilator care, or other speciality care. Barbara Landy, a South Florida nursing home expert, began her health care career in 1982. She has two masters degrees, a Master of Health Sciences in administration, and a Master of Business Administration. In addition, she is a licensed nursing home administrator and a certified health care risk manager. To determine if nursing home care is needed, Landy suggests that the following questions be answered:

- Can home health care be arranged instead?
- Can adult day care meet the patient's needs? Adult day care centers and some nursing homes provide this service.
- Is adult medical day care appropriate? Some hospitals and nursing homes provide medical day care (nursing care, activities, therapies, personal care).
- Is an over-night program appropriate? Some larger cities have over-night programs, often for persons with Alzheimer's. Some nursing homes and adult congregate living facilities (ACLFs) offer these programs.
- Is residence in an ACLF appropriate?

When visiting a nursing home, Landy suggests that it is important to note whether the facility has an odor of urine (many nursing home patients are incontinent), residents' physical appearance, whether the staff smiles and appears friendly, and whether the residents are involved in some activity between 10 a.m. and noon.

Finally, Landy says, "Be prepared for disappointments." Clothing can be given to other residents by mistake. Mealtime is seldom like it was at home. Physicians visit much less often than in a hospital and although nurses are on duty 24 hours a day, medical problems are not addressed with the same speed as in a hospital. In addition, residents may remove their shoes and socks or may shout, complain, and wander about. Some residents never are happy. One option for providing extra care to a nursing home resident is to contract with a home health agency to provide additional personal care services, or with a sitter agency for one-on-one companionship.

Determining which nursing homes to visit

Unfortunately, most people look for a nursing home at a time of crisis. But selecting a nursing home, or assisting others in that process requires analytical, clear-headed, thoughtful work.

A search for a nursing home can be conducted in three phases. The first phase is to narrow down the number of choices by examining the nursing home inventory in Appendix E and by telephoning nursing homes to learn if they have vacancies or anticipated vacancies. The second phase consists of making visits to inspect the care provided to residents. The final phase is to determine if the home has a reputation for providing good care.

In selecting a nursing home there is one other factor to consider—the best nursing homes may have no vacancies and long waiting lists. Steps to begin a search for a nursing home include:

- Examine the nursing home inventory in Appendix E to select those homes which meet your requirements. The inventory includes: the name, address, and telephone number of the facility; whether the facility is owned by a for-profit corporation, a nonprofit firm, or a government agency; the total number of beds, the number of private and semi-private rooms; and, whether the nursing home accepts Medicaid and Medicare.
- Determine the geographic area you or other family members want the nursing home to be located in.
- If Medicaid or Medicare is paying the bill, select nursing homes that accept payment from these programs. If you believe that it is likely that Medicaid will eventually pay for nursing home care, it is important to initially select a nursing home that accepts Medicaid payment. Otherwise it may be necessary to transfer the nursing home resident to another that does accept Medicaid in the future.
- Determine if a private room is needed. Private rooms may be much more expensive than semi-private rooms and are not paid for by Medicaid or Medicare.
- Contact the State Agency for Health Care Administration (AHCA) to request a copy of the *Guide to Nursing Home Charges in Florida* for your geographic area. This free publication contains useful information on nursing homes. It can be obtained by calling a toll-free number, which is answered by an answering machine. Call (800) 342-0828 and leave your name, address, and the county you live in or wish to place the patient in. Make sure to specify that you want the *Guide to Nursing Home Charges in Florida.*

- Determine if there are special needs or special medical problems. Some nursing homes do not accept residents with severe mental disorders, those who have seizures or require inhalation therapy, or certain other types of residents.
- Ask your friends, physician, clergyman, or others you trust for recommendations.
- Telephone those nursing homes in the geographic area you select to identify those homes with vacancies that both meet your requirements and have rates you can afford. Make appointments for visits.

Inspecting a nursing home

During your initial nursing home visits, meet with the administrator, the director of nurses, and the director of social services. A very important person to talk with is the chairperson or president of the resident council, this person can give you an "insider's" perspective on the nursing home.

The following nursing home checklist contains a series of important observations to make in a nursing home and important questions to ask nursing home staff.

NURSING HOME VISIT CHECKLIST

1. Resident care

—Ask if the nursing home follows federal Agency for Health Care Policy and Research clinical practice guidelines. Guidelines have been released, or are scheduled to be released, for urinary incontinence; pressure ulcers; acute pain management for operative or medical procedures, trauma, and cancer; post-stroke rehabilitation; and other medical problems.

—Observe the residents to determine if they are well cared for. Are residents clean and properly dressed? Look at fingernails and hair to determine if residents are well groomed.

—Observe how staff interacts with residents. Nursing home staff should be caring, helpful, and good natured. Residents should be treated with kindness, dignity, and respect, and should be addressed by name.

—What is the scope of mental health services provided by the facility? Research has found that many nursing home residents experience depression or other mental health problems that can be treated.

—Is the morale of the residents good? In analyzing morale, it is important to be realistic. Some residents will be alert, while others will be confused or silent. Some residents will be ambulatory; others will be in wheelchairs or bedridden.

—Does the nursing home provide restorative nursing care? Restorative nursing helps residents function at their maximum potential. Ask about the nursing home's restorative care program and if there is a nurse that specializes in restorative nursing.

—Is privacy respected? Do staff knock on doors before entering rooms? Check to see if privacy curtains are drawn when residents are being bathed or when care is being given.

—Do alert residents say they receive good care? Simply ask several residents.

—May residents choose their roommates or are residents permitted to change rooms if they are not compatible with their roommates?

—Are the visiting hours and the rules for visiting acceptable to friends and family members. Ask for the policy regarding residents being taken out occasionally by family or friends.

—What is the nursing home policy on advance medical directives?

2. *Physical environment*

—Is the nursing home free from odors? There should be no strong odor of urine or of heavy cover-up deodorants. Many nursing home residents are incontinent and signs of good care are the absence of odor and the prompt changing of sheets and diapers.

—Are resident rooms clean, attractive, cheerful and well-lit? Check for dust on the windowsills.

—Do resident rooms have nameplates indicating who resides in each room?

—May residents have their own furniture and hang pictures on the walls?

—Are resident recreation and lounge areas clean and comfortable?

—Is there an outdoor area accessible to residents in wheelchairs?

3. *Activities and daily living*

—Are residents given choices? What choices do residents have with regard to food, recreation, and daily living activities? Larger homes may offer more varied activities, but smaller homes may be more personal. Choice is a very important factor in good mental health.

—Is the food satisfactory? Observe a meal. Does the food appear appetizing? Do residents appear to be enjoying their meals, or do they leave large portions uneaten? Ask to see a weekly or monthly menu.

—Are special diets available, such as vegetarian, kosher, or low-sodium?

—Are activity calendars posted? Do the activities reflect a variety of interests? Ask how holidays are celebrated.

—Are there activities for residents who are relatively inactive or confined to their rooms?

—Are there religious services in the home? Does a clergyman visit?

—Is there an active resident council? Resident councils help govern nursing homes. Remember to speak with the chairperson or president of the resident council to learn about quality of care in the facility.

—Does the nursing home use volunteers?

Once the decision-makers have narrowed choices to two or three nursing homes, make second visits. The second visit should be at a different time of the day and unannounced, perhaps at meal time if you didn't observe a meal during your initial visit. Use the second visit to both confirm your initial impressions and to gather any information you neglected to obtain on your first visit. If you were unable to speak with the chairperson or president of the resident council on your first visit, try to do so on this visit.

Determining if a nursing home has a reputation for providing good care

Determining if a nursing home has a good reputation and provides good care takes careful consideration. Information from several sources should be evaluated. First, it is important to consider the findings of your visits and to weigh the opinions of others, particularly residents, other visitors, and volunteers who work in the nursing home. Next, the rating of the nursing home can be considered. Each year every nursing home is rated either as superior, standard, or conditional by AHCA. Finally, the district nursing home and long-term care facility ombudsman councils, which are discussed later, can be contacted to learn of any complaints against the facility.

All nursing homes are required by law to be licensed by AHCA. The agency conducts annual inspections of all nursing homes. Those homes that accept Medicaid or Medicare residents are inspected according to federal standards and are "certified" by AHCA if they meet the federal requirements. HRS County Public Health Units also inspect nursing homes to make sure they meet sanitary and health standards.

Depending upon the findings of the AHCA inspection, nursing homes are rated as either superior, standard, or conditional. The facility's license, which is required to be posted, will note if the rating is either superior or conditional. If the rating is standard, no notation appears. Ratings are generally good until the next inspection is conducted. For a facility to receive a superior rating, it must be in compliance with certain licensing and certification standards and offer services that go beyond what is required by state and federal regulations.

In evaluating nursing home ratings, it is important to remember that the rating reflects the results of an inspection at one point in time. Several years of ratings information may provide a better measure than a single year, assuming management has remained the same. It is likely that when you visit a nursing home the posted rating is for a more recent inspection. Compare the new rating with the prior ratings given in Appendix E. This will give you at least two years of ratings to evaluate. Keep in mind that the ownership of nursing homes sometimes changes, and often there is staff turnover. A nursing home may have had difficulty in the past, but with new management, or with other changes, quality of care may have improved and other problems may have been resolved.

Nursing home ratings should be considered as just one piece of evidence regarding quality of care. Your impressions, the views of nursing home residents, and the opinions of those you have confidence in are also important.

The district nursing home and long-term care facility ombudsman councils can be contacted to learn about complaints they have received. Their telephone numbers will be on the resident rights brochures that nursing homes give to all residents and they also will appear on posters in the nursing home. The Ombudsman Councils are listed in Chapter 11. When you call, ask to speak with the district ombudsman council coordinator. The coordinator will be able to tell you how many complaints have been received against a particular nursing home, the nature of the complaints, and whether they were minor or serious.

Other sources of information

The National Council of Senior Citizens has an information and referral center on long-term care. Information on nursing homes and alternative community and health services, as well as a free guide on selecting a nursing home, are available. The National Council of Senior Citizens can be reached by writing:

Nursing Home Information Service
National Council of Senior Citizens
1331 F Street, N.W.
Washington, D.C. 20004

The American Association of Retired Persons has publications on selecting a nursing home and long-term care. For a list of their publications, write to:

Health Advocacy Services
601 E Street N.W.
Washington, D.C. 20049

Three other organizations can be contacted for information regarding nursing home care:

National Consumers League
815 15th Street, N.W., Suite 928
Washington, D.C. 20005
(202) 783-2242

American Association of Homes for the Aging
901 E Street, N.W.
Washington, D.C. 2004
(202) 783-2242

American Health Care Association
1201 L Street, N.W.
Washington, D.C. 20005
(202) 842-4444

NURSING HOME RESIDENTS' RIGHTS

Florida law requires that each nursing home adopt and make public a statement of resident rights. Required provisions include:
- The right to civil and religious liberties, including knowledge of available choices and the right to make independent personal decisions and the right to encouragement and assistance from the staff of the nursing home in the fullest possible exercise of these rights;
- The right to private and uncensored communication, including access to a telephone, visiting with any person of the resident's choice during visiting hours, and overnight visitation outside the facility (within certain limitations);
- The right to present grievances, the right to recommend changes in policy, and the right to contact ombudsmen or other advocates or special interest groups;
- The right to prompt efforts by the facility to resolve grievances, including grievances with respect to the behavior of other residents;
- The right to privacy in treatment and in caring for personal needs, to close room doors, and to have staff knock before entering the room;
- The right to be treated courteously, fairly, and with the fullest measure of dignity;
- The right to be free from mental and physical abuse and from physical and chemical restraints, except those restraints authorized in writing by a physician or those needed in an emergency. Restraints may not be used in lieu of staff supervision or merely for staff convenience, for punishment, or for reasons other than for resident protection or safety;
- The right to organize and participate in resident groups in the facility;
- The right to have the resident's family meet in the facility with the families of other residents;
- The right to retain and use personal clothing and possessions as space permits;
- The right to receive adequate and appropriate health care, protective services, support services, social services, planned recreational activities, and therapeutic and rehabilitative services consistent with the resident care plan;
- The right to select a personal physician;
- The right to obtain pharmaceutical supplies from any pharmacy. If a resident chooses to use a community pharmacy and the nursing home uses a unit-dose system, the pharmacy must provide drugs in the form of unit doses;

- The right to receive a written statement and an oral explanation of the services provided by the nursing home;
- The right to be fully informed in advance of any nonemergency changes in care or treatment that may affect the resident's well-being;
- The right to refuse medication or treatment and to be informed of the consequences of such decisions, unless the resident is determined to be unable to provide informed consent under state law. When a resident refuses medication or treatment, the facility must notify the resident or the resident's legal representative of the consequences of such decision and must document the resident's decision in the medical record. The nursing home must continue to provide other services the resident agrees to in accordance with the resident's care plan;
- The right to be fully informed in writing and orally, prior to admission, of services and charges not covered by Medicaid or Medicare and of bed reservation and refund policies;
- Except when a discharge or transfer is necessary for the resident's welfare, or for the health and safety of other residents, at least 30 days written notice must be given to the resident, to a family member (if known) and to the resident's legal representative;
- A resident of any Medicaid—or Medicare—certified facility may challenge a decision to discharge or transfer the resident and is entitled to a fair hearing. The request for a hearing must be made within 90 days of the receipt of the notice for proposed discharge or transfer;
- If the request for a hearing is made with 10 days of receiving the notice, the request shall prevent the proposed transfer or discharge until there is a hearing; decision, which must be made within 90 days of receipt of a request for a fair hearing;
- If a resident fails to request a hearing within 10 days of receipt of the notice for discharge or transfer, the facility may not discharge or transfer the resident until 30 days from the date the resident receives the notice;
- The right to 15 days advance notice prior to discharge for nonpayment of a bill;
- The right to be informed of the bed reservation policy for a hospitalization. Private pay residents must have their bed reserved for up to 30 days provided the nursing home receives reimbursement. Medicaid residents shall be informed of their rights pursuant to state and federal regulations;
- The right to manage his or her own financial affairs or to delegate such responsibility to the nursing home;
- Facilities may not require a resident to deposit personal funds with the facility;
- If a resident authorizes the facility to hold personal funds, the facility must establish a separate accounting system for such funds and may not commingle these funds with any other funds;
- The right to have copies of the rules and regulations of the nursing home;
- The right to examine the results of the most recent state or federal inspection of the facility and any plan of correction; and,
- Each resident, or resident guardian, must receive a copy of the statement of resident rights at the time of admission. Each nursing home must have a written plan, and provide adequate staff training, to ensure that the statement of resident rights is enforced.

PAYING FOR NURSING HOME CARE

Nursing homes receive payment from two principal sources: Medicaid and private individuals. Although Medicare, the Veterans Administration, and some private insurance companies also pay for nursing home care, these sources pay for the care of a relatively small number of residents. According to a 1987 report on nursing homes published by the Florida Health Care Cost Containment Board, Medicaid was the largest nursing home payer, accounting for 52 percent of nursing home revenue. Thirty-nine percent of revenue was from private payment, 7 percent was from Medicare, and the remaining 2 percent was from other sources.

Nursing home charges vary substantially. Nursing homes located in urban areas, particularly South Florida, are more expensive than those in rural areas. In urban areas, it is not uncommon to find daily charges for semi-private rooms in the $90 to $110 range while $70 to $90 rates are common in rural areas. Private rooms generally are considerably more expensive than semi-private rooms. In urban areas, private room rates can range from $110 to $150 per day. In rural areas the rates are frequently lower. The average rate for all nursing homes is about $90 a day for a semi-private room.

Nursing homes have a basic charge, which usually covers meals, room, housekeeping, linen, routine nursing care, recreation, and personal care. Extra charges are made for physician and dental care, medications, physical therapy and other therapies, laboratory, radiology, and for personal services such as telephone calls, personal laundry, beauticians, and barbers.

Long-term care insurance

There are two basic types of insurance policies that pay for care in nursing homes, long-term care policies and nursing home policies. Long-term care policies cover nursing home care for a minimum of 24 months plus one year of lower level care, such as home health care or adult day care. Nursing home policies may cover either nursing home care or a combination of nursing home care and custodial care. If a policy covers care in a nursing home plus one other coverage, such as home health care or adult day care. The policy will pay benefits for one year or less.

Medicaid eligibility

The Medicaid nursing home program technically is called the Medicaid Institutional Care Program. Although eligibility for the Medicaid Institutional Care Program is complicated, in simple terms Medicaid pays for nursing care for those who do not have the resources to pay for it themselves. Another way of viewing Medicaid is to consider the program a safety net.

All persons who are admitted to nursing homes and whose bills are paid by Medicaid must be assessed by the HRS Comprehensive Assessment, Review and Evaluation Services (CARES) program. CARES teams consist of a physician, a nurse and a social worker. The teams determine if people should be placed in skilled nursing facilities, intermediate care facilities, or in community settings, such as boarding homes or retirement centers. Medicaid pays for both intermediate and skilled nursing care. The CARES program can be reached by contacting the HRS Aging and Adult Services Office in your local area. Look in the telephone book under State of Florida, Department of Health and Rehabilitative Services, Aging and Adult Services.

There are three principal factors that determine eligibility for Medicaid: the CARES team must determine that nursing home services are appropriate; monthly income must be below a certain amount; and, assets must be below a certain amount. Monthly income eligibility for nursing home care usually is revised yearly. Financial eligibility requirements are different for single and married persons.

In 1993, single persons were eligible for nursing home coverage under Medicaid if monthly income was less than $1,302 per month. Single individuals were permitted to retain $2,000 in assets unless their income was lower than $526 per month. Up to $5,000 in assets may be retained if income was below $526. Some very significant assets, however, are excluded from the limits. These include the client's home, automobile, and some life insurance.

For married persons, assets other than the homestead, automobile, and life insurance cannot exceed $70,740. The Medicaid office computes the value of the nonexempt assets. In addition, a spouse not living in a nursing home may retain a portion of monthly income. Although the amount of monthly income varies according to certain expenses, the sum a spouse could retain was generally $1,154 a month.

Medicaid residents share in the cost of nursing home care. All of their monthly income, except a personal expenses allowance of $35 per month in 1993, goes towards paying the nursing home bill. For example, if the Medicaid bill in the nursing home was $2,000 per month and the resident had income of $1,000 a month, the nursing home would have received $965 from the resident and $1,035 from Medicaid.

Some persons enter nursing homes as paying residents but become Medicaid residents when their assets become depleted. Asset depletion to become eligible for Medicaid is referred to as "spending down." To pay their nursing home bills, residents spend-down or liquidate their assets to the point that they become eligible for Medicaid.

Medicaid covers the cost of room and board, most medical supplies, prescription drugs, hospital care, medical equipment for temporary use, and routine supplies such as gowns and linens. Medicaid does not pay for personal items, such as newspapers or beauty shop charges. The $35 per month that Medicaid residents are permitted to keep may be used for personal purposes. Medicaid reimbursement to the nursing home is considered to be payment in full and the nursing home may not request or accept any additional money for a resident's care.

When individuals apply for Medicaid to pay for nursing home care, the HRS eligibility worker may request the following: bank statements, stocks, bonds, insurance policies and other financial assets, property deeds, including cemetery plots, vehicle registration, guardianship and power of attorney papers, and proof of all income.

Medicare eligibility

Medicare is a much more limited payment source for nursing home care than Medicaid. This is because Medicare is a program for short-term rehabilitative nursing, while Medicaid is a program for long-term care. As in the Medicaid nursing home program, a physician must prescribe admission to a nursing home.

Medicare will pay for up to 100 days of skilled nursing care in a semi-private room in a skilled nursing facility, provided skilled nursing care is medically necessary, there has been a hospital stay of at least three consecutive days within the previous 30 days, and care in the skilled nursing facility is for a condition that was treated in the hospital. Medicare does not pay for intermediate or custodial care in nursing homes.

Part A of Medicare pays for nursing home care. Nursing home services covered by Medicare Part A include: semi-private room; meals, including special diets; regular and rehabilitative nursing care; blood transfusions; pharmaceuticals and medical supplies; and, medical appliances such as wheelchairs. Medicare does not pay for telephones, television rental, or personal care services such as beauty or barber services.

Medicare Part B nursing home coverage pays for physician fees; laboratory and radiology; surgical dressings, splints and casts; and prosthetic implants and devices. Detailed information on Medicare coverage of nursing home care can be obtained by ordering the *Medicare Handbook*. See the Medicare section of Chapter 11.

Supplemental Security Income Medically Needy Program

A 1988 federal law established a program for persons who do not qualify for Medicaid nursing home payments but who have less than $5,000 in financial resources. The program is called the Supplemental Security Income Medically Needy Program. Although this program does not pay for room, board, and nursing care, it does pay for some services including therapies and medications. The program will help to offset the costs of nursing home care to the family. Information can be obtained from the same HRS office that determines eligibility for Medicaid.

COMPLAINTS

If there is a problem with the care that is being provided by a nursing home, the first step usually is to discuss the problem with either the director of nurses or the nursing home administrator. If the problem remains unresolved, the following organizations and agencies may be of help:

Nursing home and long-term care facility ombudsman council—Each HRS district has a Long-Term Care Ombudsman Council to assist in the resolution of complaints regarding nursing homes. Each nursing home is required to give residents an ombudsman brochure, which includes a listing of resident rights. The local ombudsman council's telephone number will appear on the brochure. Nursing homes also are required to display the telephone number of the local ombudsman council in a conspicuous place. Ombudsman Councils are listed in Chapter 11. There also is a statewide Long-Term Care Ombudsman Council:

State Long-Term Care Ombudsman Council
154 Holland Building
600 South Calhoun Street
Tallahassee, FL 32399-0001
(904) 488-6190 or
(800) 342-5772

Abuse Hotline—If you suspect that a resident has been abused or exploited, call the Abuse Hotline at (800) 342-9152 and the complaint will be investigated. All contact with the Abuse Hotline is confidential.

Area Offices of Health Facility Regulation—These offices in the state Agency for Health Care Administration (AHCA) are responsible for licensing and certifying nursing homes. Any complaint concerning the conditions in a nursing home, or the quality of care given to residents, will be investigated by area offices. All nursing homes are required to have the findings of their most recent licensure inspection posted for examination by residents and the public. The telephone number and address of the local AHCA Area Office of Health Facility Regulation will be on the inspection report or on the attached cover letter. The area offices are listed in Chapter 11. Additional information can be obtained by contacting the AHCA Office of Health Quality Assurance, 2727 Mahan Drive, Tallahassee, Florida, 32308, (904) 487-2527.

NURSING HOME CHARACTERISTICS AND RATINGS

(For information on each of Florida's nursing homes, see Appendix E.)

JCAHO-ACCREDITED LONG-TERM CARE FACILITIES

Some nursing homes are accredited by the Joint Commission on Accreditation of Healthcare Organizations. Readers should consult the "Accreditation Organizations" section of Chapter 11 for additional information. Listed below are those long term care facilities in Florida that were accredited by JCAHO as of February 22, 1993.

JCAHO-Accredited Long-Term Care Facilities
February 22, 1993

Name of Facility	City
Polk General Hospital/The Rohr Home	Bartow
VA Medical Center	Bay Pines
Mediplex Rehab-Bradenton *AC	Bradenton
Morton Plant Hospital and Nursing Center	Clearwater
VA Medical Center	Gainesville
Hollywood Hills Nursing Home	Hollywood
River Garden Hebrew Home *AC	Jacksonville
VA Medical Center	Lake City
Arbors at Lakeland *AC	Lakeland
Leesburg Regional Med Cntr Nursing Center	Leesburg
Green Briar Rehab. & Comprehensive Care Cntr	Miami
HEALTHSOUTH Regional Rehabilitation Center	Miami
Miami Jewish Home and Hospital for the Aged	Miami
VA Medical Center	Miami
West Gables Rehab Hospital & Healthcare Cntr	Miami
Bon Secours Hosp/Villa Maria Nursing Center	North Miami
Greynolds Park Manor Rehabilitation Cntr *AC	N. Miami Beach
Arbors at Orange Park Nursing/Rehab Cntr *AC	Orange Park
Tallahassee Memorial Regional Medical Center	Tallahassee
VA Medical Center	Tampa
Mediplex Rehab-Palm Beach Rehab Center *AC	W. Palm Beach
Winter Haven Hospital	Winter Haven

*AC—Accredited with Commendation on April 14, 1993

Source: JCAHO 1993.

Chapter 5
Retirement homes and communities

There are two main types of retirement facilities in Florida that provide personal care and health care services: continuing care retirement communities (CCRC) and retirement homes that are licensed as adult congregate living facilities (ACLFs). Some ACLFs have special licenses that authorize them to provide limited nursing services or limited mental health services. The principal difference between continuing care communities and ACLFs is the range of services they provide.

CCRCs usually provide, or arrange to provide, all of the residential, personal care, and health care services that a resident needs, including nursing home care. All of these services often are provided at one location. ACLFs usually provide a more limited range of services and do not provide nursing home care. Personal care services are provided by both continuing care communities and ACLFs. Personal care services include help with the activities of daily living, such as dressing, eating, and bathing.

CONTINUING CARE RETIREMENT COMMUNITIES (CCRCS)

CCRCs, often called "life care" communities, usually offer an extensive complete range of residential and health care services to elderly persons. All facilities require that a contract be signed between the resident and the facility. The contracts can differ in the services covered, and in how nursing home care is paid for. CCRCs usually provide care for as long as the resident lives and usually require both an up-front entrance fee and monthly fees.

CCRCs have three licenses—a license, one each for operation of continuing care facility, an ACLF, and a nursing home. These licenses mean that they can provide most of the services that residents may need, except for hospital care.

There are usually three levels of care in continuing care communities: apartments for independent residential living, "assisted living" units staffed to provide personal care and nursing care in a residential setting, and skilled nursing services.

Continuing care contracts

Most continuing care communities require entrance fees. These range from $30,000 to $600,000. In addition to entrance fees, there are monthly maintenance fees, which range from $115 to $6,000. Communities owned by religious organizations tend to have lower entrance and maintenance fees than other communities.

Because nursing home care is very expensive, it is important to determine whether the nursing arrangements specified in the contract are suitable. Nursing care is the most expensive service provided by continuing care communities, and continuing care contracts vary in how this service is paid for. Generally, there are three types of contracts.

* Type A. These contracts pay fully for nursing care.

- Type B. These contracts limit nursing care to a certain number of days. Days beyond this set number must be paid for by the resident.
- Type C. These contracts simply guarantee residents access to nursing home care, and the resident is responsible for paying the entire bill.

Some continuing care contracts cover food, shelter, personal services and nursing care for as long as the resident lives. Others limit or exclude certain services.

According to Florida law, continuing care community contracts must:
- Specify all services to be provided to residents, including all items they will receive. They must state whether the items will be provided for a designated time period or for life, and whether the services will be available on the premises or at another specified location. Contracts also must indicate which items, such as food, shelter, personal services, nursing care, drugs, burial, and incidentals are included in the continuing care agreement and which items are available for extra charge.
- Specify cancellation terms and conditions.
- Describe the health and financial conditions required for a person to be accepted as a resident and to continue as a resident.
- Describe how marriage and divorce will affect the contract.
- Give persons the right to rescind continuing care contracts without penalty or forfeiture within seven days after executing a contract.

Continuing care communities must provide the following to prospective residents:
- A copy of the contract;
- A summary of the last examination report from the Department of Insurance;
- A full disclosure of all ownership interests and lease agreements;
- A full disclosure of all plans for expansion or phased development for the next three years;
- Copies of the rules and regulations of the facility, including the responsibilities of the residents; and
- The facility policy with respect to admission and discharge from the various levels of health care it offers.

Because of the cost and complexity of contracting for continuing care, it may be wise to consult both a financial advisor and an attorney who has experience in continuing care contract law. The Florida Bar's "Lawyer Referral Service" can be contracted to obtain the names of attorneys who specialize in continuing care contracts, advance medical directives, Medicare, social security, and other specialized legal matters:

The Florida Bar
Lawyer Referral Service
(800) 342-8011

Florida law requires continuing care facilities to have a copy of Chapter 651 of the Florida Statutes, which governs continuing care facilities, available for inspection before an agreement is signed. Florida law also requires that the most recent financial statement of the continuing care community be available for inspection.

Continuing care resident organizations

Members of continuing care facilities may form a residents' organization, or "residents' council." According to Florida law, residents' councils have the, right to engage in concerted activities for the purpose of keeping informed on the operation of the facility which is caring for them or for the purpose of other mutual aid or protection. A member of the residents' council is entitled to attend meetings of the board of directors of the continuing care facility. If a continuing care facility does not have a residents' council, residents may elect a resident to represent them before the board of directors. According to Florida law:

- The designated resident representative must be notified at least 14 days prior to a meeting of the governing body of the continuing care facility at which proposed changes in resident fees or services will be discussed. The representative shall be invited to attend and participate in that portion of the meeting that is designated for the discussion of such changes.
- Facilities must give a copy of its annual financial statement to the head of the residents' council.
- The head of the residents' council must be notified of filings with the Department of Insurance regarding any type of new financing or proposed expansion.

Quarterly meetings

Florida law requires that the CCRC governing body hold quarterly meetings with residents. The purpose of the quarterly meeting is to discuss income, expenditures, the financial trends and problems of the facility, and proposed changes in policies, programs, and services. A new provision requires that the governing body discuss the reasons for any increase in the monthly maintenance fee that exceeds the most recently published cost of living data prior to the implementation of the fee increase.

RETIREMENT COMMUNITIES LICENSED AS ACLFS

An ACLF is a government-licensed retirement facility where adults live together and receive meals and personal care. ACLFs may be an alternative for persons who need help with the activities of daily living but do not need the 24-hour skilled nursing provided by nursing homes. Some ACLFs have a special license to provide limited nursing care.

In Florida, there are over 1,400 licensed ACLFs. All provide room, meals, and personal care services. ACLFs are different from independent living retirement homes in that they are licensed to provide personal care services.

Some elderly persons need to live in a residential setting that provides help with dressing, eating, bathing, and the taking of medications, but they do not need the intensity of nursing care provided by either nursing homes or ACLFs with limited nursing licenses. Residency in an ACLF with a standard license is an option that these persons should consider.

There are three different types of ACLFs, and each must meet different licensing criteria. ACLFs may have either a standard license, a license to provide limited nursing services, or a license to provide limited mental health services. ACLFs with limited nursing licenses meet the needs of those residents who need nursing care, but not the intensive 24-hour nursing care provided by nursing homes. Many CCRCs also have ACLF licenses.

The majority of Florida ACLFs are free standing retirement homes. ACLFs range in size from small homes that have a few residents, to large facilities that care for 250 or more residents. ACLFs sometimes may be segregated by sex, or they may specialize in the care of certain persons, such as the disabled. Some ACLFs, such as those affiliated with religious or other organizations are not open to the general public.

ACLF residents and admission requirements

ACLFs provide care to three types of residents:
- Independent Residents, who do not need personal or limited nursing services.
- Type I Residents, who require supervision of their daily living.
- Type II Residents, who require assistance with daily living activities, including security and emotional support.

State regulations require that each resident be examined by either a physician or a licensed nurse practitioner within 60 days prior to residing in the facility whenever possible. If an examination was not conducted within 60 days prior to residing in the facility, an examination must be conducted within 30 days after residence. The purpose of the examination is to determine if residency in an ACLF is appropriate or if the person should be in a nursing home. The results of the examination must be included in the resident's personal record that is maintained by each ACLF.

The following information is required to be included in the resident's personal record prior to admission:
- A physical examination report;
- A description of the physical and mental health status of the resident, including the identification of functional limitations; and
- Recommendations for care, including medications, diet, and therapy.

The requirements for continued residency are the same as for admission. Individuals with intensive medical or supervisory needs are not permitted by state regulation to reside in ACLFs. These individuals include:
- Persons who are incontinent of bladder or bowel, unless they only require assistance with personal hygiene or are able to contract with an outside individual or agency to provide this care;
- Persons who have been adjudicated incompetent, unless they have a legal guardian to make decisions on their behalf;
- Persons with apparent signs or symptoms of certain communicable diseases;
- Persons who require licensed professional care on a 24-hour basis;
- Persons who require confinement to bed for more than seven consecutive days;
- Persons who are not capable of self-preservation in an emergency situation requiring immediate evacuation with assistance from staff; and
- Persons with special dietary needs that cannot be met by the ACLF.

Services provided by ACLFs

An ACLF may be thought of as a stage between independent living and a nursing home. All ACLFs are licensed to provide housing, meals, housekeeping, laundry, recreation, and one or more personal service to residents. Personal services include assistance with eating, bathing, grooming, dressing, moving about, and the taking of medication. All ACLFs must arrange for or provide transportation to dental, medical, or mental health facilities for their residents.

ACLFs vary widely in the range of services they provide beyond housing, meals, housekeeping, laundry, planned activities, and personal services. Some ACLFs provide excellent accommodations, meals, and services and are affordable only to the very affluent. Other ACLFs provide care in modest environments that are affordable to many.

If an ACLF is licensed to provide limited nursing or limited mental health services, it will be so designated on its license. Limited nursing services include acts that may be performed by registered nurses, licensed practical nurses and advanced registered nurse practitioners while carrying out their professional duties. These professional duties include general nursing assessments, taking vital signs, administering and supervising the taking of medication, catheterization, and other nursing duties. Residents needing limited nursing services do not require the 24-hour nursing supervision provided by nursing homes. Residents in ACLFs may receive limited nursing services from ACLF staff nurses, from nurses employed by a home health agency, or from out-patient clinics. The Medicare program will reimburse for home health services in ACLFs provided the resident meets eligibility criteria.

Some ACLFs accept people with Alzheimer's disease, or who have diabetes, incontinence of bladder or bowel, or other health problems. See Chapter 7 for information on contacting local chapters of the Alzheimer's Disease and Related Disorder Association to obtain information on facilities that provide care to persons with Alzheimer's. A few ACLFs, usually larger facilities, offer rehabilitative therapy.

Paying for care in an ACLF

Most residents pay for ACLF residency from their own personal funds, including their Social Security and other retirement income. Some persons with low incomes are eligible for government assistance under the Supplemental Security Income (SSI) and Optional State Supplementation (OSS) programs. Information regarding eligibility for these programs can be obtained by contacting the local HRS Economic Services office, listed in the telephone directory under State of Florida, Department of Health and Rehabilitative Services. Another option is to contact the local "Elder Helpline" listed in Chapter 11.

ACLF contracts

All ACLF residents are required by state law to sign a contract with the facility that specifies the services they will receive, how payment will be made, advance payment and refund policies, and other conditions. Contracts with ACLFs that are not part of CCRCs must comply with the criteria listed below.

- Contracts must be executed either before admission or at the time of admission. Each resident must receive a copy of the contract.
- Each contract must contain provisions that specifically describe the services and accommodations to be provided by the ACLF, rates or charges, a provision for at least 30 days' notice of a rate increase, provisions describing the rights, duties, and obligations of the resident and any other matters either the ACLF or resident deems appropriate.
- Contracts must include a refund policy to take effect at the time of a resident's transfer, discharge, or death. The refund policy must provide that the resident or responsible party is entitled to a prorated refund based on the daily rate for any unused portion of payment beyond the termination date after all charges, including the cost of damages to the residential unit resulting from circumstances other than normal use, have been paid. Except in the case of death or a discharge due to medical reasons, the refunds must be computed in accordance with the notice of relocation requirements specified in the contract.
- Contracts must state that if an ACLF agrees to reserve a bed for a resident who is admitted to a nursing home or hospital, the resident or his responsible party must notify the ACLF of any change in status that would prevent the resident from returning. Until that notice is received, the agreed-upon daily rate may be charged by the ACLF.
- Contracts must state the purpose of advance payments and include a refund policy

for such payment, including any advance payment for meals, lodging, or personal services.

- Contracts must state whether the ACLF is affiliated with any religious organization.

Resident rights

Florida law contains specific provisions to protect the rights of ACLF residents. These provisions are known as the ACLF Resident Bill of Rights. The Resident Bill of Rights includes the following:

- The right to live in a safe and decent living environment, free from abuse and neglect;
- The right to be treated with consideration and respect with recognition of personal dignity, individuality, and the need for privacy;
- The right to retain and use personal clothing and other property in immediate living quarters unless the facility can demonstrate this would be unsafe, impractical, or an infringement upon the rights of other residents;
- The right to unrestricted private communication, including receiving and sending unopened correspondence, access to a telephone, and visiting with any person of the residents' choice, at any time between the hours of 9 a.m. and 9 p.m. Florida law requires ACLFs to extend visiting hours for caregivers and out-of-town guests, and in "other similar situations";
- The right of freedom to participate in, and benefit from, community services and activities and to achieve the highest possible level of independence, autonomy, and interaction within the community;
- The right to manage personal financial affairs unless the resident or the resident's guardian authorizes the administrator of the facility to provide safekeeping of funds;
- The right to share a room with a spouse, if both are residents;
- The right to reasonable opportunity for regular exercise and to be outdoors at regular and frequent intervals;
- The right to exercise civil and religious liberties, including the right to independent personal decisions. No religious beliefs or practices, nor any attendance at religious services, may be imposed on any resident;
- The right to access to adequate and appropriate health care consistent with established and recognized standards within the community;
- The right to receive at least 30 days notice of relocation or termination of residency from the facility unless, for medical reasons, the resident is certified by a physician to require an emergency relocation to a facility providing a more skilled level of care or in the event that the resident engages in a pattern of conduct that is harmful or offensive to other residents;
- The right to present grievances and to recommend changes in policies, procedures, and services without restraint, interference, coercion, discrimination, or reprisal. ACLFs are required to establish grievance procedures to help residents exercise this right; and
- The right to access to ombudsman volunteers and advocates and the right to be a member of, to be active in, and to associate with advocacy or special interest groups.

The ACLF Resident Bill of Rights must be posted in a prominent place in each facility and be read or explained to residents who cannot read. The name, address, and telephone numbers for the district Nursing Home and Long-Term Care Facility Ombudsman Council, as well as the telephone number for the Abuse Registry, must be available to residents. Complaints may be lodged with these organizations.

State licensing personnel may communicate with residents privately when annual inspections occur to determine if patient rights are being complied with. No ACLF may serve notice upon a resident to leave a facility or take other retaliatory action against any person who exercises any right in the ACLF Resident Bill of Rights, or appears as a witness in any hearing, or files a civil action alleging a violation of any right in the ACLF Resident Bill of Rights or notifies a state attorney or the Attorney General of a possible violation.

HOW TO CHOOSE AN ACLF

ACLFs and those continuing care communities with ACLF and nursing home licenses are regulated and inspected by the AHCA. All facilities are inspected at least annually. The most recent AHCA inspection report is required to be posted for examination.

In selecting an ACLF, it is necessary to make visits to examine the services that are provided, determine the quality of meals and other services and ascertain the dedication and capability of staff. It also is important to consider location and cost. In selecting a retirement community, it is best to attempt to determine where the resident would most like to live. People and places that are familiar to the resident may be a major consideration, also consider proximity to shopping, health care providers, senior centers, and other places of personal importance.

After you select the geographic area where the resident would most like to live, your next consideration will likely be financial. Retirement homes vary greatly in cost and services.

Before visiting an ACLF, call ahead for an appointment, and, if possible, schedule it so that you will arrive while a meal is being served. Most retirement homes will permit you to eat lunch or dinner to sample the food. You may be asked to pay for meals. Some continuing care communities have rooms for you to stay in for a few days.

Use the following checklist when you visit an ACLF retirement facility to determine whether it will meet the resident's needs.

RETIREMENT COMMUNITY VISIT CHECKLIST

1. Location

—Is the facility close to those places that are important to the resident such as churches or synagogues, senior centers, shopping, bridge clubs, beaches, and parks?

—Is the facility close to family, friends, and others that are important to the resident?

2. Cost

—Is this the best retirement home or retirement community that the resident can afford?

—Will the resident have sufficient income, after paying bills, to provide for personal needs that are not covered by the contract fees?

—Are cancellation and refund policies acceptable to the resident?

—Is the contract clear and understandable to the resident? Request a copy of the contract to take home to study or to review with your attorney, particularly if it is a continuing care or life care facility.

—If it is a CCRC, has the resident or his or her attorney or accountant examined, an audited financial statement?

—How long has the retirement home been operating and what is its track record? Is occupancy high after several years of operation?

—Is there a waiting list?

3. Meals

—Are meals well balanced and tasty? Ask to see a weekly or monthly menu.

—Does the food appear appetizing? Do residents appear to be enjoying their meals, or do they leave large portions uneaten?

—Are there choices at mealtime?

—Are special meals available?

4. Resident Care

—Observe residents to determine if they are well cared for. Are residents that receive personal care services clean and well groomed?

—Are staff considerate and helpful? Observe how staff interacts with residents. Staff should be caring, helpful, and good natured.

—Do residents say they receive good care? Simply ask several residents during your visit.

—Are the visiting hours and the rules for visiting acceptable? Ask for the policy regarding residents leaving the facility.

5. Health Care Services

—Are health care services adequate?

—If this is a continuing care facility, is the facility licensed to provide 24-hour skilled nursing home care?

—If the facility is a CCRC, determine whether all nursing care is covered under the basic contract, or whether nursing care is covered for a limited number of days and whether residents have access to nursing home care. Are these arrangements satisfactory?

—What are the physician on-call arrangements?

—Are the procedures for emergency medical care satisfactory?

6. Physical Environment

—Are rooms clean, attractive, cheerful, and well-lit?

—Are recreation and lounge areas clean and comfortable?

7. Activities and Daily Living

—What choices are there with regard to recreation and daily living activities? Larger retirement homes may offer more varied activities, but smaller ones may be more personal.

—Do the activities reflect a variety of interests?

—How are holidays celebrated?

—Are there activities for residents who are relatively inactive?

—Are religious services offered in the facility? Does a clergyman visit?

—Is there an active resident council?

8. Licensure Status/Complaints

—If the facility is licensed as an ACLF, does the facility have a standard license, a conditional license, or a provisional license? If the license is conditional or provisional, ask to see the letter from the state Agency for Health Care Administration that explains why a particular license was issued. Florida law requires that copies of the most recent licensure inspection report be provided to residents and to applicants for residency. Ask to see the report.

—Have there been complaints filed against the facility? If so, what has been the nature of the complaints? Contact the local ombudsman council listed in Chapter 11.

RETIREMENT COMMUNITY INFORMATION SOURCES

The Florida Department of Insurance is responsible for the regulation of CCRCs and the department employs examiners to monitor their financial status. The examiners can answer questions from the public regarding compliance with state regulations, including financial reporting requirements, but they cannot recommend specific facilities. Files are maintained on each CCRC and they are open to public inspection. Copies of material in facility files, including audited financial statements, can be obtained for 50 cents per page. If you have questions regarding the compliance of a specific continuing care retirement community with Department of Insurance regulations, direct your inquiry to the address below.

Bureau of Specialty Insurers
Department of Insurance
637 Larson Building
200 East Gaines Street
Tallahassee, Florida 32399-0300
(904) 487-3828.

The Florida Association of Homes for the Aging (FAHA) is an association of more than 225 retirement and health care communities, including senior housing communities, continuing care communities, and nursing homes. Member communities provide services to more than 60,000 elderly Floridians. The association publishes a directory entitled, "Florida's Retirement Housing and Nursing Home Communities," and a booklet, "Housing and Care Options for Older People In Florida." To obtain these free publications, contact:

Florida Association of Homes for the Aging
1018 Thomasville Road, Suite 200Y
Tallahassee, FL 32303
(904) 222-3562

The Retirement Housing Council is an association of proprietary ACLFs and continuing care facilities in Florida. The Council publishes Retirement Housing in Florida, which is available for $4. To obtain the publication, or other information, contact:

Retirement Housing Council
PO Box 12934
Tallahassee, FL 32317-2934
(904) 561-9162

The American Association of Homes for the Aging (AAHA) publishes a guide book for persons interested in continuing care retirement communities. The book, "The Continuing Care Retirement Community: A Guidebook for Consumers" costs $4. The AAHA also publishes the National Continuing Care Directory which is available for $19.95 ($14.50 for American Association of Retired Persons members). To obtain either publication, contact:

AAHA Publications
901 E Street, N.W., Suite 500
Washington, DC 20004-2037
(202) 783-2242

The AARP also publishes information on CCRCs. To obtain a list of publications contact:

AARP/Housing Activities
601 E Street, N.W.
Washington, DC 20049
(202) 434-2277

Some continuing care retirement communities are accredited by the Continuing Care Accreditation Commission (CCAC). Those communities that were accredited as of January 1993 are noted in the list of community care facilities that appears later in this chapter. The CCAC is an independent accrediting commission sponsored by the American Association of Homes for the Aging. Accredited facilities must meet financial, health care, and other standards. Readers should consult the "Accreditation Organizations" section of Chapter 11 for additional information. A list of accredited continuing care communities may be obtained by sending a self-addressed, stamped, legal-size envelope to:

Continuing Care Accreditation Commission
901 E Street N.W., Suite 500
Washington, DC 20004-2037
(202) 783-7286

Consumer Reports magazine published an article on continuing care retirement communities, "Communities for the Elderly," in February 1990. Most public libraries subscribe to *Consumer Reports* and would have that issue on file.

Some local health councils publish excellent guides on the retirement facilities in their geographic areas. A listing of local health councils, with their addresses and telephone numbers, appears at the end of Chapter 11.

COMPLAINTS

There are three agencies that receive and investigate complaints from residents in retirement homes with ACLF licenses:

- **District Ombudsman Councils**—There are twelve Ombudsman Councils that assist in the resolution of complaints regarding ACLFs and nursing homes. The local ombudsman council's telephone number is required to appear on a poster that is displayed in each ACLF. Ombudsman councils may tell you the number and types of complaints filed against a facility, whether they were substantiated, and whether they were minor or serious. There also is a statewide Long-Term Care Ombudsman Council which can be reached by calling (904) 488-6190. District ombudsman councils and the regions they serve are listed in Chapter 11.

- **Abuse Hotline**—In the event that an ACLF resident has been abused or exploited, call the Abuse Hotline at (800) 342-9152. All contact with the Abuse Hotline is confidential.
- **AHCA Office of Health Facility Regulation**—There are 11 area offices that are responsible for licensing ACLFs. Any complaint concerning conditions, or the quality of care given to residents will be investigated by the area offices. All ACLFs are required to have the findings of their most recent licensure inspection posted for examination by residents and the public. The telephone number and address of the area office will be on the inspection report or on the attached cover letter. The AHCA area offices of Health Facility Regulation are listed in Chapter 11.

CONTINUING CARE FACILITIES

The 68 active continuing care facilities licensed in Florida by the Department of Insurance as of March 1993 are listed below. Two additional facilities are included that did not have active licenses but had under construction nursing home facilities and independent living units. A few CCRCs have ceased marketing lifecare contracts that require entrance fees, although they continue to market ACLF contracts that require monthly payments. The licensure inspection ratings for the nursing home components of continuing care facilities are in Appendix E.

The following codes are used to describe the services provided by each continuing care facility:

CCAC = Accredited by the Continuing Care Accreditation Commission as of January 1993.

Contract = Health care delivery is by contract\

On site = Health care delivery is on site

Off site = Health care delivery is off site

AL = Assisted Living

IC = Intermediate Care

SN = Skilled Nursing

Medicare = Medicare certified nursing home beds

Medicare = Medicaid certified nursing home beds

Brevard County

Buena Vida Estates
2129 West New Haven Avenue
West Melbourne, FL 32904
(407) 724-0060

Indep. Living Units: 147
Nursing Home Beds:
Contract/IC/SN

Broward County

Covenant Village of Florida
9201 West Broward Blvd
Plantation, FL 33324
(305) 472-2860

CCAC
Indep. Living Units: 285
Nursing Home Beds: 60
On Site/AL/IC/SN/Medicare/Medicaid

John Knox Village
651 SW Sixth Street
Pompano Beach, FL 33060
(305) 782-1300

CCAC
Indep. Living Units: 639
Nursing Home Beds: 120
On Site/AL/IC/SN/Medicare/Medicaid

Margate Manor
1189 West River Dr.
Margate, FL 33063
(305) 972-0200

Indep. Living Units: 11
Nursing Home Beds: 0
On Site

The Court at Palm-Aire
2701 North Course Dr.
Pompano Beach, FL 33069
(305) 975-8900

Indep. Living Units: 236
Nursing Home Beds: 60
On Site/AL/SN/Medicare

Charlotte County
South Port Square
23023 Westchester Blvd
Port Charlotte, FL 33980
(813) 627-5111

Indep. Living Units: 440
Nursing Home Beds: 120
On Site/AL/IC/SN

Clay County
Park of the Palms
706 Palm Circle
Keystone Heights, FL 32656
(904) 473-4926

Indep. Living Units: 55
Nursing Home Beds:
On-site/AL

Collier County
Bentley Village
561 Bentley Village Court
Naples, FL 33963
(813) 923-7525

Indep. Living Units: 374
Nursing Home Beds: 93
On Site/AL/SN

The Glenview at Pelican Bay
100 Gleview Place
Naples, FL 33963
(813) 591-0011

Indep. Living Units: 140
Nursing Home Beds: 35
On site/SN

Moorings Park
120 Moorings Park Drive
Naples, FL 33942
(813) 261-1616

Indep. Living Units: 281
Nursing Home Beds: 60
On Site/SN/Medicare

Dade County
East Ridge Retirement Village
19301 SW 87th Avenue
Miami, FL 33157
(305) 238-2623

Indep. Living Units: 312
Nursing Home Beds: 60
On Site/AL/SN/Medicare

Duval County
Fleet Landing
1 Fleet Landing Blvd.
Atlantic Beach, FL 32233
904-246-9900

(Naval Personnel)
Indep. Living Units: 346
Nursing Home Beds: 42
On Site/AL/SN

Wesley Manor Retirement Village
25 State Road 13
Jacksonville, FL 32259
(904) 287-7300

Indep. Living Units: 259
Nursing Home Beds: 57
On Site/AL/IC/SN

Escambia County
Azalea Trace
10100 Hillview
Pensacola, FL 32514
(904) 478-5200

Indep. Living Units: 286
Nursing Home Beds: 90
On Site/SN/Medicare/Medicaid

Highlands County
The Palms of Sebring
725 South Pine Street
Sebring, FL 33870
(813) 385-0161

Indep. Living Units: 35
Nursing Home Beds: 120
On Site/AL/IC/SN/Medicare/Medicaid

Hillsborough County
Canterbury Towers
3501 Bayshore Blvd
Tampa, FL 33629
(813) 837-1083

Indep. Living Units: 125
Nursing Home Beds: 40
On Site/SN/Medicare

The Home Association
1203 22nd Avenue
Tampa, FL 33605
(813) 229-6901

Indep. Living Units: 96
Nursing Home Beds: 96
On Site/IC/SN/Medicaid

John Knox Village
4100 East Fletcher Avenue
Tampa, FL 33613
(813) 977-4950

Indep. Living Units: 512
Nursing Home Beds: 110
On Site/AL/IC/SN/Medicare/Medicaid

Lake Towers
101 Trinity Lakes Drive
Sun City Center, FL 33570
(813) 634-3347

Indep. Living Units: 180
Nursing Home Beds: 120
On Site/AL/IC/SN/Medicare/Medicaid

University Village
12401 North 22nd Street
Tampa, FL 33612
(813) 975-5000

Indep. Living Units: 408
Nursing Home Beds: 60
On Site/IC/SN/Medicare/Medicaid

Indian River County
Indian River Estates
2250 Indian Creek Blvd West
Vero Beach, FL 32960
(407) 562-7400

Indep. Living Units: 497
Nursing Home Beds: 60
On Site/AL/SN/Medicare

Lake County
Forester Haven
28334 Church Hill Smith Lane
Mt. Dora, FL 32757
(904) 383-6158

Indep. Living Units: 124
Nursing Home Beds: 0
Off Site/AL

Lakeview Terrace Christian
 Retirement Community
331 Raintree Drive
Altoona, FL 32702
(904) 669-2133

Indep. Living Units: 194
Nursing Home Beds: 20
On Site/AL/IC/SN/Medicare/Medicaid

Lake Port Square
701 Lake Port Blvd
Leesburg, FL 32748
(904) 728-8525
Facility was under construction in 1992

Indep. Living Units: 200
Nursing Home Beds: 60
On Site/AL/IC/SN/Medicare/Medicaid

Lee County
Calusa Harbor
2525 East First Street
Ft. Myers, FL 33901
(813) 332-3333

Indep. Living Units: 29
Nursing Home Beds: 100
On Site/AL/IC/SN/Medicare/Medicaid

Gulf Coast Village
1333 Santa Barbara Blvd
Cape Coral, FL 33991
(813) 772-1333

Indep. Living Units: 192
Nursing Home Beds: 60
On Site/AL/IC/SN/Medicare/Medicaid

Shell Point Village
15000 Shell Point Blvd
Ft. Myers, FL 339908
(813) 466-2156

CCAC
Indep. Living Units: 769
Nursing Home Beds: 180
On Site/AL/SN

Leon County
Westminster Oaks
4449 Meandering Way
Tallahassee, FL 32308
(904) 878-1136

CCAC
Indep. Living Units: 157
Nursing Home Beds: 60
On Site/AL/IC/SN/Medicare/Medicaid

Manatee County
Westminster Asbury Towers
1533 Fourth Ave. West
Bradenton, FL 34205
(813) 747-1881

Indep. Living Units: 95
Nursing Home Beds: 34
On Site/AL/IC/SN/Medicare/Medicaid

Westminster Asbury Manor
1700 21st Avenue West
Bradenton, FL 33505
(813) 748-4161

CCAC
Indep. Living Units: 132
Nursing Home Beds: 60
On Site/AL/IC/SN/Medicare/Medicaid

Freedom Village
6501 17th Avenue West
Bradenton, FL 34209
(813) 798-8190

Indep. Living Units: 442
Nursing Home Beds: 120
On Site/AL/IC/SN/Medicare/Medicaid

Orange County
Central Park Village
9309 S. Highway 441
Orlando, FL 32821
(407) 859-7990

Indep. Living Units: 37
Nursing Home Beds: 120
SN/Medicare/Medicaid

The Mayflower
1620 Mayflower Court
Winter Park, FL 32792
(407) 672-1620

Indep. Living Units: 240
Nursing Home Beds: 60
On Site/SN

Orlando Lutheran Towers
300 East Church Street
Orlando, FL 32801
(407) 425-1033

Indep. Living Units: 244
Nursing Home Beds: 60
On Site/AL/SN/Medicaid/Medicare

Westminster Towers
70 West Lucerne Circle
Orlando, FL 32801
(407) 841-1310

CCAC
Indep. Living Units: 290
Nursing Home Beds: 120
On Site/AL/IC/SN/Medicaid/Medicare

Winter Park Towers
1111 South Lakemont Avenue
Winter Park, FL 32792
(407) 647-4083

CCAC
Indep. Living Units: 303
Nursing Home Beds: 121
On Site/AL/IC/SN/Medicare/Medicaid

Palm Beach County
Abbey Delray
2000 Lowson Boulevard
Delray Beach, FL 33445
(407) 278-3249

Indep. Living Units: 360
Nursing Home Beds: 100
On Site/SN/Medicare/Medicaid

Abbey Delray South
1717 Homewood Blvd
Delray Beach, FL 33445
(407) 272-9600

Indep. Living Units: 286
Nursing Home Beds: 60
On Site/SN/Medicare/Medicaid

Bishop Gray Inn, Lake Worth
4445 Pine Forest Drive
Lake Worth, FL 33463
(407) 965-5954

Indep. Living Units: 73
Nursing Home Beds: 60
On Site/SN/Medicare

Edgewater Pointe Estates
23315 Blue Water Circle
Boca Raton, FL 33433
(407) 391-6305

Indep. Living Units: 359
Nursing Home Beds: 60
On Site/AL/SN/Medicare

Harbour's Edge
401 East Linton Blvd
Delray Beach, FL 33483
(407) 272-7979

Indep. Living Units: 276
Nursing Home Beds: 54
On Site/SN/Medicare

St. Andrews Estates
6152 North Verde Trail
Boca Raton, FL 33433
(407) 487-5500

Indep. Living Units: 602
Nursing Home Beds: 120
On Site/AL/SN/Medicare/Medicaid

The Waterford
601 South U.S. Highway 1
Juno Beach, FL 33408
(407) 627-3800

Indep. Living Units: 300
Nursing Home Beds: 60
On Site/SN/Medicare/Medicaid

Pinellas County
Bayview Gardens
2833 Gulf-To-Bay Blvd
Clearwater, FL 34619
(813) 797-7400

Indep. Living Units: 327
Nursing Home Beds: 0
Off site/AL

College Harbor
4600 54th Avenue South
St. Petersburg, FL 33711
(813) 866-3124

Indep. Living Units: 109
Nursing Home Beds: 60
On Site/AL/SN/Medicare

Freedom Square
7800 Liberty Lane
Seminole, FL 34642
(813) 398-0166

Indep. Living Units: 383
Nursing Home Beds: 240
On Site/IC/SN

Majestic Towers
1255 Pasadena Avenue South
St. Petersburg, FL 34707
(813) 381-5411

Indep. Living Units: 374
Nursing Home Beds: 150
On Site/AL/IC/SN/Medicare/Medicaid

Masonic Homes of Florida
3201 First Street Northeast
St. Petersburg, FL 33704
(813) 821-5062

Indep. Living Units: 102
Nursing Home Beds: 85
On Site/AL/SN/

Mease Manor
700 Mease Plaza
Dunedin, FL 33698
(813) 733-1161

Indep. Living Units: 260
Nursing Home Beds: 100
On Site/SN/Medicare/Medicaid

Oak Bluffs
420 Bay Avenue
Clearwater, FL 34616
(813) 445-4700

Indep. Living Units: 94
Nursing Home Beds: 60
On Site/IC/SN/Medicare/Medicaid

Oak Cove
210 South Osceola Avenue
Clearwater, FL 34616
(813) 441-3763

Indep. Living Units: 93
Nursing Home Beds: 56
On Site/IC/SN/Medicare/Medicaid

Palm Shores
830 North Shore Drive
St. Petersburg, FL 33701
(813) 894-2102

Indep. Living Units: 159
Nursing Home Beds: 42
On Site/AL/IC/SN

Regency Oaks
2751 Regency Oaks Blvd
Clearwater, FL 34619
(813) 791-3381
Under construction in March 1993

Indep. Living Units: 200
Nursing Home Beds: 60
On Site/AL/IC/SN

St. Mark Village
2655 Nebraska Avenue
Palm Harbor, FL 34684
(813) 785-2577

CCAC
Indep. Living Units: 323
Nursing Home Beds: 80
On Site/AL/IC/SN/Medicare

Suncoast Manor
6909 9th Street South
St. Petersburg, FL 33705
(813) 867-1131

Indep. Living Units: 246
Nursing Home Beds: 208
On Site/SN

Westminster Shores
125 Fifty Sixth Avenue South
St. Petersburg, FL 33705
(813) 867-9663

Indep. Living Units: 193
Nursing Home Beds: 120
On Site/AL/SN/Medicaid/Medicare

Polk County
Florida Presbyterian Homes
16 Lake Hunter Drive
Lakeland, FL 33803
(813) 682-7787,

Indep. Living Units: 129
Nursing Home Beds: 185
Off Site/AL/IC/SN/Medicare/Medicaid

Bishop Gray Inn—Davenport
206 West Orange St
Davenport, FL 33837
(813) 422-4961

Indep. Living Units: 75
Nursing Home Beds: 60
On Site/AL/SN/Medicare/Medicaid

Carpenter's Home Estate
1001 Carpenter's Way
Lakeland, FL 33809
(813) 858-3847

Indep. Living Units: 340
Nursing Home Beds: 60
On Site/AL/IC/SN/Medicare/Medicaid

Saint Johns County
Vicar's Landing
1000 Vicar's Landing Way
Ponte Vedra Beach, FL 32082
(904) 273-1700

Indep. Living Units: 229
Nursing Home Beds: 30
On site/AL/SN/Medicare

Sarasota County
Bay Village of Sarasota
8400 Vamo Road
Sarasota, FL 34231
(813) 966-5611

CCAC
Indep. Living Units: 328
Nursing Home Beds: 107
IC/SN

Lakehouse East
4540 Bee Ridge Road
Sarasota, FL 34233
(813) 377-0102

Indep. Living Units: 164
Nursing Home Beds: 0
Off Site

Lakehouse West
3435 Fox Run Road
Sarasota, FL 34231
(813) 923-7525

Indep. Living Units: 168
Nursing Home Beds: 0
Off Site

Lake Pointe Woods
7979 South Tamiami Trail
Sarasota, FL 34231
(813) 923-4944

Indep. Living Units: 188
Nursing Home Beds: 113
On site/AL/IC/SN

Plymouth Harbor
700 John Ringling Blvd
Sarasota, FL 34236
(813) 365-2600

Indep. Living Units: 238
Nursing Home Beds: 60
On site/AL/SN

Southwest Fla Retirement Center
950 South Tamiami Trail
Venice, FL 34285
(813) 484-9753

Indep. Living Units: 229
Nursing Home Beds: 60
On Site/AL/IC/SN/Medicare/Medicaid

Seminole County
Village on the Green
500 Village Place
Longwood, FL 33779
(305) 682-0230

Indep. Living Units: 242
Nursing Home Beds: 60
On Site/SN/Medicare

Volusia County
Alliance Retirement Cntr
600 South Florida Avenue
DeLand, FL 32720
(904) 734-3481

Indep. Living Units: 111
Nursing Home Beds: 60
AL/IC/SN/Medicare/Medicaid

Florida Lutheran Retirement Center
450 N. McDonald Avenue
DeLand, FL 32724
(904) 736-5800

Indep. Living Units: 114
Nursing Home Beds: 0
AL

John Knox Village
101 Northlake Drive
Orange City, FL 32763
(904) 775-3840

Indep. Living Units: 492
Nursing Home Beds: 120
On Site/AL/IC/SN/Medicare/Medicaid

ACLFS WITH LIMITED NURSING SERVICES

There are over 1,400 ACLFs licensed in Florida. Those ACLFs which were licensed as of January 1993 with standard or provisional licenses to provide limited nursing services are listed below. Some of these facilities are also licensed as continuing care facilities.

Alachua County
High Springs Care Center
201 N.E. 1st Avenue
High Spring, FL 32643
(904) 454-5000
Capacity—60

Brevard County
Meadowbrook Terrace of Melbourne
85 Bulldog Boulevard
Melbourne, FL 32901
(407) 984-7966
Capacity—100

Broward County
Abbe West, Inc.
459 Pompano Park Place
Pompano Beach, FL 33060
(305) 942-6000
Capacity—80

Bernadette's ACLF
520 Northwest 2nd Avenue
Hallandale, FL 33009
(305) 458-8005
Capacity—8

Broward House
417 S.E. 18th Court
Ft. Lauderdale, FL 33316
(305) 522-4749
Capacity—52

The Court at Palm-Aire
2701 N. Course Drive
Pompano Beach, FL 33069
(305) 975-8900
Capacity—100

Forum at Deer Creek
3001 Deer Creek Country Club Blvd.
Deerfield Beach, FL 33442
(305) 698-6269
Capacity—70

Horizon Club (The)
1208 S. Military Trail
Deerfield Beach, FL 33442
(305) 481-2304
Capacity—68

Westchester (The)
9701 West Oakland Park Blvd
Sunrise, FL 33351
(305) 572-4444
Capacity—124

Williamsburg Landing
1776 Northeast 26th Street
Fort Lauderdale, FL 33305
(305) 566-1775
Capacity—100

Woodsetter Retirement Club
4700 NW 3rd Avenue
Pompano Beach, FL 33064
(305) 942-2233
Capacity—220

Collier County
Arbor Trace
14551 Vanderbilt Drive
Naples, FL 33963
(813) 598-1155
Capacity—40

Canterbury House
10 Seventh Street
Bonita Springs, FL 33923
(813) 597-1322
Capacity—38

Renaissance of Naples
900 Imperial Golf Course Blvd.
Naples, FL 33942
(813) 591-4800
Capacity—60

Dade County
Camelot Care Center
25268 S.W. 134th Avenue
Princeton, FL 33032
(305) 258-2222
Capacity—196

Duval County
Cypress Village
4600 Middleton Park Circle, West
Jacksonville, FL 32224
(904) 223-6185
Capacity—38

Fleet Landing
One Fleet Landing Boulevard
Atlantic Beach, FL 32333
(904) 246-9900
Capacity—30

Mandarin Manor Retirement Village
10680 Old St. Augustine Road
Jacksonville, FL 32223
(904) 268-4953
Capacity—300

Regents Woods
7130 Southside Blvd
Jacksonville, FL 32216
(904) 642-7300
Capacity—102

Wyndham Lakes
10680 Old St. Augustine Road
Jacksonville, FL 32257
(904) 262-4600
Capacity—95

Escambia County
Bayou Villas
201 South Stillman St.
Pensacola, FL 32505
(904) 434-1504
Capacity—148

Carpenter's Creek Community
5918 North Davis Highway
Pensacola, FL 32503
(904) 477-8998
Capacity—125

Homestead Village Retirement Center
7830 Pine Forest Road
Pensacola, FL 32526
(904) 944-4366
Capacity—50

Hillsborough County
Rosemont Retirement Residence
722 Bowing Oak Drive
Brandon, FL 33511
(813) 654-1080
Capacity—41

Tampa Bay Retirement Center
11722 North 17th Street
Tampa, FL 33612
(813) 971-8072
Capacity—116

Indian River County
Indian River Estates
2200 Indian Creek Blvd.
Vero Beach, FL 32966
(407) 562-8700
Capacity—48

Lake County
Lake Port Inn
701 Lake Port Boulevard
Leesburg, FL 34748
(904) 728-8525
Capacity—70

Mayfield Retirement Center
460 Newell Hill Road
Leesburg, FL 34748
(904) 365-6011
Capacity—49

Somerset On Lake Sauders
15330 Dora Avenue
Tavares, FL 32778
(904) 343-4464
Capacity—24

Lee County
Cross Key Manor
1550 Lee Boulevard
Lehigh Acres, FL 33936
(813) 369-2194
Capacity—32

Leon County
Meadowbrook Terrace of Tallahassee
1978 Village Green Way
Tallahassee, FL 32308
(904) 385-4533
Capacity—120

Manatee County
The Shores
1700 3rd Avenue West
Bradenton, FL 33505
(813) 748-1700
Capacity—310

Orange County
Noble Care
1201 Noble Place
Orlando, FL 32801
(407) 894-6325
Capacity—7

Osceola County
Happy Acres Home for the Aged
2411 Fortune Road
Kissimmee, FL 34744
(407) 348-6100
Capacity—34

Palm Beach County
Colonial Inn at Heritage Park
14565 Sims Road
Delray Beach, Fl 33484
(407) 499-2300
Capacity—60

Edgewater Pointe Estates
23315 Blue Water Circle
Boca Raton, FL 33433
(407) 391-6305
Capacity—44

Meadowbrook Manor of Boca Cove
1130 N.W. 15th Street
Boca Raton, FL 33486
(407) 394-6282
Capacity—73

St. Andrews Estates South
6051 South Verde Trail
Boca Raton, FL 33433
(407) 487-6200
Capacity—40

The Village at Manor Park
3005 South Congress Avenue
Boynton Beach, FL 33426
(407) 738-4777
Capacity—120

Whitehall Boca Raton
7300 Del Prado South
Boca Raton, FL 33433
(407) 392-3000
Capacity—114

Pasco County
Forest Glen Lodges
7435 Plathe Road
New Port Richey, FL 34653
(813) 845-0609
Capacity—72

LTC Care Center
2201 Dairy Road
Zephryhills, FL 33540
(813) 782-4417
Capacity—160

Meadowbrook Terrace of NPR
7220 Ballie Drive
New Port Richey, FL 34653
(813) 842-9899
Capacity—176

Pinehill Village
5905 Pinehill Road
Port Richey, FL 34668
(813) 845-0527
Capacity—230

Pinellas County
College Harbor Inc.
4600 54th Avenue South
St. Petersburg, FL 33711
(813) 866-3124
Capacity—40

Coral Oaks ACLF
2650 West Lake Road
Palm Harbor, FL 34684
(813) 787-3333
Capacity—32

The Village at Manor Park
880 Patricia Avenue
Dunedin, FL 34698
(813) 734-4696

Polk County
Florida Presbyterian Homes
16 Lake Hunter Drive
Lakeland, FL 33803
(813) 688-5521
Capacity—150

Lake Howard Heights
650 N. Lake Howard Drive
Winter Haven, FL 33881
(813) 293-3171
Capacity—180

Lime Plaza
400 S. Florida Avenue
Lakeland, FL 33801
(813) 682-7327
Capacity—71

Meadowbrook Terrace of Winter Haven
5890 Cypress Garden Blvd
Winter Haven, FL 33884
(904) 385-4533
Capacity—176

T.L.C. Retirement Residence
747 Bon Air Street
Lakeland, FL 33805
(813) 688-1196
Capacity—39

Sarasota County
Barrington Woods
7850 Beneva Road
Sarasota, FL 34238
(813) 924-1711
Capacity—110

Hacienda-La-Grande
671 Bradenton Road
Venice, FL 34293
(813) 497-2937
Capacity—4

Southwest Fla Retirement Center
950 S. Tamiami Trail
Venice, FL 33595
(813) 484-9753
Capacity—571

The Village at Manor Park
5501 Swift Road
Sarasota, FL 34231
(813) 922-8778
Capacity—120

Seminole County
Better Living Center of Seminole County
201 Sunset Drive
Casselberry, FL 32707
(407) 699-5002
Capacity—80

Lakewood Adult Care Facility
8511 La Amistad Cove
Fern Park, FL 32730
(904) 332-1711
Capacity—24

Volusia County
Woodland Towers
113 Chipola Avenue
Deland, FL 32720
(904) 738-2700
Capacity—170

CHAPTER 6
Birth centers, hospices & home health agencies

Birth centers, hospice programs, and home health agencies provide health care services in non-institutional settings. Birth centers and hospices are relatively new health care providers, and both emphasize using family members as supportive caregivers.

Birth centers are an option available to women at low risk for complications who want to deliver their babies in a more personal and less technologically intensive environment than in a hospital. Hospice programs provide care for the terminally ill and their families. Hospices care is provided both in the home and in health care facilities. Home health agencies provide a range of health care and personal care services to persons who can be cared for at home. These services help many elderly persons live at home for longer periods of time, thus delaying or avoiding residing in a nursing home.

BIRTH CENTERS

Birth centers offer an alternative to hospital delivery for low-risk pregnant women who are in good health, who are sustaining a normal pregnancy, and who are highly motived to have a natural birth without intervention. Birth centers provide a home-like and natural environment for delivery, and family members may be present at the time of birth.

Birth centers differ with regard to the types of professionals who deliver babies. In Florida, most birth centers use either physicians or certified nurse midwives. A small number use licensed lay midwives. All birth centers must have either a physician on staff or have a physician consultant who provides advice and services to the birth center. In Florida, birth centers must meet the following requirements:

- Before admission to a birth center, patients must sign a written agreement to receive prenatal care by the birth center. Patients are required to be informed of the qualifications of the staff, the benefits and risks related to out-of-hospital childbirth, and the possibility of referral or transfer if complications arise during pregnancy or labor.
- General health status and risk assessments are completed for each patient. This must be determined by a physician, certified nurse midwife, or advanced registered nurse practitioner. Women must be at low risk for a poor pregnancy outcome, and they must be evaluated regularly during their pregnancies to ensure that they remain at low risk. The risk assessment must be included in the patient's medical record.
- Birth center contracts typically include the costs patients are expected to pay for birth center services, which include prenatal, delivery, and postpartum care and contain provisions for paying for hospital care if hospital care is required.
- As part of the course of prenatal care, patients receive counseling and instruction to prepare them for childbirth including, nutritional needs, good health habits, danger signs of pre-term labor, and what to expect during labor and delivery.

- Birth centers must have arrangements to transport the patient to a hospital in the event of an emergency.

The National Birth Center Study, the largest and most rigorous ever undertaken of birth centers, examined 11,814 women who delivered in 84 free-standing birth centers from mid-1985 to 1987 (Rooks et al. 1989). Certified nurse midwives delivered at 60 of the 84 centers, obstetrician-gynecologists delivered in 11, family practitioners or other physicians delivered in six, and licensed or lay midwives delivered in three. The principal findings of the National Birth Center Study were:
- Certified nurse midwives or nurse midwifery students delivered approximately 80 percent of the women.
- The overall cesarean section rate was 4.4 percent.
- 15.8 percent of women were transferred to hospitals, and 7.9 percent had serious emergency complications at the time of labor and delivery or soon thereafter.
- Patient satisfaction was very high, even among women who were transferred to hospitals to deliver.

The study found that, "Few innovations in health service promise lower cost, greater availability, and a high degree of satisfaction with a comparable degree of safety. The results of this study suggest that modern birth centers can identify women who are at low risk for obstetrical complications and can care for them in a way that provides these benefits." The authors concluded by stating, "we conclude that birth centers offer a safe and acceptable alternative to hospital confinement for selected pregnant women, particularly those who have previously had children, and that such care leads to relatively few cesarean sections."

Sources of Information on Birth Centers

Florida Alliance of Birth Centers
260 East 6th Avenue
Tallahassee, FL 32303
(904) 224-0490

National Association of Childbearing Centers
3123 Gottschall Road
Perkiomenville, PA 18074
(215) 234-8068

American College of Nurse-Midwives
1522 K Street, N.W., Suite 1000
Washington, D.C. 20005
(202) 289-0171

Florida birth centers licensed as of February, 1993 were:

North Florida
Milton Memorial Birthing Center
Route 2, Box 124
Laurel Hill, FL 32567
(904) 834-2946

Physicians Alternate Birthing Home
100 Saint Augustine South Drive
St. Augustine, FL 32086
(904) 797-3785

The Tallahassee Birth Centre
260 East 6th Avenue
Tallahassee, FL 32303
(904) 378-2882

Patience Corner Nurse-Midwifery Center
717 S.W. 4th Avenue
Gainesville, FL 32601
(904) 378-2882

The Birth Center of Gainesville
218 N.W. 2nd Avenue
Gainesville, FL 32601
(904) 372-4784

Central Florida
Brevard Birthing Center
190 S. Sykes Creek Parkway
Merritt Island, FL 32954
(407) 453-0562

Family Birth Center
211 W. Warren Avenue
Longwood, FL 32750
(407) 331-4437

Physicians Birthing Center
521 W. State Road 434
Longwood, FL 32750
(407) 322-6611

Orlando Birthing Center
3765 N. John Young Parkway
Orlando, FL 32804
(407) 292-7500

Special Beginnings Birth and Gynecology
   Center
1010 Arthur Avenue
Orlando, FL 32804
(407) 291-4777

Birthing Cottage of Winter Park
120 Benmore Drive
Winter Park, FL 32792
(407) 644-5567

Labor of Love Childbirth Services
1525 Edgewater Beach Drive
Lakeland, FL 33805
(813) 680-2229

Birthing and Baby Center
7275 Estapona Circle
Fern Park, FL 32730
(407) 339-1611

Special Delivery Birthing Center
1095 N. Washington Avenue
Titusville, FL 32796
(407) 264-1614

The Women's Center of Martin County
448 East Osceola Street
Stuart, FL 34994
(407) 283-5909

West Coast
Labor of Love Childbirth
   Services of Dunedin
204 Scotland Street
Dunedin, FL 34698
(813) 734-2229

New Beginnings Natural Childbirth
   Center
609 Deleon Street
Tampa, FL 33606
(813) 254-2796

Countryside Birthing Place
3060 Jones Lane
Clearwater, FL 34619
(813) 797-3443

Florida West Coast Birthing Center
4400 South Tamiami Trail
Sarasota, FL 34231
(813) 366-2229

Venice Obstetrics Clinic
5001 South Tamiami Trail
Venice, FL 34293
(813) 493-5301

Collier Childbirth Center
803 Vanderbilt Beach Road
Naples, FL 33963
(813) 597-9444

HOSPICE CARE

Hospice and hospitality are derived from the same root word. In medieval Europe, hospices gave shelter to traveling pilgrims. Today, hospice programs provide comfort and care to terminally ill persons and their families during the final stages of illness when curative treatment is not appropriate. The vast majority of hospice patients have terminal cancer (84% according to one study). The modern concept of hospice originated in Great Britain, with the founding of St. Christopher's Hospice, in 1967. The first hospice program in the U. S. began in 1974.

Hospice services

The goal of hospice care is, "To provide a dignified, comfortable death for the terminally ill and to care for the patient and family together" (Rhymes 1990). Many hospices receive substantial charitable donations, and all use volunteers. An article in the *New England Journal of Medicine* on hospice care (Bulkin and Lukashok 1988) concludes that,

> "*Most of us, doctors and patients alike, fear death far less than we fear a long and painful dying that leaves us incapacitated, helpless, totally dependent on the good will of strangers—bereft of dignity, comfort, and human warmth.*"

Hospice care is intended to ameliorate these fears by caring for both the patient and family members. The main responsibilities of health care professionals are to control the patient's symptoms, particularly pain. An interdisciplinary team of professional caregivers cares for the psychological, social, and spiritual needs of the patient and the family.

Bonnie Wood, a nursing home and hospice administrator in Arizona, suggests that hospice care can provide insights into the meaning of life (Wood, 1993). According to Wood,

> "*The gifts of dying can be precious, for when the social masks slip away, the dying are often able to communicate on a deeper level with those around them. It is extremely valuable for the living to see life from a different perspective, to experience it from a more timeless vantage point. Those who have witnessed a peaceful death are less fearful of their own life's end and accept death more naturally. There is much we can learn about life from the dying, thus comes the basic hospice concept of the patient as giver as well as receiver.*"

In Florida, hospice programs are licensed to provide palliative and supportive care to patients with terminal illnesses with a life expectancy of a year or less. Although hospice care is usually provided at home, hospice care also may be provided in adult congregate living facilities (ACLFs), nursing homes, and hospice residential units. Hospice patients also may receive short-term inpatient hospital care for pain control, symptom management, or caregiver respite.

Hospice care is provided by a "hospice care team" that consists of qualified professionals and volunteers who collectively assess, coordinate, and provide palliative and supportive care to patients and their families. The control and relief of pain and other symptoms of distress, and providing comfort to the patient and family, are the primary goals of care. Services provided by licensed hospices in Florida include physician services, nursing services, dietary counseling, home health aid services, social work services, patient care training for family members and Pastoral or counseling services to relieve emotional stress.

Florida requires that the interdisciplinary hospice care team include a physician, registered nurse, social worker, clergy person or counselor, and a volunteer. The overall program of hospice care is coordinated by a registered nurse who acts as the "patient and family care coordinator." A physician establishes written protocols for the control of pain, nausea, and other symptoms. The physician may be the patient's family physician or the medical director of the hospice. Volunteers provide companionship, friendship, and respite for caregivers.

The interdisciplinary team develops a written care plan which is based on an assessment of the needs of the both the patient and the family. Care plans include skilled palliative care to control physical pain and other symptoms, and skilled psychosocial, spiritual and bereavement counseling for both the patient and the family. Care plans must be reviewed regularly by the professional care team.

Hospice care, including physician care, nursing care, and counseling must be available 24 hours a day, seven days a week. Sometimes it is necessary for the hospice patient to be moved from home to a hospital. This may occur when it is necessary to better manage symptoms such as pain, or if the family caregiver becomes unable to continue to provide care. Designated inpatient hospice beds may also exist in hospitals of other facilities.

Hospice benefits under Medicare

The Medicare program pays for hospice care when: a doctor certifies the patient has a terminal illness; the patient chooses Medicare hospice benefits rather than standard Medicare benefits for the terminal illness; and the hospice is recognized by Medicare. Hospice services are covered under Medicare Part A and include nursing and physician care; drugs, including outpatient drugs for pain relief and symptom control; physical therapy, occupational therapy and speech language pathology; home health aid and homemaker services; medical social services, medical supplies and appliances; short-term inpatient care, including respite care; and counseling. There are no deductibles and the only out-of-pocket costs are small coinsurance amounts for outpatient drugs and inpatient respite care. Hospice patients remain eligible for standard Medicare benefits that are not related to the treatment of the terminal illness.

Research on care for persons with terminal illnesses

Research on hospice care for patients with terminal cancer in Great Britain suggests that pain management and symptom control may be better in hospitals (Parkes 1985) and that hospice patients are less depressed and anxious (Hinton 1979).

Research findings in the U.S. are similar to those in Great Britain (Rhymes 1990). Rhymes reviewed studies of hospice care that were conducted in the U.S. and concluded that, "Overall, patient and caregiver satisfaction with hospice care was at least comparable to conventional care. Hospice programs offering hospital services may be more successful at reducing patient pain and caregiver stress than home care-based programs."

The H. Lee Moffitt Cancer Center and the University of South Florida conducted a survival and cost-effectiveness analysis of all cancer patients who were admitted to the intensive care unit (ICU) between July 1988 and June 1990 (Schapira et al. 1993). The study, published in the *Journal of the American Medical Association*, included 86 patients with solid tumors and 64 patients with hematologic cancers (leukemia and lymphoma).

Of the 86 patients with solid tumors, 40 percent died in the hospital and 60 percent died at home. Of the 64 patients with hematologic cancers, half died in the hospital and half at home. Mean survival was similar for both groups of patients, 4.8 months for patients with solid tumors and five months for those with hematologic cancers. More than three-fourths of the patients in both groups spent less than three months at home before dying. According to the authors,

> *"Despite the potential for prolonged survival, once patients became critically ill and required admission to the ICU, their prognosis was poor. Attempts to save these patients incur considerable costs that may affect the families of these patients."*

The study found that the cost for each year of life gained was $82,845 for patients with solid tumors and $189,339 for those with hematologic cancers. For patients with solid tumors, the cost per year of life gained at home was $95,142 and $449,544 for those with hematologic cancers.

The Moffit study recommended that before the patient becomes critically ill, the physician, the patient, and the family should discuss and agree on a "reasonable strategy" involving the admission to an ICU, the use of mechanical ventilatory assistance, and the withdrawal of resources. The authors wrote that,

> *"Physicians must be prepared to advise that resources be withdrawn when a clinical scenario appears hopeless. An increasing number of alternative forms of health care have become available for patients during their last months of life, aimed at providing them with less invasive, less aggressive, less costly care."*

A study published in *Medical Care* examined the views of 335 relatives of persons with terminal cancer who died in Majorca, Spain between 1984 and 1986 (Catalan-Fernandez, et al. 1991). The study included interviews with the relatives of 184 persons who died in hospitals (55 percent) and 151 persons who died at home (45 percent). Those who died at home were cared for by relatives, rather than by organized hospice or home health care programs.

The findings of the study offer interesting perspectives on care for the terminally ill. It found marked differences in how relatives perceived deaths that occurred at home versus those that occurred in a hospital. Based on interviews with the surviving relatives of those who died of terminal cancer, the authors wrote, "It can be concluded that hospitals are not the best places in which to die of cancer. Greater technical assistance is provided in an environment that increases the family's distress. In most cases, the quality of life is much better at home, and there is no evidence to show that a decision one way or another improves the quality of death."

Sources of information on hospice care

Several national organizations can be contacted for information about hospice care.

Foundation for Hospice and Home Care
519 C Street, N.E.
Washington, D.C. 20002
(202) 547-7424

Hospice Education Institute
5 Essex Square, Suite 3-B
Essex, CT 06426
(800) 331-1620

National Hospice Organization
1901 North Moore Street, Suite 901
Alexandria, VA 22209
(800) 658-8898 or (703) 243-5900

Children's Hospice International
901 N. Washington Street, Suite 700
Alexandria, VA 22314
(800) 242-4453

Licensed hospice programs

Some hospices are accredited by the Joint Commission on Accreditation of Healthcare Organizations (JCAHO). Readers should consult the "Accreditation Organizations" section of Chapter 11 for additional information regarding accredited facilities. Those hospices with accreditation as of February 22, 1993 are indicated with the statement "JCAHO Accredited (February 1993)."

Alachua County
Hospice of North Central Florida
720 S.W. 2nd Avenue, Suite 506
Gainesville 32601
JCAHO Accredited (February 1993)
Serves: Alachua, Bradford, Columbia,
Dixie, Gilchrist, Hamilton, Levy,
Putnam, Union, Suwannee, Lafayette

Bay County
Bay Medical Center Hospice
615 North Bonita Avenue
Panama City 32401
(904) 769-1511
Serves: Bay, Calhoun, Gulf, Homes,
Jackson, Washington

Brevard County
Brevard Hospice
110 Longwood Ave
Rockledge 32956-0965
(407)-636-2211

Holmes Regional Hospice
1900 Dairy Road
West Melbourne 32904

Hospice of St. Francis
9 South Palm Avenue
Titusville 32783

Broward County
Hospice Care of Broward County
309 Southeast 18th Street
Fort Lauderdale 33316
(305) 467-7423

Hospice of Gold Coast Home Health
  Services
911 East Atlantic Boulevard, #200
Pompano Beach 33060
(305) 785-2990
Serves: Broward, Palm Beach

VITAS Healthcare Corporation
3323 W. Commercial Blvd.
Fort Lauderdale 33309

Charlotte County
Hospice of Charlotte
3280-17 Tamiami Trail
Port Charlotte 33952
(813) 625-9992
Serves: Charlotte, Desoto

Citrus County
Hospice of Citrus County
565 Gulf to Lake Highway
Lecanto 32651-0368

Collier County
Hospice of Naples
850 6th Ave North
Naples 33940
(813) 261-4404

Dade County
The Catholic Hospice
Suite 370
14100 Palmetto Frontage Rd
Miami Lakes 33016
(305) 822-2380

Hospice Care of South Florida
7270 N.W. 12th Street, 33126
Miami 33126

VITAS Healthcare Corporation
4770 Biscayne Blvd., Suite 200
Miami 33137

Duval County
Hospice of Northeast Florida
One Prudential Plaza
841 Prudential Drive
Jacksonville 32207-8331
(904) 398-4724
Serves: Baker, Clay, Duval Nassau, Saint
Johns

Methodist Hospital Hospice
580 West Eighth Street
Jacksonville 32205
(904) 798-8340
Serves: Baker, Clay, Duval, Nassau, Saint
Johns

Escambia County
Hospice of Northwest Florida
2001 North Palafox Street
Pensacola 32501
(904) 433-2155
*Serves: Escambia, Okaloosa, Santa Rosa,
Walton*

Highlands County
Good Shepherd Hospice of Mid-Florida
245 South Commerce
Sebring 33870

Hillsborough County
Hospice of Hillsborough
3010 West Azeele Street
Tampa 33609
(813) 877-2200
JCAHO Accredited (February 1993)

Indian River County
VNA Hospice of Indian River
1111 36th Street
Vero Beach 32960
(407)-569-1444

Lake County
Hospice of Lake & Sumter
12300 Lane Park Road
Tavares 32778-9660
(904) 383-0794
Serves: Lake, Sumter

Lee County
Hope Hospice
8290 College Parkway, #100
Fort Myers 33919
(813) 936-1157
Serves: Lee, Glades, Hendry

Leon County
Big Bend Hospice
1932 Miccosukee Rd
Tallahassee 32308-5308
(904) 878-5310
*Serves: Leon, Madison, Taylor, Franklin,
Jefferson, Gadsden, Liberty, Wakulla*

Marion County
Hospice of Marion County
P.O. Box 4860
Ocala 32678-4860
(904) 351-4610
JCAHO Accredited (February 1993)

Martin County
Hospice Of Martin
2300 S.E. Ocean Blvd.
Stuart 34996
(407) 287-7860

Monroe County
Hospice of the Florida Keys
724 Truman Ave
Key West 33041
(305) 294-8812

Okeechobee County
Hospice of Okeechobee
210 West North Park Street
Okeechobee 34973

Orange County
Hospice of Central Florida
Suite 300
2500 Maitland Center Parkway
Maitland 32751
(407)-647-2523
Serves: Orange, Osceola, Seminole

Osceola County
Hospice of Osceola County
419 Broadway
Kissimmee 32742

Palm Beach County
Hospice by the Sea
1531 W. Palmetto Park Rd.
Boca Raton 33486
(407)-395-5031
Serves: Broward, Palm Beach

Hospice of Palm Beach County
5300 East Ave
West Palm Beach 33407
(407)-848-5200

Pasco County
Central Gulfside Hospice
7716 Massachusetts Ave
New Port Richey 34653
(813) 845-5707

Hernando-Pasco Hospice
12107 Majestic Boulevard
Hundson 34667
Serves: Hernando and Pasco

Pinellas County
Hospice of the Florida Suncoast
300 East Bay Drive
Largo 34640
(813) 586-4432

Polk County
Good Shepherd Hospice of Mid-Florida
1201 1st Street South
Winter Haven 33883
(813) 293-6737

St. Lucie County
Hospice of the Treasure Coast
PO Box 1742
Fort Pierce 34954
(407)-461-4000

Sarasota County
Hospice of Southwest Florida
6055 Rand Boulevard
Sarasota 34238
(813) 923-5822

Seminole County
Hospice of the Comforter
841 Douglas Avenue, #101
Altamonte Springs 32714

Volusia County
Hospice of Volusia and Flagler
655 N. Clyde Morris Blvd.
Daytona Beach 32114
(904) 254-4237
Serves: Flagler and Volusia

HOME HEALTH CARE

Many persons with illnesses and disabilities can live at home, rather than in a nursing home or other residential facility, if they receive services from a home health agency.

Home health agencies develop care plans to meet the specific needs of individual patients. Some may need relatively minor assistance, while others may need more intensive services. Services range from skilled nursing care to help with shopping and other homemaker chores. In addition, home health agencies can relieve the strain and stress of caregiving by family and friends.

Three different types of agencies provide care to persons in their homes:

Homemaker agencies

These agencies do not employ nurses or other health care professionals and they are not licensed to provide health care services. Homemaker services include domestic maid services, companion or "sitter" services, and help with money management, home maintenance, shopping, chores, and preparing meals. Agencies that provide these services do not need a home health agency license unless they also provide home health services.

Home health agencies

Home health agencies provide health care services and employ nurses and other health care professionals. They provide care to persons who are recovering from surgery or other medical treatment, and to persons with either temporary or chronic medical problems. Frequently, home health care services can prevent or delay nursing home or other institutional care. In Florida, patients must have treatment plans prepared by a physician, and patient care plans prepared by registered nurses in cooperation with other health care professionals who are involved in providing care.

In Florida, there are two types of home health agencies-certified and not certified. Certified agencies may bill Medicare; non-certified agencies may not. However, the services provided by both types of agency are the same, and both must meet the same licensing standards. The Medicare program will pay for part-time intermittent nursing care to homebound people 65 or older and for certain disabled people. Medicare will not pay for full-time nursing care, for home delivered meals, or for homemaker services.

Some home health agencies provide technologically advanced health care services, such as treatment with infusion pumps and ventilators, home dialysis, I.V. therapy, and parenteral nutrition. Home health agencies are licensed to provide: nursing care; physical, occupational, or speech therapy; medical social services; nutritional and dietary guidance; home dialysis services, respiratory therapy, infusion therapy, and other therapies; certain medical supplies (such as drugs) prescribed by a physician; and home health aide services. Care is provided by registered nurses, licensed practical nurses, physical therapists, occupational therapists, speech therapists, medical social workers, and home health aids. Home health aides provide personal care services, such as help with eating, bathing, and toileting.

Nurse registries

Nurse registries refer nurses who "list" with the registry. Most nurses who list with registries provide care to elderly persons in their homes, although some work for hospitals and other health care facilities. Nurses who list with nurse registries typically work under contract, and bill clients directly for the services they provide. A change in Florida law allows nurse registries to provide the services of certified nursing assistants, homemakers, companions, and sitters.

In 1992, there were about 25 to 30 nurse registries in Florida. The cost of obtaining nursing services from nurse registries compared with home health agencies is estimated to be from 10 to 30 percent less than home health agencies since nurse registries have less overhead and therefore lower administrative costs. The services of nurse registries are not covered by Medicare.

Selecting a home health agency

Home health agencies are operated either on a profit-making or non-profit basis. Several large national companies operate home health agencies. Local non-profit agencies also provide home health services, and some use sliding fee scales that are based on income. In selecting a home health agency, physicians, hospital discharge planners, nurses, clergy, and local senior citizen organizations often are good sources of advice.

According to the Foundation for Hospice and Homecare, a national organization devoted to helping advance the quality of home care nationwide, better home care agencies will:

- Develop a plan based on individual health, social and financial needs;
- Provide only needed services; and
- Supervise all personnel who provide care or services in the home.

Both the federal General Accounting Office (GAO, October 1989) and Office of Technology Assessment (OTA, May 1992) have examined the provision of home drug infusion therapy. Drug infusion therapy intravenously releases drugs, such as antibiotics, anticancer drugs, and pain medications, slowly into the body. Both agencies concluded that quality standards are very important for this therapy. The GAO called for the development of specific training and experience requirements for personnel who perform home drug infusion therapy. OTA concluded that, "Drug infusion therapy can be provided safely and effectively at home, but only if patients are carefully selected and providers offer coordinated, high-quality care."

CONSIDERATIONS IN SELECTING A HOME HEALTH AGENCY

1. Selecting a Home Health Agency
—Is the agency affiliated with the better health care providers in the community? Which hospitals, nursing homes, physicians, and retirement homes refer patients to the agency?

—If drug infusion therapy or another high-technology medical service is needed, what are the qualifications (training and experience) of the personnel who provide this therapy?

—Does the agency provide written material that explains the services that are provided?

—If services are needed that the agency does not provide directly, does the agency make arrangements or refer persons to other providers that furnish the needed services?

—If care will be provided by home health aides, how often will a supervisor visit? Poor supervision of home health aides was found to be the principal cause of inadequate care in a 1987 study by the federal government.

—If home health aides are providing care, what is the extent of their training? Some are graduates of training programs conducted by vocational schools and hospitals. Others complete a minimum of forty hours of training that may be provided by a home health agency.

—Are all health care professionals licensed and bonded?

—Does the agency provide information that describes the fees and the insurance that is accepted?

—Are satisfactory procedures in place to handle complaints and problems?

—Is the agency licensed by the State of Florida?

—Does the agency have liability insurance? Florida law requires that home health agencies have liability insurance. The exact amount of liability insurance is established by administrative rule, but must be at least $250,000 per claim.

2. *Assessing the Quality of Home Health Care*

—Is the patient receiving the health care and other services that you need?

—Was a "plan of care" prepared by a physician within 48 hours after services began? Did the plan include diagnosis, permitted activities, dietary requirements, medication, treatment, required equipment, and other needed services.

—If the patient has been receiving home health services for more than 60 days, was the treatment plan reviewed by a physician? If the illness requires more frequent review, the treatment plan should be reviewed as required.

—Is the patient receiving adequate instruction in health care at home, including the operation of medical equipment?

—Does the patient receive a prompt response to requests for assistance?

—Is there a 24-hour telephone number to call when help is needed?

—Do the agency's health care professionals and home health aids have good work habits? Do they arrive on time? Are they courteous?

—Are patients given the Patient Bill of Rights and Responsibilities?

—Are the patients given information regarding the patient abuse toll-free telephone hotline as required by state law? If the patient has been abused, neglected, or exploited, call the Abuse Hotline at (800) 342-9152. All contact with the Hotline is confidential.

Sources of information on home health care

Two national organizations provide information on home health care.

National League for Nursing
350 Hudson Street
New York, New York 10014
(212) 989-9393

Foundation for Hospice and Home Care
519 C Street, N.E.
Washington, D.C. 20002
(202) 547-7424

Visiting Nurse Associations (VNAs) are nonprofit home health care providers. As of May 1993, there were VNA agencies in Jacksonville, Fort Myers, Key West, Miami, Orlando, Stuart, Vero Beach, West Palm Beach, and Wachula. The Visiting Nurse Associations of America has an information service and makes available a fact sheet about VNAs.

Visiting Nurse Associations of America
Suite 900
3801 East Florida
Denver, CO 80210
(800) 426-2547

Accredited home health agencies

Three national organizations accredit home health agencies and each will tell you if a particular agency is accredited by them. The accreditation organizations are:

Community Health Accreditation Program
(800) 669-1656

Joint Commission on Accreditation of Healthcare Organizations,
Customer Service Center
(708) 916-5800

National League for Nursing
American Public Health Association, Home Care
(212) 989-9393

Community Health Accreditation Program

The Community Health Accreditation Program (CHAP) is a subsidiary of the National League for Nursing and is devoted solely to accrediting organizations involved in home care. According to CHAP, the organization's purpose is, "To employ accreditation to elevate the quality of home care in this country and to counter public fears about a quality crisis in this increasingly crucial health care area." In September 1989, CHAP received a three-year $1.2 million dollar grant from the W.K. Kellogg Foundation to develop the first-ever outcome measures of patient care quality. Readers should consult the "Accreditation Organizations" section of Chapter 11 for additional information.

CHAP-Accredited Home Health Agencies
November 1992

Tri-County Home Health Care Services
210 North University Drive, Suite 200
Coral Springs, FL 33071
(800) 841-9374

Home Intensive Care of Florida
3375 NW 55th Street, Bldg. 12
Fort Lauderdale, FL 33309
(305) 486-2883

Home Intensive Care of Florida
445 Nova Road
Ormond Beach, FL 32176
(904) 672-9982

Home Intensive Care of Florida
6308 Benjamin Road, Suite 705
Tampa, FL 33634
(813) 884-8849

Visiting Nurse Assoc. of Palm Beach
560 Village Boulevard
West Palm Beach, FL 33409
(407) 689-7862

Joint Commission on Accreditation of Healthcare Organizations (JCAHO)

The following list of home health agencies includes those that were accredited by the JCAHO as of April, 1993. Twenty-three of the 130 home health agencies (18 percent) were accredited with commendation. Readers should consult the "Accreditation Organizations" section of Chapter 11 for additional information.

JCAHO-Accredited Home Health Agencies
April, 1993

Caremark, Inc.
380 South North Lake Boulevard,
    Suite 1032
Altamonte Springs, FL 32701
(407) 830-1505
Accreditation Codes: 1-3-9
Accredited With Commendation

Healthdyne Perinatal Services
222 South Westmonte Drive, Suite 206
Altamonte Springs, FL 32714-4269
(407) 862-6000
Accreditation Codes: 1-3-9

HealthInfusion
718 South North Lake Blvd, Suite 1020
Altamonte Springs, FL 32701
(407) 841-8888
Accreditation Codes: 1-3-9
Accredited With Commendation

Desoto Memorial Home Health Care
900 North Robert Avenue
Arcadia, FL 33821-2180
(813) 494-8401
Accreditation Codes: 1-6

Aldencare, Inc.
1225 Broken Sound Parkway, NW,
    Suite A
Boca Raton, FL 33487
(407) 994-8585
Accreditation Codes: 1-3-9

HealthInfusion, Inc.
902 Clint Moore Road, Suite 110
Boca Raton, FL 33487
(407) 241-7660
Accreditation Codes: 1-3-9
Accredited with Commendation

Bethesda Care
2815 South Seacrest Boulevard
Boynton Beach, FL 33435
(407) 737-7733
Accreditation Codes: 1-6
Accredited with Commendation

Pharmacy Corporation of America
2102 Corporate Drive
Boynton Beach, FL 33426
(407) 736-4400
Accreditation Codes: 1-3-9

Florida Home Health Services Manasota
1111 Third Avenue West
Bradenton, FL 34205
(813) 746-5111
Accreditation Codes: 1-6

HCA Blake Home Health
1886 59th Street West
Bradenton FL 34209
(813) 798-6111
Accreditation Codes: 1-6
Accredited with Commendation

Memorial Hospital—Flagler
Star Route 1, Box 2
Bunnell, FL 32110
(904) 437-2211
Accreditation Codes: 1

Cape Coral Hospital Home Health
636 Del Prado Boulevard
Cape Coral FL 33990
(813) 574-2323
Accreditation Codes: 1-6

Northwest Florida Community Hospital
PO Box K
Chipley, FL 32428
(904) 638-1610
Accreditation Codes: 1-6

Independent HH Services
1020 Lakeview Road
Clearwater, FL 34616
(813) 462-7000
Accreditation Codes: 1-6

Lincare Inc.
19337 U.S. 19, North, Suite 400
Clearwater, FL 34624
(813) 530-7800
Accreditation Codes: 4

Mercury Medical
11300A 49th Street North
Clearwater, FL 34622-4800
(813) 573-0088
Accreditation Codes: 1-3-4

Olsten Healthcare
220 South Ridgewood Avenue
Daytona Beach FL 32114
Accreditation Codes: 1-6-7

NMC Homecare
664A South Military Trail
Deerfield Beach, FL 33442
(305) 427-7200
Accreditation Codes: 1-3-9

Waterman Medical Center—HHA
1 West Park Avenue
Eustis, FL 32727
(904) 589-3333
Accreditation Codes: 1-6

Curaflex Infusion Services
3330 Northwest 53rd Street
Fort Lauderdale, FL 33309
(305) 486-0636
Accreditation Codes: 1-3-9

H.M.S.S. of Texas, Inc.
1770 NW 64th Street, Suite 620
Fort Lauderdale, FL 33309
(305) 351-0880
Accreditation Codes: 1-3-9

Home Nutritional Services, Inc.
5249 NW 33rd Ave, Building #6
Fort Lauderdale, FL 33309
(305) 735-5080
Accreditation Codes: 1-3-9
Accredited with Commendation

Homecare Medical Associates, Inc.
6001 Northwest 29th Avenue, Suite B
Fort Lauderdale, FL 33309
(305) 971-6404
Accreditation Codes: 4

Kimberly Quality Care
3201 West Commercial Blvd, Suite 102
Fort Lauderdale, FL 33309
(305) 733-2222
Accreditation Codes: 1-3-4-6-7

Sunrise Systems
10401 Northwest 53rd Street
Fort Lauderdale, FL 33351
(305) 748-5533
Accreditation Codes: 1-3-4

Florida Home Health Services/Home Care
2776 Cleveland Ave.
Fort Myers, FL 33901
(813) 332-1111
Accreditation Codes: 1-4-6-7

United Health Care Services, Inc.
3805 Fowler Street, Suite 3
Fort Myers, FL 33901
(813) 936-1800
Accreditation Codes: 5

Gresham Healthcare
916 Northwest 66th Street
Gainesville FL 32605
(904) 331-1112
Accreditation Codes: 5

SantaFe Homecare
816 Southwest Fourth Avenue
Gainesville, FL 32601
(904) 372-4321
Accreditation Codes: 1-6

Shands Homecare
1600 Southwest Archer Road
Gainesville, FL 32610
(904) 395-0141
Accreditation Codes: 1

Caremark, Inc.
3011 Greene Street
Hollywood, FL 33020
(305) 921-6011
Accreditation Codes: 1-3-9

Bayonet Point Oxygen Services
13910 Fivay Road, Number 17
Hudson, FL 34667
(813) 862-4644
Accreditation Codes: 5

Citrus Memorial Home Health
502 Highland Boulevard
Inverness, FL 32652
(904) 726-1551
Accreditation Codes: 1

Lake City, FL 32056
(904) 755-3200
Accreditation Codes: 1-6

Palm Home Care
1005 Tenth Street
Lake Park, FL 33403
(407) 844-5336
Accreditation Codes: 5
Accredited with Commendation

State Oxygen Servs Home Med Equip
4830 Highway 92 East
Lakeland, FL 33801
(813) 956-3525
Accreditation Codes: 4

CompCare of, Florida, Inc.
3779 Northwest 16th Street
Lauderhill, FL 33311
(305) 583-0587
Accreditation Codes: 5

Home Health Corporation Of America
3172 N Andrews Ave Extension
Pompano Beach, FL 33064
(305) 971-9888
Accreditation Codes: 1-3-4-6

LRMC Home Health Services, Inc
734 North Third Street, Suite 310
Leesburg, FL 34748
(904) 365-4505
Accreditation Codes: 1-2-6

NMC Homecare
976, Florida Central Parkway, Suite 112
Longwood, FL 32750
(407) 339-8648
Accreditation Codes: 1-3-9

Pharmacy Corporation of America
735 West Highway 434, Suite A
Longwood, FL 32750
(407) 767-9010
Accreditation Codes: 1-3-4

Olsten Healthcare
PO Box 2607
Maitland,, FL 32751
(407) 661-1116
Accreditation Codes: 1-6-7

Abbey Home Healthcare
274 North Wickham
Melbourne, FL 32935
(407) 533-0400
Accreditation Codes: 4

Baptist Hospital of Miami Home Health
8900 North Kendall Drive
Miami, FL 33176-2197
(305) 596-1960
Accreditation Codes: 1-3-4

Bay Shore Home Health, Inc.
1100 Northwest 95th Street
Miami, FL 33150
(305) 835-6000
Accreditation Codes: 1-6-9

Complete Care Home Health Agency
9495 Sunset Drive Suite B-280
Miami, FL 33173
(305) 693-6100
Accreditation Codes: 1-2-6

Florida Home Health Services, Inc.
1321 Northwest 14th Street
Miami, FL 33136
(305) 325-4515
Accreditation Codes: 1-6

HealthInfusion, Inc.
1921 NW 82nd Avenue
Miami, FL 33126
(305) 592-1177
Accreditation Codes: 1-3-9
Accredited with Commendation

Mercy Hospital Home Health Dept
3663 South Miami Avenue
Miami, FL 33133
(305) 854-4400
Accreditation Codes: 1-6

Option Care Home Pharmacy, Inc
8323 NW 12th St, Suite 109
Miami, FL 33126
(305) 594-9000
Accreditation Codes: 1-3-9

Pan American Home Health Services
815 NW 57th Avenue, Suite 120
Miami, FL 33126
(305) 267-1515
Accreditation Codes: 1-3-6

Professional Oxygen Service
7280 Northwest 58th Street
Miami, FL 33166
(305) 592-5920
Accreditation Codes: 5

Roche Prof Service Cntrs of Miami
1000 Park Ctr. Blvd., Suite 128
Miami, FL 33169
(305) 628-4316
Accreditation Codes: 1-3-9
Accredited with Commendation

South Miami Hospital Home Care
6250 Sunset Drive
Miami, FL 33143
(305) 661-4611
Accreditation Codes: 1-2-4-6-7

Vamedical Center
1201 Northwest 16th Street
Miami, FL 33125
(305) 324-4455
Accreditation Codes: 1-2-4

Tokos Medical Corporation
8000 Governors Square Boulevard,
   Suite 300
Miami Lakes, FL 33016
(305) 557-2220
Accreditation Codes: 1-3-9

Critical Care America
10102 USAToday Way, Suite 101
Miramar, FL 33025
(305) 436-0400
Accreditation Codes: 1-3-9
Accredited with Commendation

Community Home Services, Inc.
851 Fifth Avenue North
Naples, FL 33940
(813) 263-7113
Accreditation Codes: 1-6
Accredited with Commendation

Option Care of Southwest Florida
3666 Tamiami Trail, North Suite 201
Naples, FL 33940
(813) 261-6353
Accreditation Codes: 1-3-9

Olsten Healthcare
660 Ninth Street North
Naples, FL 33940
(813) 649-7078
Accreditation Codes: 1-6-7

Fish Memorial Hospital Home Health
401 Palmetto Street
New Smyrna Beach, FL 32168
(904) 427-3401
Accreditation Codes: 1-6

Central Florida Home Therapeutics
345 West Michigan Street, Suite 104
Orlando, FL 32806
(407) 648-5408
Accreditation Codes: 1-3-9
Accredited with Commendation

Colonial Medical Supplies
915 South Orange Avenue
Orlando, FL 32806
(407) 849-6455
Accreditation Codes: 5

Florida Hospital Home Care Services
2608 North Orange Avenue Suite 102
Orlando, FL 32804-7604
(407) 897-1646
Accreditation Codes: 1-6

Healthcare Equipment And Supplies
2404 North Orange Avenue
Orlando, FL 32804
(407) 898-6004
Accreditation Codes: 4

The Hug Center
1200 Fairbanks
Orlando, FL 32804
(407) 298-8810
Accreditation Codes: 1-3-4
Accredited with Commendation

Medical Options, Inc
2116 South Orange Avenue
Orlando, FL 32806
(407) 841-9999
Accreditation Codes: 4

Orlando Regional Home Health
601 West Michigan Avenue
Orlando, FL 32805
(407) 841-5111
Accreditation Codes: 1-2-6-9

West Medical
2321 Silver Star Road
Orlando, FL 32804
(407) 297-0100
Accreditation Codes: 5

East Coast Option Care
593 South Yonge Street
Ormond Beach, FL 32174
(904) 673-4511
Accreditation Codes: 1-3-9

Interim Health Care of Palm Beach
50 Cocoanut Row, Suite 120
Palm Beach, FL 33480
(407) 655-8622
Accreditation Codes: 1-6-7

High Tech Home Health, Inc.
10800 North Military Trail, Suite 106
Palm Beach Gardens, FL 33410
(407) 624-0606
Accreditation Codes: 1-4-6

Bay Medical Center Home Health Care
615 North Bonita Avenue
PO Box 2515
Panama City, FL 32401
(904) 769-1511
Accreditation Codes: 1-6

West, Florida Home Health Care
PO Box 109
Panama City, FL 32402-0591
(904) 769-5688
Accreditation Codes: 1-4

American Home Patient Centers, Inc.
2114 Airport Boulevard, Suite 1000
Pensacola, FL 32504
(904) 478-4822
Accreditation Codes: 1-3-4

Home Health Care of Pensacola, Inc.
1717 North E Street, Suite 422
Pensacola, FL 32501
(904) 434-4559
Accreditation Codes: 1-3-4-6-7

Northwest, Florida Home Health Agency
4700 Bayou Boulevard, Suite 4A
Pensacola, FL 32503
(904) 477-5800
Accreditation Codes: 1-6

Pfeiffer Home Health Care of Pensacola
715 North "S" Street
Pensacola, FL 32505
(904) 432-2405
Accreditation Codes: 5

Pharmathera Home Health Agency
826 Creighton Road, Suite A102
Pensacola, FL 32504
(904) 484-2844
Accreditation Codes: 1-3-9

Women's Intervention Srvs Lakeview
  Cntr
1221 West Lakeview Avenue
Pensacola, FL 32501
(904) 432-1222
Accreditation Codes: 1-6

South Fla Baptist Hospital Home Health
301 North Alexander Street
Plant City, FL 33566
(813) 757-1200
Accreditation Codes: 1-6

Gold Coast Home Health Services
911 East Atlantic Boulevard, Suite 200
Pompano Beach, FL 33060
(305) 786-6950
Accreditation Codes: 1-3-6

Primedica Home Health
3600 Essential Park Blvd, Suite 3670
Pompano Beach, FL 33064-2209
(305) 968-6897
Accredited with Commendation

Olsten Healthcare
949 Tamiami Trail
Port Charlotte, FL 33953
(813) 629-4066
Accreditation Codes: 1

Brevard Homecare
PO Box 5002
Rockledge, FL 32956-5002
(407) 636-2211
Accreditation Codes: 1-6-7

Doctors Home Health Service
1217 East Avenue South, Suite 201
Sarasota, FL 34239
(813) 366-1411
Accreditation Codes: 1-6

Florida Home Health Care
6075 Rand Boulevard
Sarasota, FL 34238
(813) 955-1111
Accreditation Codes: 1-6

Sarasota Home Therapeutics
7220 Beneva Road South
Sarasota, FL 34238
(813) 924-9596
Accreditation Codes: 1-3-9

Community Home Health Care
400 Health Park Boulevard
St. Augustine, FL 32086
(904) 829-5155
Accreditation Codes: 1-6

HealthInfusion, Inc.
9505 International Ct, North
St. Petersburg, FL 33716
(813) 228-0044
Accreditation Codes: 1-3-9
Accredited with Commendation

Kimberly Quality Care
10901-A Roosevelt, Building A, Suite 500
St. Petersburg, FL 33716
(813) 579-9847
Accreditation Codes: 1-3-7-6-9

NMC Homecare/Infusion Care
10901 Roosevelt Boulevard
St. Petersburg, FL 33716
(813) 576-7070
Accreditation Codes: 1-3-9

St. Anthony's Home Health Services
1600 Ninth Street North
St. Petersburg, FL 33704
(813) 825-1100
Accreditation Codes: 1-6-7

Visiting Nurse Assoc Martin/St. Lucie
633 East Fifth Street
Stuart, FL 34994
(407) 286-1844
Accreditation Codes: 1-6

Enteral and Parenteral Support Services
8322 West Oakland Park Boulevard
Sunrise, FL 33351
(305) 741-1111
Accreditation Codes: 1-3-4-6

Lincare
2522 Capital Circle Northeast at Canopy
   Lane, Suite 6
Tallahassee, FL 32308
(904) 385-6594
Accreditation Codes: 4

Tallahassee Memorial Home Hlth Care
1617-1619 Physicians Drive
Tallahassee, FL 32308
(904) 942-7222
Accreditation Codes: 1-6

American Homepatient
6313 Benjamin Road, Suite 106
Tampa, FL 33614
(813) 885-9578
Accreditation Codes: 1-3-4

Caremark
6301 Benjamin Road, Suite 105
Tampa, FL 33634
(813) 884-6987
Accreditation Codes: 3
Accredited with Commendation

Critical Care America
8509-A Benjamin Road
Tampa, FL 33634-1224
(813) 888-7545
Accreditation Codes: 1-3-9

Excellence, Inc.
3001 North Rocky Point Road East
   Suite 350
Tampa, FL 33607
(813) 289-6565
Accreditation Codes: 1-3-9

HMSS, Inc.
5670 West Cypress Street, Suite D
Tampa, FL 33607
(813) 289-6364
Accreditation Codes: 1-3-9

Home Nutritional Services, Inc
5402 Beaumont Center Blvd, Suite 114
Tampa, FL 33634
(813) 882-0083
Accreditation Codes: 1-3-9

Interim Healthcare, Inc.
4730 North Habanna, Suite 101
Tampa, FL 33614-7114
(813) 877-9444
Accreditation Codes: 1-3-4-6-7
Accredited with Commendation

Payors Home Care Systems Inc.
6103 Johns Road, Suite 1
Tampa, FL 33634-4412
(813) 885-1312
Accreditation Codes: 1-3-9

Pharmacy Corporation Of America
3925 Coconut Palm Drive, Suite 115
Tampa, FL 33619
(813) 623-3521
Accreditation Codes: 3

Roche Professional Service Centers
6408 North Armenia Avenue
Tampa, FL 33604
(813) 933-5862
Accreditation Codes: 3

St. Joseph's Hospital
PO Box 4227
Tampa, FL 33677-4227
(813) 870-4020
Accreditation Codes: 1-4-6

Tokos Medical Corporation
3109 West Buffalo Avenue, Suite 80
Tampa, FL 33607
(813) 878-2593
Accreditation Codes: 1-3-4

University Community Hosp Home
   Health
3100 East, Fletcher Avenue
Tampa, FL 33613
(813) 979-7326
Accreditation Codes: 1-6

Lincare, Inc.
48 Royal Palm Boulevard
Vero Beach, FL 32960
(813) 576-1231
Accreditation Codes: 4

Nurse's House Call
3975 20th Street, Suite D
Vero Beach, FL 32960
(407) 562-0215
Accreditation Codes: 1-6-7

Visiting Nurse Assoc Treasure Coast
1111 36th Street
Vero Beach, FL 32960
(407) 567-5551
Accreditation Codes: 1-6
Accredited with Commendation

Signature Home Care Services
Oakwood Square, 1950 Dairy Road
West Melbourne, FL 32904
(407) 723-4044
Accreditation Codes: 1-3-4-6

Hospicare
5300 East Avenue
West Palm Beach, FL 33407
(407) 844-0405
Accreditation Codes: 1-6
Accredited with Commendation

St. Mary's Hospital Home Health Agency
901 45th Street
West Palm Beach, FL 33407-2495
(407) 881-2865
Accreditation Codes: 1-6

U.S. Homecare Certified Corp of S. Fla
701 Northpoint Parkway, Suite 515
West Palm Beach, FL 33407
(407) 687-2442
Accreditation Codes: 1

Mid-Florida Home Health Services, Inc.
1201 First Street South
Winter Haven, FL 33881
(813) 297-1871
Accreditation Codes: 1-6

Infusion Therapies, Inc
450 North Lakemont Avenue, Suite 2000
Winter Park, FL 32792
(407) 678-3381
Accreditation Codes: 1-3-9

Winter Park Home Health Care
200 North Lakemont Avenue
Winter Park, FL 32792
(305) 646-7495
Accreditation Codes: 1-6

National Medicare Equipment Centers
90 First Street, Southeast
Winter Haven, FL 33880
(813) 294-7534
Accreditation Codes: 4

ACCREDITATION CODES:

1 Home Health Care Services

3 Pharmaceutical Services

4 Home Equipment Management

5 Home Equipment Management,
   Respiratory

6 Personal Care Services

7 Support Services

9 Durable Medical Equipment,
   100% Infusion

Source: JCAHO.

CHAPTER 7
Mental health and substance abuse treatment

As in other areas of medicine, a revolution is occurring in psychiatry. An article that reviewed the recent literature on psychiatry states that psychiatry has "shifted from a model of psychiatric disorders based on maladaptive psychological process to one based on medical diseases" (Michels and Marzuk 1993). Researchers are concentrating on the brain, rather than the mind, to learn the medical basis of disorders. Genetics has been found to be a factor in several major psychiatric disorders, and researchers are increasingly investigating biochemical and other medical factors. Some believe that by the end of the decade neuroscience will better identify the genetic basis of many disorders, and this will lead to new treatments.

Although studies have found that a large numbers of adults need mental health treatment, relatively few receive it. The largest and most detailed national study of mental health problems found that only 28.5 percent of persons with a mental health or substance abuse disorder received help over a 12-month period. Persons with severe disorders were found to be more likely to seek and receive help than persons with disorders that were not severe. The study found that 14.5 percent of the population nationwide uses outpatient mental health services in a 12-month period.

There are many treatment options for persons with mental health problems, including outpatient programs and self-help organizations. Mental health experts believe that treatment on an outpatient basis is appropriate for the vast majority of persons with health problems. A prestigious national study estimated that approximately 95 percent of all persons with psychiatric and substance abuse problems can be treated as outpatients.

PREVALENCE OF MENTAL DISORDERS

Sizeable proportions of adults experience mental disorders and abuse alcohol and drugs. To estimate prevalence rates of mental disorders and alcohol and drug abuse, the National Institute of Mental Health (NIMH) sponsored an Epidemiologic Catchment Area (ECA) study that interviewed 18,571 persons age 18 and older between 1980 and 1984 in New Haven, Connecticut, Baltimore, Maryland, St. Louis, Missouri, Durham, North Carolina, and Los Angeles, California (Regier et al. 1988). Disorders were classified according to the NIMH's Diagnostic Interview Schedule.

The authors state that the study, "may provide more confident projections to the nation than could be made previously." A major objective was to provide the "best estimates" of prevalence rates for the United States for mental and substance abuse disorders.

The study found that at any time during a one-month time frame, 15.4 percent of adults (14 percent of males and 16.6 percent of females) experience symptoms of a mental or substance disorder. The most common mental health disorders are anxiety disorders (phobias, panic, and obsessive-compulsive disorders) and affective disorders (depression, manic-depression, and dysthymia).

The following table from the Regier study, which includes six-month and lifetime prevalence rates that were reported in earlier NIMH Epidemiologic Catchment Area studies, shows that the overall one-month prevalence rate of 15.4 percent for any mental disorder increases to 19.1 percent during a six-month period and to 32.2 percent over a lifetime.

Estimates on Prevalence Rates of
Mental Disorders in Adult Population
Disorders per 100 Persons

Condition	1 month	6 months	Lifetime
Any Disorder	15.4	19.1	32.2
Any except substance abuse	12.6	14.8	22.1
Any except phobia	11.2	14.0	25.2
Substance abuse	3.8	6.0	16.4
Alcohol abuse	2.8	4.7	13.3
Drug abuse	1.3	2.0	5.9
Schizophrenia	0.6	0.8	1.3
Affective disorders	5.1	5.8	8.3
Manic episode	0.4	0.5	0.8
Major depression	2.2	3.0	5.8
Dysthymia*	3.3	3.3	3.3
Anxiety Disorders	7.3	8.9	14.6
Phobia	6.2	7.7	12.5
Panic	0.5	0.8	1.6
Obsessive-compulsive	1.3	1.5	2.5
Antisocial personality	0.5	0.8	2.5
Severe Cognitive Impairment*	1.3	1.3	1.3

*The authors note that cognitive impairment was assessed only when study participants were interviewed and that dysthymia was determined as a lifetime disorder because diagnosis requires a two-year duration of symptoms.

Source: Regier et al. "One-Month Prevalence of Mental Disorders in the United States." *Archives of General Psychiatry*, Vol. 45, p. 981 (November, 1988). Reprinted by permission of the American Medical Association, Copyright 1988.

The Regier study also derived estimates of one-month prevalence rates of mental disorders for adult men and women by age group. The study found that:
- Alcohol and drug abuse is most common in younger age groups. Men have much higher monthly prevalence rates of substance abuse than women; between the ages of 18 and 24, 9.3 percent of men and 4.5 percent of women have a substance abuse disorder. Between age 25 and 44, substance abuse disorders decline only slightly for men, to 7.9 percent; for women, the decline is steep, to 1.8 percent.
- The monthly prevalence rate for women for both affective and anxiety disorders is about twice that for men, with 6.6 percent of women and 3.5 percent of men reporting affective disorders, and 9.7 percent of women and 4.7 percent of men reporting anxiety disorders.

A 1993 study by Regier found that relatively few persons with mental disorders receive help over the course of a given year (Regier et al. 1993). Regier determined that only 28.5 percent of persons with any disorder received some professional or voluntary help for mental health or substance abuse problems. Those with severe disorders such as somatization, schizophrenia, and bipolar disorders were more likely to seek help than persons with addictive disorders or those with severe cognitive impairment. Regier found that 23.6 percent of those with addictive disorders and 45.7 percent of those with affective disorders received treatment. In addition, Regier found that:

- 14.5 percent of the population nationwide used outpatient mental health services over a 12-month period and some received help in more than one setting;
- 6.4 percent received outpatient help from general medical practitioners;
- 5.6 percent received outpatient help from speciality mental health and addiction providers;
- 3 percent received outpatient help from human services professionals; and,
- Less than 1 percent received inpatient care.

Regier and his colleagues are continuing to analyze the ECA survey data to identify the characteristics of people who most need treatment for mental disorders. In addition, the survey data will be analyzed to determine the average duration and chances for recurrence of specific disorders (Bower 1993).

**Estimates on Monthly Prevalence Rates of
Mental Disorders in Adult Population
Disorders per 100 Persons**

	Any disorder	*Alcohol abuse*	*Drug abuse*	*Affective disorder*	*Anxiety disorder*
Men					
All ages	14.0	5.0	1.8	3.5	4.7
18–24	16.5	6.0	4.8	3.4	4.9
25–44	15.4	6.2	2.3	4.5	4.7
45–64	11.9	4.0	0.1	3.1	5.1
65+	10.5	1.8	0.0	1.4	3.6
Women					
All ages	16.6	0.9	0.7	6.6	9.7
18–24	17.3	2.3	2.4	5.3	10.4
25–44	19.2	1.1	0.8	8.2	11.7
45–64	14.6	0.3	0.0	7.2	8.0
65+	13.6	0.3	0.0	3.3	6.8

Source: Regier et al. "One-Month Prevalence of Mental Disorders in the United States." *Archives of General Psychiatry*, vol. 45, p. 982–983 (November 1988). Reprinted by permission of the American Medical Association, Copyright 1988.

TREATMENT METHODS

There is a consensus of opinion in the research literature that mental health services should be provided in the least restrictive setting appropriate to the treatment needs of the patient. Outpatient care is the least restrictive setting; hospitalization is the most restrictive. A national study estimated that about 95 percent of all persons with psychiatric and substance abuse problems can be treated as outpatients (Graduate Medical Education National Advisory Committee 1981).

There are three basic approaches to treatment that may help a person overcome mental health problems-biomedical therapy, behavioral therapy, and psychotherapy. There are, however, many specific types of therapies that may be used alone or in various combinations.

Treatment may have one or more goals. According to the National Institute of Mental Health (NIMH 1987), these goals include reducing symptoms of emotional disorders, improving personal and social functioning, correcting distorted thinking, developing and strengthening coping skills, and promoting behavior that makes a person's life better.

Sometimes therapy for mental and emotional problems works, sometimes it doesn't. Success depends on the patient and the therapist. According to the NIMH, it is important for patients to share concerns in a serious, sincere, and open manner. There are times when a patient may not "click" with a particular therapist or therapy. If this should happen, it is best to find a different therapist. Each therapist has particular therapies that he or she specializes in.

Biomedical therapies

According to the NIMH, many persons have benefited from drug treatment for emotional, behavioral, and mental disorders. Drug treatment often is combined with psychotherapy.

Behavioral therapy

This therapy uses learning principles to systematically change troublesome thinking patterns and behaviors. Specific skills are learned to obtain rewards and satisfaction. This therapy may involve the cooperation of important persons in the patient's life, and a range of methods such as stress management, biofeedback, and relaxation training.

Psychotherapy

In psychotherapy, a therapist helps the patient discuss and resolve troubling personal problems. Psychotherapy can be short or long-term. According to the NIMH, the goal of the therapist is to help the patient resolve his or her problem as quickly as possible. Problems that result from a stressful life event such as a death in the family, divorce, or physical illness, are handled in short-term psychotherapy. The study of underlying problems that started in childhood are handled in long-term psychotherapy.

The following descriptions of the principal types of psychotherapy has been published by the NIMH.

- Psychoanalysis is a long-term therapy that emphasizes how the patient's unconscious motivations and early patterns of resolving issues are important influences in his or her current actions and feelings.
- Psychodynamic psychotherapy examines important relationships and experiences from early childhood to the present. The purpose is to analyze and change unsettling or destructive behaviors, and to resolve emotional problems.
- Cognitive therapy seeks to identify and correct distorted thinking patterns that can lead to troublesome feelings and behaviors.
- Family therapy involves discussions and problem-solving sessions with every member of a family, either as a group or individual..
- Couple therapy aims to develop a rewarding relationship and minimize problems through understanding how individual conflicts are expressed in a couple's interactions.
- Group therapy involves a small group of people who, with the guidance of a therapist, discuss individual issues and help each other with problems.

- Play therapy is a technique used for establishing communication and resolving problems with young children.

ALZHEIMER'S DISEASE

The most common cause for memory disorder in old age is Alzheimer's disease. The disease was identified by Alois Alzheimer, a German physician, in the early 1900s. Alzheimer's disease is a type of dementia in which brain cells die prematurely. The result is progressive memory impairment and intellectual decline. Dementia is not a result of normal aging and the cause of Alzheimer's is not yet known, although there are many theories. Scientists believe that some people with a particular gene may develop Alzheimer's. At present, there is no cure.

Studies have found different prevalence rates of Alzheimer's in the elderly. These may be due to population differences or may stem from the difficulty of diagnosing Alzheimer's (Larson 1993). Studies do agree, however, that the incidence of Alzheimer's increases with age. Prevalence is particularly high among those 85 years of age and older. Two recent studies, one in the US and one in Sweden, examined the prevalence of Alzheimer's. The US study, published in the *Journal of the American Medical Association* (Evans et al. 1989) found that the prevalence rates for persons with probable Alzheimer's disease increase sharply with age from 3 percent for persons 65 to 74 years of age, to 18.7 percent for persons age 75 to 84, to 47.2 percent for persons 85 years of age or older. The study examined a sample of 467 non-institutionalized persons living in East Boston, Massachusetts. The Swedish study, published in the *New England Journal of Medicine* (Skoog et al. 1993) examined 147 85 year olds. That study found that the prevalence rate for all dementia was 29.8 percent. Just over 8 percent had mild cases of dementia, 10.3 percent had moderate cases, and 11.1 percent had severe cases. The prevalence rate for Alzheimer's was 12.9 percent. Of those with dementia, 43.5 percent had Alzheimer's, 46.9 percent had vascular dementia, and 9.5 percent had dementia from other causes.

Besides Alzheimer's, there are other causes of memory loss in elderly persons, some of which are reversible. The only way to be certain of an Alzheimer's diagnosis is to conduct a brain autopsy at the time of death to determine whether there are amyloid plaque deposits. It is important to correctly diagnose Alzheimer's because confused behavior may result from stress, depression, or from other causes that are treatable and reversible. According to the University of South Florida Suncoast Gerontology Center, a complete medical, neurological, and psycho-social evaluation, including either a CT scan or a Magnetic Resonance Imaging (MRI) scan, is necessary to rule out other causes of memory loss and to render a "probable" diagnosis of Alzheimer's. "Probable" diagnoses of Alzheimer's are usually 85 percent to 90 percent accurate.

Although Alzheimer's cannot be cured, medications can be prescribed to treat symptoms of depression, anxiety, agitation, and hostility. Family members should receive counseling and instruction regarding how to care for Alzheimer's patients. The most important components of care are symptom management, family involvement and environmental adaption.

During the early stages of the disease, patients generally can live at home with family support. Although Alzheimer's affects patients differently, those at the latter stages of the disease may experience severe personality changes, develop eating and sleeping disorders, and be profoundly disoriented. Patients with advanced Alzheimer's require assistance in almost all activities of daily living activities. Some nursing homes have special facilities or programs for Alzheimer's patients. The Suncoast Gerontology Center offers a directory of facilities that offer specialized care to Alzheimer's patients.

This directory is discussed later in this chapter. In addition, local Florida chapters of the Alzheimer's Disease and Related Disorder Association can be contacted for information and referrals.

Memory disorder clinics

Florida has five clinics that have been established by the Florida Legislature under the Alzheimer's Disease Initiative. All are affiliated with medical schools. The clinics have staff specially trained in the diagnosis and treatment of patients with memory problems and provide ongoing management to patients with memory problems. They are also consult physicians, and provide information and counseling. Medicare and supplemental insurance covers most of the cost of diagnostic evaluations for elderly persons. The clinics are:

University of South Florida Memory
  Disorder Clinic
Suncoast Gerontology Center
USF Div. of Geriatric Medicine and USF
  Department of Neurology
Tampa, Fl
(813) 974-3100

J.H. Miller Health Center
University of Florida
Department of Neurology
Gainesville, Fl 32610
(904) 291-3491

Memory Disorder Clinic
University of Miami School of Medicine
1500 NW 12 Avenue, Suite 1103
Miami, Fl 33136
(305) 547-5883

Wien Center for Alzheimer's Disease
  and Memory Disorders
Mount Sinai Medical Center
4300 Alton Road
Miami Beach, Fl 33140
(305) 674-2543

East Central Florida Memory Disorder
  Clinic
1322 S Oak Street
Melbourne, Fl 32901-3111
(407) 768-9575

Suncoast Gerontology Center

The Suncoast Gerontology Center in Tampa provides comprehensive information and assistance regarding Alzheimer's disease. This nationally recognized center offers a variety of services:
- Memory disorder clinic;
- National Resource Center on Alzheimer's Disease. This center is one of six in the nation that is funded by the federal government to conduct research and provide training, technical assistance, and information to regional, state, and local agencies to develop programs for Alzheimer's patients and their caregivers;
- Geriatric Education Center to train faculty and practitioners in geriatrics and gerontology;
- Publications and videotapes on Alzheimer's disease, including a *Statewide Community Resource Directory* which lists Alzheimer's disease evaluation and research clinics, adult day care and in-home respite care programs, adult congregate living facilities, dementia-specific nursing home care units, family support groups, Alzheimer's Association chapters, and other Alzheimer's disease resource directors and information clearinghouses; and,
- A resource library, a quarterly newsletter, and a toll-free telephone line for information on Alzheimer's.

Suncoast Gerontology Center
University of South Florida Health Sciences Center
MDC 50
12901 Bruce B. Downs Blvd.
Tampa, Florida 33612

Suncoast Alzheimer's Information Line
(800) 633-4563

The Florida brain bank program

The Florida Brain Bank Program is engaged in scientific research to learn how to prevent and treat Alzheimer's. The program conducts brain autopsies at the time of death to examine the brains of individuals with Alzheimer's. Participation in this program helps advance science and, in the future may help other individuals with Alzheimer's in the future. The program is supported by the State of Florida and by Florida's medical schools. To obtain information regarding the Florida Brain Bank Program, contact the Mount Sinai Medical Center in Miami, the University of Florida in Gainesville, the University of Miami, or the University of South Florida in Tampa.

Other sources of information on Alzheimer's disease

The Alzheimer's Disease and Related Disorders Association (ADRDA) is a national organization, with more than 200 local chapters, that promotes education and research for health care professionals and families of persons with Alzheimer's. The association offers a wide range of publications on Alzheimer's disease, including publications for caregivers. In addition, the association publishes a quarterly newsletter for 700,000 readers nationwide and operates a toll-free referral help line. The help line provides information on Alzheimer's, including information for caregivers, and makes referrals to local chapters for help in locating physicians, nursing homes, adult congregate living facilities, and other facilities and providers that care for persons with Alzheimer's. For information contact:

Alzheimer's Disease and Related Disorders Association
919 North Michigan Avenue, Suite 1000
Chicago, Illinois 60601-1676
(800) 272-3900 or (312) 335-8700

The Alzheimer's Disease Education and Referral Center is a service of the National Institute on Aging. The Center can be contacted to ask questions about Alzheimer's Disease, to learn about clinical trials sponsored by the National Institute on Aging; and to order free publications, such as the "Progress Report on Alzheimer's Disease: Discoveries in Health for Aging Americans." The Alzheimer's Disease Education and Referral Center can be reached at:

Alzheimer's Disease Education and Referral Center
P.O. Box 8250
Silver Spring, MD 20907-8250
(800) 438-4380

Florida chapters of the Alzheimer's Disease and Related Disorder Association

The Alzheimer's Disease and Related Disorders Association has 15 chartered local chapters in Florida that can be contacted to obtain information on local adult day care centers, nursing homes, adult congregate living facilities, and other providers. Adult day care centers, many of which have special programs for Alzheimer's patients, provide custodial care to adults during the day. Florida law authorizes adult day care centers to provide "....a protective setting, social activities, leisure-time activities, self-care training, rest, nutritional services, and, when possible, speech and physical therapy."

In addition to providing help with referrals, local chapters also offer a range of informational and supportive services. Florida's local chapters are:

Broward County Chapter
8333 McNab Road, Suite 203
Tamarac, FL 33321
(305) 726-0002

Charlotte and Desoto Counties Chapter
118 Sullivan St.
Punta Gorda, FL 33950
(813) 624-5727

East Central FL Chapter
1250 South Harbor City Blvd., Suite 7
Melbourne, FL 32901
(407) 729-8536

Greater Miami Chapter
1133 Kane Concourse
Bay Harbor Islands, FL 33154
(305) 864-5866

Greater Orlando Chapter
PO Box 3107
Orlando, FL 32802-3107
(407) 422-9595

Greater Palm Beach Chapter
3200 North Federal Highway, Suite 226
Boca Raton, FL 33431
(407) 392-1363

Highlands County Chapter
74 Hickory Hills Circle
Lake Placid, FL 33852
(813) 465-7266

Manatee/Sarasota Chapter
Happiness House
350 Braden Avenue
Sarasota, FL 34243
(813) 355-7637

North Central Florida Chapter
502 N.W. 75th Street
Gainesville, FL 32607-1799
(904) 372-6266

Northeastern Florida Chapter
2131 Mango Place
Jacksonville, FL 32207
(904) 398-5193

Northwest Florida Chapter
310 E. Government Street
Pensacola, FL 32501
(904) 435-1558

Southwest Florida Chapter
660 Tamiami Trail North, Suite 37
Naples, FL 33940
(813) 262-8388

Tampa Bay Chapter
MacDill-Columbus Plaza
2700 North MacDill Avenue, Suite 205
Tampa, FL 33607
(813) 875-7766

Volusia/Flagler Counties Chapter
310 N. Nova Road
Ormond Beach, FL 321-5126
(904) 673-8833

West Central Florida Chapter
P.O. Box 2070
New Port Richey, FL 34656-2070
(813) 848-8888

COMMUNITY MENTAL HEALTH CENTERS

Most Florida counties have community mental health centers. These centers offer a range of mental health services that includes individual and group treatment for mental health problems and treatment for alcohol and drug dependency. Several community mental health centers are licensed as specialty hospitals and provide 24-hour care. Many provide residential treatment.

Community mental health centers are supported, in part, by public funds. Patients are billed according to sliding fee scales which take income into account. Persons with very low income receive free treatment. Although some community health centers provide a greater range of services than others, services typically provided include: outpatient care; 24-hour emergency services for persons in crisis situations; partial hospitalization; inpatient care; consultation, education, and prevention services for schools, community organizations, institutions, and business that assist them in dealing with mentally ill persons; developing programs that help prevent emotional disorders; treatment services for substance abusers, children with emotional disturbances, and families of persons with mental illnesses; and conducting outreach programs for the elderly.

Some community mental health centers have been accredited by either the Joint Commission on the Accreditation of Healthcare Organizations (JCAHO) or by the Commission on Accreditation of Rehabilitation Facilities (CARF). Those community mental health centers that have accredited programs in mental health and substance are listed later in this chapter in the JCAHO and CARF sections. In addition to mental health and substance abuse programs, CARF also accredits organizations that provide rehabilitative services to persons with mental disorders. Community mental health centers with CARF-accredited rehabilitation programs are listed below. Readers should consult the "Accreditation Organizations" section of Chapter 11 for additional information regarding accredited facilities.

Community Mental Health Centers with
CARF Accredited Rehabilitation Programs
December 4, 1992

ACT Corporation/Enrichment Industries
771 Fentress Boulevard
Daytona Beach, FL 32114
(904) 274-1150

New Horizons of the Treasure Coast
415 Avenue A, Suite 306
Fort Pierce, FL 34950
(407) 468-5670

Boley, Inc
1236 Ninth Street North
St. Petersburg, FL 33705
(813) 821-4819

Mary R. Koening Center
647 34th Avenue, South
St. Petersburg, FL 33705
(813) 824-5774

Northside Centers, Inc.
Community Support Center
13001 Bruce B. Downs Boulevard
Tampa, FL 33612
(813) 977-8700

Source: CARF.

HOSPITAL AND RESIDENTIAL TREATMENT

Both general hospitals and specialty hospitals provide psychiatric treatment. In general hospitals, psychiatric care is provided in discrete units staffed with nurses skilled in the care of persons with psychiatric disorders.

As the severity of illness increases, residential or inpatient hospital care becomes more appropriate. According to the research literature, residential or inpatient hospital treatment for psychiatric and substance abuse problems is appropriate for those persons with the most severe problems—those believed to be a threat to themselves or to others. Those in need of 24-hour supervision, or those treatment requiring constant monitoring. Patients diagnosed with serious mental disorders such as schizophrenia, organic brain syndrome, and profound mental retardation may be hospitalized for most, if not all, of their lives. Florida law (The Baker Act) provides for the involuntary confinement of persons who pose a threat to themselves or others.

Recent research studies concerning the treatment of persons with mental illnesses were examined by Geoffrey M. Margo, M.D., and John M. Manring, M.D. (Margo and Manring 1989). After examining 36 psychiatric studies, they found that:
- Hospital care should be crisis-oriented. The goal of hospital treatment should be to stabilize the patient and return the patient to outpatient care.
- It is important that outpatient treatment be provided after discharge from a hospital. Treatment success can be increased with quality aftercare.
- The most widely practiced treatment uses interdisciplinary teams that include psychiatrists, psychologists, nurses, social workers, occupational therapists, and recreational therapists.

The 1989 Florida Health Care Cost Containment Board's Annual Report contained patient data for Florida's psychiatric specialty hospitals for 1988. The data do not include patients treated in general hospitals with psychiatric units or state hospitals. In 1988, the average length of stay in psychiatric specialty hospitals was 20 days for adults and 35 days for children. The table below shows the distribution of patients by principal diagnosis and age.

Patient Discharges by Diagnosis
Psychiatric Specialty Hospital
1988

Diagnosis	Children	Adults
Affective Psychosis	25.8 percent	32.1 percent
Schizophrenic Psychosis	3.1 percent	17.7 percent
Neurotic Disorders	16.7 percent	8.0 percent
Adjustment Reaction	12.4 percent	7.4 percent
Alcohol Dependence	0.9 percent	9.0 percent
Disturbance of Conduct	17.1 percent	0.4 percent
Other	24.0 percent	25.4 percent

Source: 1989 Annual Report. Florida Health Care Cost Containment Board (1990).

Over the past two decades there has been a steady increase in the admission of children and adolescents to hospital treatment programs. Explanations for the increase are controversial. One argument is that much of the increase is attributable to hospital marketing programs directed toward children with minor behavioral problems and "conduct disorders." Another argument is that there is a growing need for mental health services for children and teenagers. According to a 1986 University of South Florida study, children with emotional or behavioral problems should make greater use of outpatient treatment (Friedman and Kutash 1986).

SOURCES OF INFORMATION

The National Institute of Mental Health makes available numerous publications on mental health problems to professionals and the public. The topics of these publications include Alzheimer's disease; AIDS; attitudes toward mental illness; basic sciences and mental health research; mental health problems of children, adolescents, adults, and families; general mental health; panic disorders; depressive disorders; schizophrenia; minorities; and special populations. Spanish language publications are available for some topics. In addition, treatment guidelines, including consensus development conference statements, and treatment issues in medical settings, are available. To receive a list of all of their free publications, write:

Information Resources & Inquiries Branch
Office of Scientific Information
National Institute of Mental Health
5600 Fishers Lane, Room 15C-05
Rockville, Maryland 20857

Professional organizations

Some professional societies publish member directories or will provide information on their members. These societies include:

American Psychiatric Association
(202) 682-6000

American Psychological Association
(202) 336-5500

National Association of Social Workers
(202) 408-8600

American Society of Clinical Hypnosis
2200 East Devon Avenue, Suite 291
Des Plaines, Illinois 60018

Society for Clinical and Experimental Hypnosis
128-A Kingspark Drive
Liverpool, New York 13090

Biofeedback Certification Institute of America
10200 West 44th Ave, Suite 304
Wheatridge, Colorado 800033

The Florida Department of Business and Professional Regulation (DBPR) can be contacted to learn if a practitioner is licensed in the State of Florida. The DBPR medical quality assurance boards were scheduled to be transferred to the state Agency for Health Care Administration (AHCA) July 1, 1994.

Florida Department of Business and Professional Regulation
(904) 487-2252

Self-help organizations

The underlying philosophy of self-help organizations is that the best helpers often are those who have experienced similar problems. These groups provide emotional support and practical help for dealing with problems that their members have in common. Self-help or mutual support groups provide assistance for particular problems such as phobias, bereavement, obsessive-compulsive disorder, anorexia, bulimia, and AIDS. Information about self-help groups can be obtained from:

Alcoholics Anonymous
(check your local telephone directory)

Anxiety Disorders Association of
  America
6000 Executive Blvd., Suite 200
Rockville, MD 20852

The National Alliance for the Mentally Ill
1901 North Fort Myer Drive
Suite 500
Arlington, VA 22209
(703) 524-7600

National Alliance of Mental Patients
PO Box 618
Sioux Falls, SD 57101
(605) 334-4067

National Depressive and Manic
  Depressive Association
730 North Franklin Street, Suite 501
Chicago, Illinois 60610
(312) 642-0049

National Foundation for Depressive
  Illness, Inc.
20 Charles St.
New York, NY 10014
(212)924-9171
(800) 248-4344

National Mental Health Association
1021 Prince Street
Alexandria, VA 22314-2971
(703) 684-7722

The National Mental Health Consumer's
  Association
311 South Juniper St., Room 903
Philadelphia, PA 19107
(215) 735-2465

National Self-Help Clearinghouse
Graduate School & University Center
City University of New York
33 West 42nd St.
New York, NY 10036
(212) 625-7101

Obsessive-Compulsive Foundation
PO Box 9573
New Haven, CT 06535
(203) 772-0565

Recovery, Inc.
802 North Dearborn St.
Chicago, Illinois 60610
(312) 337-5661

Self-Help Clearinghouse
St. Claires—Riverside Medical Center
25 Pocono Road, Denville, N.J. 07834
Denville, NJ 07834
(201) 625-7101

Self-Help Center
1600 Dodge Ave.
Suite S-122
Evanston, IL 60201
(312) 328-0470

JCAHO-ACCREDITED MENTAL HEALTH AND ALCOHOL/ DRUG TREATMENT PROGRAMS

The Joint Commission on the Accreditation of Healthcare Organizations (JCAHO) accredits inpatient, outpatient, and residential programs in adult mental health, child/ adolescent mental health, and alcohol/drug treatment. Readers should consult the "Accreditation Organizations" section of Chapter 11 for additional information. Florida facilities that were JCAHO-accredited in Florida by the JCAHO are listed below. The first table lists facilities accredited under the JCAHO mental health accreditation program. The second table lists facilities accredited under the hospital accreditation program.

JCAHO-Accredited
Inpatient and Outpatient
Mental Health and Substance Abuse Programs
February, 1993
(Accredited with Commendation as of April, 1993)

Name of facility & telephone	*City*	*Facility & service Codes*
Alternatives in Treatment (407) 998-0866 Accredited with commendation	Boca Raton	35 75
American Day Treatment Centers (407) 241-7741	Boca Raton	31 32 65
Interphase Recovery Program (407) 487-5400	Boca Raton	35 65
Lifeskills/Boca Raton (407) 392-1199	Boca Raton	31 35 75
National Recover Institutes Group (407) 392-8444 Accredited with commendation	Boca Raton	35 77
Renaissance Institute of Palm Beach Inc. (407) 241-7977	Boca Raton	35 66
Charter Hospital (813) 792-2222	Bradenton	32 67
Manatee Glens Corp. (813) 741-3111	Bradenton	31 32 35 71 72 66
Manatee Palms Adolescent Spec Hospital (813) 746-1388	Bradenton	32 35 64 67
Outreach, Inc. (813) 574-4357	Cape Coral	35 65
The Shores (904) 697-3375	Carrabelle	N/A
Fairwinds Treatment Center (813) 449-0300 Accredited with commendation	Clearwater	32 35 64

The Renfrew Center of Florida (305) 698-9222	Coconut Creek	31 32 63
High Point (305) 680-2700	Cooper City	31 35 64 71
Care Unit of Coral Springs (305) 753-5200	Coral Springs	35 72
Seafield Center South (305) 321-9400	Davie	35 63
ACT Corporation (904) 255-6538	Daytona Beach	31 32 35 72 77 C M1
Leon Stewart/Hal Marchman Center (904) 255-0447	Daytona Beach	35 72
The Beachcomber (407) 734-1818	Delray Beach	35 64
Pathways to Recovery (407) 496-7532	Delray Beach	35 73
South County Mental Health Center (407) 495-0522	Delray Beach	31 32 35 69 71 72
Harbor Oaks Hospital (904) 863-4160	Fort Walton Beach	32 64
Mental Health Services of N. Central Fla (904) 374-5670	Gainesville	31 32 35 71 72
The Friary, Inc. (904) 932-9375 Accredited with commendation	Gulf Breeze	31 35 72 75
Montanari Residential Treatment Center (305) 887-7543	Hialeah	32 64
Northwest. Dade Center (530) 582-5030	Hialeah	31 32 35 71 72 77 C
Parkside Lodge of Florida (407) 841-7071 Accredited with commendation	Intercession City	35 71
Daniel Memorial Hospital (904) 737-1677	Jacksonville	32 74
Mental Health Resource Center (904) 642-9100	Jacksonville	31 32 35 69 72 75 C F
Oak Center (904) 725-7073	Jacksonville	31 32 35 64 77
Growing Together, Inc. (407) 585-0892	Lake Worth	35 73
Florida Camelot, Inc. (813) 949-7491 Accredited with commendation	Land O'Lakes	32 73

Bay Harbor Residential Treatment Center (813) 587-1000	Largo	32 35 64
Prof. Comprehensive Addiction Services (813) 530-1420	Largo	35 71
Lake Sumter Mental Health Center & Hospital (904) 787-9178	Leesburg	31 32 35 72 76
La Amistad Residential Treatment Center (407) 647-0660	Maitland	31 32 64
Devereux Hospital & Children's Center (305) 242-9100	Melbourne	32 37 64
Heritage Family Treatment Center (407) 725-5222	Melbourne	35 63
HCA Grant Center Hospital (305) 251-0710	Miami	32 64
South Florida Evaluation and Treatment Center (305) 637-2511	Miami	38 63
Spectrum Programs (305) 653-8288	Miami	35 72 77
The Village South (305) 573-3784	Miami	35 74
David Lawrence Center (813) 455-1031	Naples	31 32 35 72 76
The Willough at Naples (813) 775-4500	Naples	31 35 64 73
Twelve Oaks (904) 939-1200	Navarre	35 77
Marion Citrus Mental Health Center (904) 629-8893	Ocala	31 32 35 71 72 74
Laurel Oaks Residential Treatment Center (407) 363-7700 Accredited with commendation	Orlando	32 64
CPC Palm Bay Hospital (407) 729-0500	Palm Bay	2 64
Recovery Corner of West Palm Beach (407) 626-1411	Palm Beach Gardens	35 66
Crossroads/Recovery Center (904) 784-0869	Panama City	35 63
Rivendell Psychiatric Center (904) 763-0017	Panama City	32 63
Lakeview Center, Inc. (904) 432-1222	Pensacola	31 32 35 72 76 77
The Cloisters at Pine Island (813) 283-1019 Accredited with commendation	Pineland	35 67

Personal Enrichment Through Mental Health (813) 545-5636	Pinellas Park	31 32 63 70 C DD GG
Apalachee Center for Human Services (904) 487-2930	Tallahassee	31 32 35 69 72 74 C F
DISC Village (904) 575-4388	Tallahassee	35 74
Careunit South Florida (813) 978-0879	Tampa	31 32 35 64 77
Florida Mental Health Institute (813) 974-4533 Accredited with commendation	Tampa	31 32 35 77 66
Mental Health Care, Inc. (813) 237-3914	Tampa	31 32 69 76
Northside Centers, Inc. (813) 977-8700	Tampa	31 32 69 72 C Q CC DD GG
Tampa Bay Academy (813) 677-6700 Accredited with commendation	Tampa	32 73
Turning Point of Tampa (813) 882-3003	Tampa	31 35 65
45th St. Mental Health Center (305) 844-9741	W Palm Beach	31 32 68 72
Hanley/Hazelden Center at St. Mary's (407) 848-1666	W Palm Beach	35 71
The Palm Beach Institute (407) 833-7553	W Palm Beach	35 70
Mainstream of Winter Park (407) 629-0629	Winter Park	31 32 35 65

(Code legend appears on page 150)

Hospital Accreditation Program
February 1993

Name of facility	City	Facility and service codes
Charter Hospital of Bradenton	Bradenton	32 70 C DD
Greenbrier Hospital	Brooksville	31 32 63
The Shores	Carrabelle	32 67 C FF
Horizon Hospital	Clearwater	31 32 35 63 63 C F L BB CC DD FF GG
Atlantic Shores Hospital	Daytona Beach	31 32 35 68 68 63
Fair Oaks Hospital	Delray Beach	31 32 35 63 63 C F GG
C.P.C. Ft. Lauderdale Hospital	Ft. Lauderdale	31 32 35 63 C F CC GG
Coral Ridge Psychiatric Hospital	Ft. Lauderdale	31 35 63 C F DD GG
Charter Glade Hospital	Ft. Myers	31 32 35 68 68 68 C F Q DD GG
Harbor Oaks Hospital	Ft. Walton Beach	32 67
Glenbeigh Hospital of Miami	Hialeah	31 35 68 76 F
Southern Winds Hospital	Hialeah	31 63 C CC DD GG
CPC St. Johns River Hospital	Jacksonville	31 32 35 63 68 C E F DD GG
Charter Hospital	Jacksonville	32 35 63 68 C F M1 M2 O Q R S DD FF GG
Charter Hospital Orlando South	Kissimmee	31 32 35 63 69
Medfield Hospital	Largo	31 32 68 68 C F Q CC DD GG
Heritage Gulf Shore Institute	Lecanto	31 35 69
HCA West Lake Hospital	Longwood	31 32 35 63
Charter Hospital of Pasco	Lutz	31 32 35 69 76 C F
Circles of Care	Melbourne	31 35 69 72 C F CC
Devereux Hospital/Children's Center	Melbourne	32 63 C
Charter Hospital of Miami	Miami	31 32 76 C L O Q R S BB CC DD FF NN

HCA Grant Center Hospital	Miami	31 32 66 76 C CC DD FF GG
Harbor View Hospital	Miami	31 32 63 C F BB CC DD FF GG
Charter Springs Hospital	Ocala	31 32 35 69 76 C F Q BB CC DD FF GG
Crossroads/University Behavioral Center	Orlando	31 32 68 68 C L Q CC DD FF GG NN
Glenbeigh Hospital of Orlando	Orlando	31 32 35 75 76 C F Q CC DD GG
Laurel Oaks Hospital	Orlando	32 35 68 63 C CC DD GG
CPC Palm Bay Hospital	Palm Bay	32 70 C GG
Rivendell Psychiatric Center	Panama City	31 63
Savannas Hospital	Port St. Lucie	31 32 35 63 68 C F DD
St. Augustine Psychiatric Center	St. Augustine	31 32 63 C DD
Sarasota Palms Hospital	Sarasota	31 32 68 68 C L O Q BB CC DD GG
The Retreat	Sunrise	31 32 35 63 68 C F
Charter Hospital of Tampa Bay	Tampa	31 32 35 63
Glenbeigh Hospital of Tampa	Tampa	31 32 35 63 69
Anclote Manor Hospital	Tarpon Springs	32 39 68 65
Charter Hospital	W Palm Beach	32 63
Glenbeigh Hospital	W Palm Beach	31 32 35 69 75 C
Winter Park Pavilion	Winter Park	31 35 63 C F

JCAHO Accreditation Facility and Service Codes:

31 Adult mental health
32 Child/adolescent mental health
35 Alcohol/drug mental health
63 Inpatient services
64 Residential services
65 Partial hospitalization services
66 Outpatient services
67 Inpatient/residential services
69 Inpatient/outpatient services
70 Inpatient/residential/partial hosp.
71 Inpatient/residential/outpatient

72 Inpatient/res/outpat/partial hospital
73 Residential/partial hospital
75 Outpatient/partial hospital
76 Inpatient/outpatient/partial hospital
77 Residential/outpatient/partial hospital
C Psychiatric, acute care
DD Recreational therapy
F Alcoholism/other drug services
GG Psychiatric educational services
MI Emergency department

Source: JCAHO 1993.

SUBSTANCE ABUSE TREATMENT

Substance abuse programs treat persons who are dependent on alcohol, illegal drugs, or prescription drugs. As with psychiatric programs, outpatient and residential treatment programs are available that are less expensive than hospital programs.

An article that reviewed the recent research literature on psychiatry stated that there are three general principals in effective alcohol treatment programs (Michels and Marzuk 1993). According to the authors:

- Because those patients who cannot control drinking without a relapse cannot be readily identified, complete abstinence is a feature of most programs.
- There are different goals in each phase of treatment: prevention of complications during detoxification, achievement of abstinence during rehabilitation, and consolidation of abstinence and reduced craving during longer-term treatment.
- Treatment must address occupational, family, psychiatric, and medical problems.

The Michels and Marzuk literature review concluded that outpatient detoxification programs are safe for some alcoholics, but alcoholics with serious medical illness, a history of serious withdrawal symptoms or seizures, mental-status changes, or marked autonomic lability probably are best treated as inpatients.

The National Clearinghouse for Alcohol and Drug Information (NCADI) makes available numerous publications on substance abuse disorders, and answers questions from both health care professionals and the public on drug and alcohol abuse treatment and prevention.

**National Clearinghouse for Drug
and Alcohol Information
P.O. Box 2345
Rockville, Maryland 20852
(800) 729-6686**

CARF-accredited outpatient substance abuse programs

The Commission on Accreditation of Rehabilitation Facilities (CARF) accredits substance abuse, mental health, and other facilities that meet its national standards. According to CARF, one of the purposes of the Commission is to "develop and maintain current, state-of-the-art standards which can be used by organizations to measure their level of performance, to promote consumer-responsiveness, and to strengthen their programs." CARF has numerous sponsoring and associate members, including the American Psychological Association, the National Association of Addiction Treatment Providers, the National Association of Alcoholism and Drug Abuse Counselors, and 35 other national organizations.

Readers should consult the "Accreditation Organizations" section of Chapter 11 for additional information regarding accredited facilities.

CARF-Accredited Alcoholism & Drug Dependency Programs
December 4, 1992

Chautauqua Offices of Psychotherapy and
   Evaluation, Inc.
C.O.P.E.
112-A West Nelson Avenue
DeFuniak Springs, FL 32433
(904) 892-8035

Osceola Counseling Center/Center for
   Drug Free Living
1200 North Central Avenue
Kissimmee, FL 34741

Center for Drug-Free Living, Inc.
100 West Columbia Street
Orlando, FL 32806
(407) 423-6606

Men's Residential Treatment Center/
   Center fro Drug-Free Living
8301 East Colonial Drive
Orlando, FL 32817
(407) 273-4970

Women's Residential Treatment Center/
   Center for Drug-Free Living
1780 Mercy Drive
Orlando, FL 32808
(407) 297-2010

LIST OF PSYCHIATRIC AND SUBSTANCE ABUSE SPECIALTY HOSPITALS

Bay County
Rivendell of Bay County
1940 Harrison Ave
Panama City 32405
(904) 763-0017

Brevard County
Circles of Care
400 East Sheridan Road
Melbourne 32901
(407) 723-3920

CPC Palm Bay Hospital
4400 Dixie Highway N.E.
Palm Bay 32905
(407) 729-0500

Devereux Hospital and Children's Center
8000 Devereaux Drive
Melbourne 32936
(407) 242-9100

Broward County
Coral Ridge Psychiatric Hospital
4545 North Federal Highway
Fort Lauderdale 33308
(305) 771-2711

CPC Fort Lauderdale Hospital
1601 East Las Olas Blvd
Fort Lauderdale 33301
(305) 463-4321

Hollywood Pavilion
1201 North 37th Ave
Hollywood 33021
(305) 962-1355

The Retreat
555 S.W. 148th Ave
Sunrise 33325
(305) 370-0200

University Pavilion Hospital
7425 University Drive
Tamarac 33321
(305) 722-9933

Citrus County
Heritage Hospital-Beverly Hills
PO Box 550
Beverly Hills, FL 32665
(904) 746-9000

Collier County
The Willough at Naples
9001 Tamiami Trail
Naples 33962
(813) 775-4500

Dade County
Charter Hospital of Miami
11100 N.W. 27th Street
Miami 33172
(305) 591-3230

Glenbeigh Hospital of Miami
4425 W. 20th Ave
Hialeah 33012
(305) 558-9999

Grant Center Hospital
20601 S.W. 157th Ave
Miami 33187
(305) 251-0710

Harbor View
1861 N.W. South River Drive
Miami 33125
(305) 642-3555

Southern Winds Hospital
4225 W. 20th Ave
Hialeah 33012
(305) 558-9700

Duval County
Charter Hospital of Jacksonville
3947 Salisbury Road
Jacksonville 32216
(904) 731-2447

Daniel Memorial Hospital (IRFT)
3725 Belfort Road
Jacksonville 32216
(904) 737-1677

Methodist Pathway Center
580 West 8th Street
Jacksonville 32209
(904) 798-8250

Saint Johns River Hospital
6300 Beach Blvd
Jacksonville 32216
(904) 724-9202

Franklin County
The Shores
Star Route Box 73
Carrabelle 32322
(904) 697-3375

Hernando County
Greenbrier Hospital
7007 Grove Road
Brooksville, Fl 34605
(904) 596-4306

Hillsborough County
Charter Hospital of Tampa Bay
4004 North Riverside Drive
Tampa 33603
(813) 238-8671

Glenbeigh Hospital of Tampa
3102 E. 138th Avenue
Tampa 33613
(813) 971-5000

Northside Community Mental Health
 Center
13301 Bruce B. Downs Blvd.
Tampa 33612
(813) 977-8700

University of South Florida Psychiatric
 Center
3515 East Fletcher Ave
Tampa 33613
(813) 972-3000

Lake County
Lake/Sumter CMHC & Hospital
2020 Tally Road
Leesburg, Fl 34748
(904) 787-9178

Lee County
Charter Glade Hospital
3550 Colonial Blvd
Fort Myers 33906
(813) 939-0403

Leon County
Eastside Psychiatric Hospital
2634-B Capital Circle, NE
Tallahassee 32308
(904) 487-0300

Wateroak Adolescent Hospital
2634-G Capital Circle, NE
Tallahassee 32308
(904) 487-2930

Manatee County
Charter Hospital of Bradenton
4480 51st Street West
Bradenton 34209
(813) 792-2222

Glen Oaks Hospital
2020 26th Ave East
Bradenton 33506
(813) 747-8648

Manatee Palms Adolescent Specialty
    Hospital
1324 37th Avenue East
Bradenton, Fl 33508
(813) 746-1388

Marion County
Charter Springs Hospital
3130 S.W. 27th Ave
Ocala 32678
(904) 237-7293

Martin County
Sandypines
11301 S.E. Tequesta Terrace
Tequesta, Fl 33469
(407) 743-0224

Okaloosa County
Harbor Oaks Hospital
1015 Mar-walt Drive
Fort Walton Beach 32548
(904) 863-4160

Orange County
Crossroads University Behavioral Center
2500 Discovery Drive
Orlando 32826
(407) 281-7000

Glenbeigh Hospital-Orlando
7450 Sand Lake Commons Blvd
Orlando 32819
(407) 352-6550

La Amistad Psychiatric Treatment Center
201 Alpine Drive
Maitland 32751
(407) 647-0660

Laurel Oaks Hospital
6601 Central Florida Parkway
Orlando 32821
(407) 352-7000

Laurel Oaks Residential Treatment Center
6849 Sea Harbor Drive
Orlando 32821
(407) 363-7700

Osceola County
Charter Hospital of Orlando South
206 Park Place Blvd
Kissimmee 32741
(407) 846-0444

Palm Beach County
Charter Hospital of West Palm Beach
1950 Benoist Farms Road
West Palm Beach 33411
(407) 687-1511

Fair Oaks Hospital
5440 Linton Blvd
Delray Beach 33445
(407) 495-1000

45th Street Mental Health Center
1041 45th Street
West Palm Beach 33(407)
(407) 844-9741

Glenbeigh Hospitals of Palm Beaches
4700 Congress Ave
West Palm Beach 33(407)
(407) 848-5500

Pasco County
Charter Hospital of Pasco
21808 State Road 7
Lutz, FL 33549
(813) 948-2441

Pinellas County
Horizon Hospital
11300 U.S. 19 South
Clearwater 33546
(813) 541-2646

Medfield Hospital
12891 Seminole Blvd
Largo 34648
(813) 581-8757

The Manors
1527 Riverside Drive
Tarpon Springs 34689
(813) 937-4211

Polk County
Palmview Hospital
2510 North Florida Ave
Lakeland 33805
(813) 682-6105

St Johns County
St. Augustine Psychiatric Center
200 River Haven Way
St. Augustine 32086
(904) 482-9800

St Lucie County
Savannas Hospital
2550 Walton Road
Port St. Lucie 34952
(407) 335-0400

Sarasota County
Sarasota Palms Hospital
1650 South Osprey Ave
Sarasota 33579
(813) 366-6070

Seminole County
HCA West Lake Hospital
589 W. Sanlando Springs Dr.
Longwood 32750
(407) 834-0900

Winter Park Pavilion
1600 Dodd Road
Winter Park 32792
(407) 677-6842

Volusia County
Atlantic Shores Hospital
841 Jimmy Ann Drive
Daytona Beach 32117
(904) 274-5333

CHAPTER 8
Veterans Administration health care services

The Veterans Administration (VA) has five hospitals, five nursing homes, nine outpatient clinics, one domiciliary facility, and ten VET centers in Florida. Eligibility for VA health care services varies, depending on whether a veteran has a service-related disability, annual income, and other factors. Because of limited funding, a priority system is used to provide health care services.

ELIGIBILITY FOR VA HOSPITAL AND NURSING HOME CARE

The VA has two eligibility categories, "mandatory" and "discretionary." Veterans in the mandatory category are not subject to income eligibility requirements and are assured treatment. Veterans in the discretionary category are subject to income eligibility requirements and may receive care if resources are available. For the purpose of hospital and nursing home care, all veterans with disabilities, regardless of age, are divided into two groups.

Mandatory

Hospital care is mandatory if the veteran is in one of the groups listed in the chart below or if the patient has a nonservice-connected disability and has an annual income of $19,408 or less if single with no dependents, ($23,290 or less if married or single with one dependent, plus $1,295 for each additional dependent). Income eligibility amounts are increased each year on January 1 by the same amount as the rate at which VA pension rates are increased. These income limits are for 1993.

Discretionary

Hospital care is discretionary if the veteran has a nonservice-connected disability and has annual income above $18,844 if single with no dependents, ($22,613 if married or single with one dependent, plus $1,258 for each additional dependent). Veterans in the discretionary group must agree to pay for a small part of the cost of their care. Payment is based on the Medicare deductible plus a small daily charge. In 1993, veterans paid $676 for the first 90 days of hospital or nursing home care during any 365-day period. For each additional 90 days of care, veterans were charged $338. The daily charges were $10 for hospital care and $5 for nursing home care. The chart below shows mandatory eligibility for hospital and nursing home care.

VA Hospital and Nursing Home Care
Mandatory Eligibility
Not Subject to Income Requirements
1993

- Veterans with service-connected disabilities.
- Veterans who are former prisoners of war.
- Veterans receiving VA pensions.
- Veterans in need of treatment for a condition related to exposure to ionizing radiation from participating in nuclear tests or in the occupation of Hiroshima or Nagasaki.
- Veterans in need of treatment for a condition related to exposure to dioxin or other toxic substances, such as Agent Orange, while in Vietnam.
- Veterans of the Spanish American War, the Mexican Border Period, World War I, or World War II veterans eligible for Medicaid.

The most common reasons for admission to VA hospitals in 1988 were: psychoses, alcohol dependence, pulmonary obstruction, and respiratory neoplasm. Nearly 95 percent of the veterans who were admitted to VA hospitals in Florida in 1988 were mandatory admissions. Veterans with bona fide medical emergencies are admitted immediately without regard to which priority category they are in. A bona fide medical emergency is defined as a situation in which a delay in treatment would result in a serious threat to life or health.

VA Hospital Medical Centers in Florida 1993

City	Hospital beds
Bay Pines	671
Gainesville	461
Lake City	322
Miami	622
Tampa	604

Note: All five VA medical centers were accredited by the Joint Commission on the Accreditation of Healthcare Organizations (JCAHO) in 1993.

ELIGIBILITY FOR VA OUTPATIENT CARE

Although the VA has official eligibility requirements for outpatient care, in actual practice eligibility requirements vary substantially. A 1993 report by the General Accounting Office (GAO) reviewed the 158 VA outpatient centers across the country and found that they interpret eligibility criteria differently (GAO 1993). The report also found that the VA medical centers use different methods to ration care. This means that a veteran can be found to be eligible for services at one outpatient center, but not at another.

Outpatient health care services are provided "within the limits of VA facilities." Services include medical examination and related medical services, drugs and medicines, rehabilitation, counseling, mental health services, and home health care. There are four eligibility categories:

Outpatient care **must** be furnished for any disability to:
- Veterans with service-connected disabilities;
- Veterans with a 30 to 40 percent service-connected disability;
- Veterans who have suffered an injury as a result of VA hospitalization; or
- Veterans in a VA-approved vocational rehabilitation program.

Outpatient care **must** be furnished for any condition to eliminate the need for hospital care, to prepare for hospitalization, or to treat a condition for which the veteran was hospitalized to:
- Veterans with a 30% to 40% service-connected disability; or
- Veterans whose annual income is not greater than the maximum pension rate of a veteran in need of "regular aid and attendance" by another person.

The VA **may** provide outpatient care to:
- Veterans in a VA-approved vocational rehabilitation program;
- Former prisoners of war;
- World War I or Mexican Border Period veterans; or
- Veterans who receive increased pensions or compensation that is based on the need for regular aid and attendance of another person, or who are permanently homebound.

The VA **may** provide outpatient care to eliminate the need for hospitalization, to prepare for hospitalization, or for a condition for which the veteran was hospitalized to:
- Veterans with up to 20 percent service-connected disability;
- Mandatory category veterans whose income is more than the pension rate of veterans in need of regular aid and attendance;
- Discretionary category veterans, subject to a copayment of $26 per outpatient visit; or
- Beneficiaries of other specified federal programs.

VA NURSING HOMES

Eligibility for VA nursing home care is essentially the same as eligibility for hospital care. Normally, VA nursing home care will not be provided for more than six months unless the veteran has a service-connected disability, or the veteran was hospitalized primarily for the treatment of a service-connected disability. Nursing home care for veterans with a disability that is not service-connected, and whose income exceeds the income threshold amount applicable to hospital care eligibility, may be authorized only if the veteran agrees to pay a copayment. Veterans who have a service-connected disability are given first priority for admission to VA nursing home care.

The VA will pay for care in private nursing homes if the veteran requires nursing care for a service-connected disability after medical determination by the VA or the veteran has been discharged from a VA medical center and is receiving VA medical center-based home health services.

Florida's five VA nursing homes are located at the same sites as the five VA hospitals.

VA Nursing Homes in Florida 1989

City	Nursing home beds
Bay Pines	240
Gainesville	120
Lake City	120
Miami	240
Tampa	120

VA DOMICILIARY CARE

Domiciliary care is available at only one VA facility in Florida, the VA Medical Center complex at Bay Pines in Pinellas County. The Bay Pines facility has 200 domiciliary beds. Eligibility is limited to veterans with annual incomes that do not exceed the amount of the maximum annual VA pension and to veterans the Secretary of Veterans Affairs determines have no adequate means of support. Prior approval is needed by the VA for placement in a domiciliary care facility. Veterans can apply at any VA office.

OTHER VA HEALTH CARE BENEFITS

The Veterans Administration provides outpatient dental treatment, reimbursement for certain medically related travel, medical examinations for veterans exposed to Agent Orange or to radiation, alcohol and drug dependence treatment, prosthetic appliances, blind aids and services, and readjustment counseling at Vet Centers.

Although eligibility for the services mentioned above varies, a service-connected disability is usually necessary to receive care. Eligibility may sometimes be found where the veteran meets income eligibility criteria or the veteran makes a copayment for services. Any of the VA facilities listed at the end of this chapter can assist with determining eligibility for these services.

NAMES AND ADDRESSES OF VA FACILITIES AND VET CENTERS

The following listing of VA health care facilities was published in 1992 by the Veterans Administration.

Facility	Services
Bay Pines 1000 Bay Pines Blvd, North (813) 398-6661	Hospital, Domiciliary, Nursing Home, Outpatient
Daytona Beach 1900 Mason Avenue (904) 274-4600	Outpatient
Fort Myers 2070 Carrell Road (813) 939-3939	Outpatient
Gainesville 1601 SW Archer Road (904) 376-1611	Hospital, Nursing Home
Jacksonville 1833 Boulevard (904) 791-2712	Outpatient
Key West 1111 12th Street, Suite 207 (305) 536-6696	Outpatient
Lake City 801 S. Marion Street (904) 755-3016	Hospital, Nursing Home

Miami   Hospital, Nursing Home
1201 N.W. 16th Street
(305) 324-4455

Oakland Park   Outpatient
(Ft. Lauderdale)
5599 N. Dixie Highway
(305) 771-2101

Orlando   Outpatient
83 W. Columbia St.
(407) 425-7521

Pensacola   Outpatient
312 Kenmore Road
(904) 476-1100

Port Richey   Outpatient
Plaza Medical Center
8911 Ponderosa Avenue
(813) 869-3203

Riviera Beach   Outpatient
Exec. Plaza
301 Broadway
(407) 845-2800

Tampa   Hospital, Nursing Home
13000 N. 30th Street
(813) 972-2000

Benefit Information
Statewide
(800) 827-1000

Vet Centers
Ft. Lauderdale   (305) 356-7926

Jacksonville   (904) 791-3621

Lake Worth   (407) 585-0441

Miami   (305) 859-8387

Orlando   (407) 648-6151

Pensacola   (904) 479-6665

Sarasota   (813) 952-9406

St. Petersburg   (813) 893-3791

Tallahassee   (904) 942-8810

Tampa   (813) 228-2621

ADDITIONAL SOURCES OF INFORMATION

Federal Benefits for Veterans and Dependents, VA Pamphlet 80-92-1, Department of Veterans Affairs, 1992. Department of Veterans Affairs, Washington DC 20420. This publication is revised annually.

Disabled American Veteran Magazine. Write to DAV Magazine, 807 Maine Ave. SW, Washington, DC 20024.

CHAPTER 9
Health care options and decision-making
in the last years of life

Planning for the last years of life involves making decisions that are based on financial and health care considerations. This chapter includes information from many sources that shed light on aging and health care decision-making. In reviewing the information that is discussed in this chapter, it is important to keep in mind that researchers have found that people age differently and that changes occur gradually over time. Averages, of course, do not apply to all people.

This chapter begins with brief discussions of health care options—home health care, residence in an assisted living facilities, and nursing home care. Other chapters discuss these options in greater detail.

A sizeable proportion, but not the majority, of elderly persons will spend some time in a nursing home. Women are much more likely to spend time in a nursing home and for much longer periods of time than men. Research indicates that about 22 percent of males and 41 percent of females who reach age 65 will spend at least three months in a nursing home. On average, men who reach age 65 and require nursing home care spend about eight months in a nursing home, women in the same situation will spend an average of about 20 months in a nursing home.

Studies have found that persons in good health will, on average, spend more time in nursing homes than persons in poor health. This is because persons in poor health die sooner. Research has also found that, on average, the longer a person lives, the greater the time spent in a nursing home. For example, persons who die between age 65 and 70 spend, on average, only about a month in nursing homes, while persons who live past age 95 spend about three and one-third years in nursing homes.

HOME CARE, ACLF, CONTINUING CARE FACILITY OR NURSING HOME?

When help is needed to deal with declining health, it is often difficult to decide what course of action to take. This is because the problem often has many dimensions. In addition to making a decision on how to meet health care needs, there can be other problems such as housing, help with meals, shopping, transportation, and assistance with other daily living activities such as bathing. If there is a terminal illness, the problem is even more difficult. In Florida there are four main residential health care options:
1. Residing at home. Depending upon individual needs, there are a range of options that include receiving home health care or nursing services, adult day care or adult medical day care, homemaker services, sitter services, and hospice care.
2. Residing in an adult congregate living facility (ACLF).
3. Residing in a continuing care retirement community (CCRC).
4. Residing in a nursing home.

When choosing among options, it is important to carefully consider both present and future health care needs, personal care needs, quality of life, costs, and insurance coverage. Physicians, hospital discharge planners, and medical social workers probably are the most knowledgeable health care professionals in this area. They have considerable knowledge of how to meet both health care needs and the problems of daily living. In addition, they also are a good source of information regarding the quality of local health care facilities and local programs that provide home care and other services. They also are familiar with costs, insurance coverage, and public programs that provide assistance.

In choosing among the four options, key questions to consider include:
- To what extent is help needed for personal care such as bathing, cooking, and other aspects of daily living?
- What setting will help promote the most independence and the best quality of life for the longest period?
- Is living at home practical if supplemented with home health services, homemaker services, adult day care, or respite care?
- What family considerations are there?
- What future needs are anticipated?
- To what extent is skilled nursing care needed?
- In the case of a terminal illness, is hospice care desirable?
- What are the costs, and how will the bill be paid?

Option 1—Living at home

Nursing care, and other related services are provided in the home by home health agencies, nurse registries, and hospice programs. Home health agencies employ persons who provide a range of nursing and personal care services that permit older persons to live at home for as long as possible. Nurse registries accomplish the same end by serving as a source of referrals of professionals and paraprofessionals who will work in the direct employ of the individual receiving care or a family member. Hospices provide care to persons with terminal illnesses and their families through an interdisciplinary team of physicians, nurses, and other care givers.

Many people prefer living at home and contracting with a home health care agency for nursing services and help with activities of daily living. Living at home often can provide the greatest independence and be the least costly option. Home health agencies employ homemakers, certified nursing assistants, physical therapists, nurses and others to provide a range of services. Some home health agencies provide technologically advanced health care services, such as treatment with infusion pumps and ventilators, home dialysis, I.V. therapy, and parenteral nutrition. Home health aides, under the supervision of a nurse or other health care professional, provide personal care services, such as assistance with eating, bathing and toileting.

In Florida, home health care agencies must meet certain standards to be licensed. A physician must prepare a treatment plan, and a registered nurse must prepare a plan of care. Medicare and Medicaid pay for home health care under certain circumstances. Some private health insurance also pays for home health care.

Nurse registries refer nurses who "list" with the registry to persons who want care at home. It is estimated that the costs of nursing services from nurse registries is 10 percent to 30 percent less than those provided by home health agencies. A recent change in Florida law allows nurse registries to provide homemaker, companion and sitter services. Individuals who hire through nurse registries are responsible for paying them directly and for calculating federal taxes and withholding and reporting that information to the federal government. They also assume liability for injuries that may affect the home health worker.

If nursing and other health care services are not needed, there are agencies that provide "homemaker" assistance. These agencies provide domestic maid services, sitter services, companion services, and services such as cooking, shopping, money management, and laundry. Home health agencies can be either private for-profit companies or non-profit agencies. Some non-profit agencies are supported by the United Way or by religious organizations.

Another option is to subscribe to a home medical emergency response service, such as "Lifeline." This service often is provided by hospitals. When a "help button" that is worn around the subscriber's neck is pressed, a radio signal to a telephone notifies a dispatcher who then arranges for an ambulance if circumstances warrant.

Other options for providing relief for caregivers, include arranging for adult day care services and 24-hour short-term respite care. Adult day care centers and some nursing homes provide care for persons during the day. Some nursing homes provide 24-hour short-term respite care. See Chapter 6 for a detailed discussion of home health care.

Hospice care for persons with terminal illnesses

Hospices provide care to persons with terminal illnesses and their families. An interdisciplinary team of caregivers cares for the psychological, social, and spiritual needs of the patient and the family. The team develops a written care plan based on an assessment of the needs of the patient and the family. The main health care responsibility is to control the patient's symptoms, particularly pain. Medicare pays for hospice care.

A study of patients with terminal cancer admitted to the H. Lee Moffitt Cancer Center in Tampa suggests that physicians discuss options with the patient and their family before the patient becomes critically ill and aggressive measures are taken. The authors noted that alternative forms of health care, such as hospices, provide "less invasive, less aggressive, less costly care" than hospital intensive care units (Schapia et al. 1993). Hospices are discussed in greater detail in Chapter 6.

Option 2—Living in an ACLF

The term "Adult congregate living facility" (ACLF) is government licensing jargon for a "board and care" home or a "home for the aged." ACLFs can be found in the yellow pages of the telephone directory under "retirement homes." An ACLF may have a regular license, a license to provide limited nursing services, or a license to provided limited mental health services.

ACLFs provide housing, meals, recreation, and personal care services to residents in home like settings. Personal care services include help with eating, bathing, grooming, moving about, and the supervision of self-administered medication.

State regulations require that all ACLF residents be examined by a physician or licensed nurse practitioner within 60 days prior to residing in the facility "when possible." The examination must include an assessment of the appropriateness of placement in the facility.

If nursing care is needed there are two options: residing in an ACLF that has a limited nursing license; or contracting with a home health agency or nurse registry for nursing care to be provided at the ACLF. Hospice care also may be provided in ACLFs.

ACLFs range from the modest to the very expensive and exclusive. Neither Medicaid, Medicare, or private insurance pays for the cost of living in an ACLF. There are, however, two possible sources of financial assistance for persons with low incomes, the Optional State Supplementation (OSS) and Supplemental Security Income (SSI) programs. Paying for care in an ACLF is discussed in more detail in Chapter 5.

Option 3—Living in a continuing care retirement community

Continuing care retirement communities (CCRCs) often are called "life care" communities. With the exception of hospital care, continuing care communities usually provide a complete range of health care services in additional to residential services. They provide all of the services that ACLFs provide—housing, meals, recreation, and personal care services—and usually they also usually either provide or arrange for nursing home care when it is needed. Many have independent living units in addition to congregate living facilities. A continuing care community will often have at least three licenses: an ACLF license, a nursing home license, and a continuing care facility license.

When CCRC residents need more assistance with health and personal care needs, they move from independent living to assisted living to nursing home care. These are often referred to as "levels" of care. Not all continuing care facilities provide a complete range of services, however and there are differences in how nursing home care is paid for and arranged. Hospice care may also be provided to residents of CCRCs.

Careful consideration is a must before signing a contract. Residents usually pay an entrance fee in addition to monthly maintenance fees. Florida law requires that continuing care contracts contain certain provisions. Because of the costs and complexities associated with continuing care community contracts, it is often prudent to consult with an attorney before signing a contract. Continuing care communities are discussed in greater detail in Chapter 5.

Option 4—Living in a nursing home

Nursing homes care for persons who need 24-hour skilled nursing care both in the short and long-term. Short-term residents include persons needing rehabilitative care when recovering from accidents, strokes, surgery, or illnesses. Long-term residents comprise the majority of nursing home residents, and, for most, a nursing home is their final place of residence.

Admission to a nursing home must be ordered by a physician. After admission, residents remain under the care of a physician. Medicare pays for up to 100 days of nursing home care, provided certain criteria are met. For Medicaid to pay for nursing home care, a person must be screened by the CARES program and meet Medicaid financial criteria. Nursing homes are discussed in greater detail in Chapter 4.

The American Council of Life Insurance publishes "Health Care and Finances: A Guide for Adult Children and Their Parents." This excellent guide discusses health care choices, financial planning, and lists resources to obtain further information. The guide can be obtained by contacting:

American Council of Life Insurance
Health Insurance Association of America
External Affairs
1001 Pennsylvania Avenue, NW
Washington, D.C. 20004-2599

LIFE EXPECTANCY AND DISABILITY AFTER AGE 65

Several recent national studies have examined the health status, longevity, and nursing home use of people as they grow older. The largest and most complex study was undertaken by researchers from the Urban Institute, the Duke University Center for Demographic Studies, and the National Institutes of Health. The study examined data from three nationally representative surveys to estimate life expectancy and disability for persons who reach age 65 (Liu, Manton and Liu 1990). The surveys included data for elderly persons regarding disability, health status and nursing home use. This research was conducted to produce actuarial information for long-term care insurance financing.

The table below, reproduced from the Liu study, shows estimates for life expectancy and disability for persons who reach age 65. In examining the table, it is important to keep in mind that the table shows averages for persons of all races and income levels. Many researchers have found that persons in high income groups have longer life expectancies and enjoy better health than persons in low income groups (Feinstein 1993).

The Liu study contains detailed estimates of disability for males and females for five-year age groups. Although the likelihood of increased physical impairment and institutionalization increases with age, Liu and Manton state that the projections of health statistics in the table are conservative. Other statistical methods of estimating show "both longer overall life expectancy and greater proportions of life expectancy to be spent in active status."

The table shows that 65 percent of males who reach age 65 will reach age 75; 27 percent of males who reach age 75 will reach 85; and 3 percent of males who reach age 85 will reach age 95. In addition, the table shows that 93 percent of males who reach age 65 will not have any type of disability, while 7 percent will experience some type of disability. Not shown in the table, but included in the Liu study, are data showing that the 7 percent of males that reach age 65 who will experience disability include persons in six categories: light physical impairment and early dementia (1 percent); light impairment and early cardiopulmonary problems (1 percent); cardiopulmonary and moderate physical impairment (1 percent); hip fracture, moderate physical impairment and self-care needs (2 percent); the highly frail (2 percent); and persons who are institutionalized (1 percent).

The table also shows that males at age 65 are estimated to have an average of 14.3 years of remaining life, with 12.0 years expected to be lived in a non-disabled condition.

Estimates of Life Expectancy and Disability
Males and Females Who Reach Age 65

Age	Percent surviving	Percent non-chronically disabled	Remaining life expectancy	Expected years of life, non-chronically disabled
Males				
65	100.0%	93%	14.3	12.0
75	65.0%	88%	9.2	6.9
85	26.8%	68%	5.2	3.0
95	3.1%	48%	3.1	1.6
Females				
65	100.0%	91%	18.4	13.5
75	79.4%	82%	11.8	7.0
85	46.4%	51%	6.3	2.3
95	9.1%	21%	3.5	.8

Rounding prevents the percentages from totaling to exactly 100%

Source: Liu, K., K.G. Manton and B.M. Liu. "Morbidity, Disability, and Long-term Care of the Elderly: Implications for Insurance Financing." *The Milbank Quarterly*, Vol. 68., No. 3, 1990. Reprinted with permission from the Milbank Quarterly.

NURSING HOME USE AFTER AGE 65

The federal Agency for Health Care Policy and Research in the Public Health Service conducted a study that estimated nursing home use (Kemper, Murtaugh and Spillman 1991). The survey data was based on interviews with the next of kin of 9,181 persons who were at least 65 years of age when they died. The study used data from 1986.

The following table from the Kemper study indicates that men who reach age 65 spent an average of 0.69 years (about 8 months) in nursing homes, while women spent an average of 1.66 years (about 20 months) in nursing homes. Other findings include:

- The longer a person lives, the greater the time spent in a nursing home. Persons who die between ages 65 and 70 spend, on average, 0.1 year (slightly over a month) in a nursing homes, persons who live past age 95 spend 3.3 years there.
- Those in good health will spend more time in nursing homes, on average, than persons in poor health; this is because persons in poor health die sooner.
- Persons with serious medical conditions at age 65 (except for men who have had a stroke), heavy smokers, heavy drinkers, women who are obese, and persons with walking limitations at age 65, on average, use less nursing home care and die sooner than the general population.
- Nursing home use is lower in Florida than the national average.

Mean Years of Remaining Lifetime Nursing Home Use and Survival after Age 65 by Health and Functional Limitations at Age 65 National Data

| | Men | | Women | |
	Nursing home use	Survival	Nursing home use	Survival
All Persons[1]	.69	15.5	1.66	19.7
Medical Conditions				
Cancer	.10	4.7	.76	8.4
Diabetes	.43	9.5	.83	9.7
Heart Attack	.26	9.7	.80	12.8
Lung Condition[2]	.45	10.5	.80	13.0
Stroke	.85	9.1	1.24	13.5
Life Style				
Heavy Smoker[3]	.39	11.5	.68	10.8
Heavy Drinker[4]	.50	10.4	.97	11.0
Obese[5]	1.07	12.5	1.09	15.3
Functional Limitation				
Walking	.46	7.1	1.05	6.4
Activities of Daily Living[6]	.73	5.3	1.92	7.4

[1]For both sexes, the average time spent in nursing homes for persons at age 65 in Florida was .87 years compared with 1.22 years nationally.

[2]Persons with emphysema or chronic obstructive pulmonary disease.

[3]Persons smoking at age 65 who smoked 25 or more cigarettes a day when the smoked the most.

[4]Persons who consumed, on average, 4 or more drinks per day.

[5]Persons 50 percent or more above their ideal body mass based on usual adult weight and height.

[6]Activities of daily living include eating, toileting, dressing, and bathing.

Note: Persons can be in multiple categories.

Source: Kemper, P., C.M. Murtaugh and B.C. Spillman. (1991, June) "Nursing Home Use After Age 65 in the United States: Differences in Remaining Lifetime Use Among Subgroups and States." Rockville, MD: Agency for Health Care Policy and Research, Public Health Service.

Another article by Kemper and Murtaugh on nursing home use was published in *The New England Journal of Medicine* (Kemper and Murtaugh 1991). This article contained estimates on the projected use of nursing homes by persons who reached 65 years of age in 1990. Kemper and Murtaugh projected that 33 percent of males and 52 percent of females who reached the age of 65 in 1990 will spend some time in a nursing home before they die. The authors write that, "Those who incur extremely high nursing home costs will be predominantly women. Almost 8 of 10 persons using at least five years of nursing home care will be women." The table below was derived from the Kemper and Murtaugh article:

**Projected Nursing Home Use for Persons
Who Reached 65 Years of Age in 1990
National Data**

Time in nursing home	Men	Women
Any admission	33%	52%
3 months or more	22%	41%
1 year or more	14%	31%
5 years or more	4%	13%

Source: Kemper, Peter and C. M. Murtaugh. "Lifetime Use of Nursing Home Care." *The New England Journal of Medicine.* Vol. 324, No. 9 (February 28, 1991). Reprinted, by permission of the *New England Journal of Medicine.*

The statistical probabilities reported in the Kemper study were derived from a large national sample. Some of the factors that influence whether or not an individual enters a nursing home include:
- Personal health status (genetics, lifestyle habits, and environmental factors).
- Extent of functional disability and intensity of impairment. The likelihood of nursing home use increases as impairment with activities of daily living increases.
- The availability of a family member or other informal caregiver to provide care.
- The amount of personal financial resources which, if sufficient, could be used for private duty nursing in the home or in another setting.

AGING

The most comprehensive study of aging ever undertaken in the United States, the Baltimore Longitudinal Study of Aging, began more than 30 years ago with 1,800 participants. About 1,000 men and women are now participating in the on-going study to better understand the dynamics of aging. Every two years participants spend two and one-half days undergoing a battery of extensive physical and mental examinations.

Scientists are learning that aging, by itself, has a small impact on mortality. According to Nathan W. Shock, M.D., the former scientific director of the National Institute on Aging, "The things that get you are those darned diseases." (National Institutes of Health 1989). Baltimore study researchers have found that:

- Aging is not a disease. Aging does not cause a general decline in physical and psychological functions.
- People age differently, even organs within an individual have different rates of decline, and there is no "single, simple pattern of aging."
- Changes occur gradually with age. Researchers found that, "Any unusual change in physical and/or psychological abilities is more likely to be due to disease that to age."
- Our personalities remain relatively stable throughout life. People do not become "mellow" or "grouchy" as a result of aging. People who were cheerful when young remain so, and those who were grouchy when young are grouchy when they are old.
- Mental performance may be even more important than physical ability in determining longevity. The Baltimore study found that men in their 70s who remained proficient at problem solving tended to live longer. Other studies also have found a relationship between mental performance and longevity.

The Baltimore findings, and findings from other studies, suggest that diet is important in preventing disease. Men who died of heart disease ate less fiber and more saturated fat than men without heart disease. Men who did not have colon polyps ate more carbohydrates and fiber and drank less alcohol than men who developed colon polyps. The Dietary Guidelines for Americans, published by the U.S. Department of Agriculture and the U.S. Department of Health and Human Services, recommend diets low in saturated fat and cholesterol; that diets include plenty of vegetables, fruits and grain products; and that sugars, salt and sodium be used only in moderation.

In addition to diet, many researchers point to the need to "use it or loose it." This adage applies to both the body and the mind. Numerous studies have found that regular exercise yields substantial health benefits. Researchers also have found that persons who continue to challenge themselves mentally tend to be sharper than those who don't.

The concluding message of the Baltimore study is:

> *"Live the years of your life with vigor and exuberance, and the chances are you will enjoy your golden years."*

A very interesting study of the oldest of the old, the *Georgia Centenarian Study*, examined demographic, personality, health, mental health, nutritional, social, and other characteristics of persons who reached the age of 100 years (Poon et al. 1992, Poon et al. 1992, Martin et al. 1992 and Johnson et al. 1992). The *Georgia Centenarian Study* included 88 persons in each of three age groups: over 100 years old, between 80 and 89, and between 60 and 70. Participants were randomly selected to reflect the sex and racial characteristics of residents of Georgia for each age group. All were cognitively intact and were either self-sufficient or partially self-sufficient and living at home or in other non-institutional settings.

About one in 10,000 people lives to be a centenarian, and only 38 percent of centenarians "maintain some level of independence by living in their own homes and within their community." The authors noted that the centenarians in the study included "a number of extraordinary persons who write, publish, perform musically, give daily guided tours of a historical landmark, invest in the stock market, earn a living, and manipulate the environment in the face of poor support systems." Among the centenarians studied, a large number stated that throughout their lives they had "rarely been sick." Alcohol consumption was very low.

The study found that centenarians, compared to the other age groups in the study, "Consumed breakfast more regularly, avoided weight loss diets and large fluctuations in body weight, [and] consumed slightly more vegetables." Younger age groups were found more likely to eat diets that conform to nutritional standards. Centenarians were found less likely to eat diets low in fat, possibly because they ate the same foods they did when they were younger, before nutritional standards were widely publicized. The results of personality tests indicated that centenarians, compared with other age groups, scored higher on dominance, suspiciousness, and imagination and lower on intelligence, emotional stability, and conformity.

The cognitive findings are perhaps the most interesting. Although centenarians performed lower on intelligence and memory tests, "When cognitive activities were dependent on everyday experiences, no age-related problem-solving decline was found." The authors also found that cognitive performance increased with physical health, and that persons with higher fluid intelligence, and those who were less depressed, were the most successful in maintaining independence. The authors concluded that, "Cognitive resources are important contributors to the successful adaptation of the oldest-old."

The National Institute of Aging has published an excellent summary of research on the genetic, biochemical, and physiological processes of aging (NIH 1993). Researchers believe that humans may have a maximum life span of 120 years. A Japanese man, Shirechiyo Izumi is believed to be the person who has lived the longest, reaching the age of 120 years and 237 days when he died in 1986. Researchers believe that genetics, lifestyle, and environment all affect how long we live. Maintaining a strong immune system, adequate nutrition, and exercise are thought to be important factors. Studies of laboratory animals have shown that a restricted calorie, nutritionally-complete diet can significantly extend life.

The following general statements about normal aging are reprinted almost verbatim from the NIH publication "In Search of the Secrets of Aging." The National Institute on Aging cautions that the statements below do not apply to all people.

Heart—It grows slightly with age. Maximal oxygen consumption during exercise declines in men by about 10 percent with each decade of adult life and in women, by about 7.5 percent. However cardiac output stays nearly the same as the heart pumps more efficiently.

Lungs—Maximum breathing (vital) capacity may decline by about 40 percent between the ages of 20 and 70.

Brain—With age, the brain loses some cells (neurons) and others become damaged. However, it adapts by increasing the number of connections between cells (synapses) and by regrowing the branch-like extensions, dendrites and axons, that carry messages in the brain.

Kidneys—They gradually become less efficient at extracting wastes from the blood. Bladder capacity declines. Urinary incontinence, which may occur after tissues atrophy, often can be managed through exercise and behavioral techniques.

Body fat—The body does not lose fat with age but redistributes it from just under the skin to deeper parts of the body. Women are more likely to store it in the Hips and thighs and men in the abdominal area.

Muscles—Without exercise, estimated muscle mass declines 22 percent for women and 23 percent for men between the ages of 30 and 70. Exercise can prevent this loss.

Sight—Difficulty focusing close up may begin in the 40s; the ability to distinguish fine details may begin to decline in the 70s. From 50 on, there is increased susceptibility to glare, greater difficulty in seeing at low levels of illumination, and more difficulty in detecting moving targets.

Hearing—It becomes more difficult to hear higher frequencies with age. Hearing declines more quickly in men than in women.

Personality—After about age 30, personality is stable. Sudden changes in personality sometimes suggest disease processes.

Source: "In Search of the Secrets of Aging" National Institutes of Health. NIH Publication No. 93-2756. (May 1993). This publication is free and may be obtained by calling:

National Institute on Aging
Information Center
(800) 222-4225

THE YEAR BEFORE DEATH

An article in the *American Journal of Public Health* examined 5,582 persons who died during 1986 to determine how well people functioned during the last 12 months of life (Lentzner et al. 1992). The Lentzner study confirmed findings from other studies that found differences between the functional status of males and females before death. Males have shorter life expectancies and are less likely than females to have functional impairments before death. Lentzner found that:

- "In the last year of life, women were about 40 percent less likely than men to have been fully functional and 70 percent more likely to have been severely restricted;"
- During their last year of life, 15 percent of persons who died between age 65 and 74 had trouble knowing where they were, 13 percent had trouble remembering the year, and 10 percent had trouble recognizing family or good friends;
- Persons with a history of stroke were more likely to be severely restricted in their last year of life; and
- At age 85 and over, 9.8 percent of men and 4 percent of women were fully functional during their last year of life.

The table below is from the Lentzner study. It shows that 23.9 percent of men between the ages of 65 and 74 are fully functional while only 1.8 percent are severely restricted. The remaining 74.3 percent of males fall between being fully functional and severely restricted, with many needing help with eating or bathing.

Functional Status During Last 12 Months of Life
By Age at Death
1986 National Data

	65–74	75–84	85+
Men			
Fully functional	23.9%	16.7%	9.8%
Severely restricted	1.8%	5.6%	12.8%
Women			
Fully functional	16.5%	12.7%	4.0%
Severely restricted	4.2%	12.5%	25.8%
Both Sexes			
Needed help with eating	30.9%	36.6%	48.5%
Needed help with bathing	49.6%	59.4%	78.3%
Difficulty knowing where they were	14.5%	24.6%	39.8%

Source: Lentzner et al. "The Quality of Life in the Year Before Death." *American Journal of Public Health.* Vol. 82, No. 8 (August 1992).

Another National Institute on Aging study examined the deaths of people in Fairfield County, Connecticut (Brock and Foley 1985, 1988). This study found that:
- 40 percent died in their sleep (data were not available for 13 percent).
- 53 percent were free of pain on the day before they died (data were not available for 17 percent).
- 38 percent died in a hospital; 38 percent died in a private residence; and 23 percent died in a nursing home.
- On the day before they died, 13 percent could walk, 28 percent could feed themselves, 51 percent knew who and where they were, and 43 percent could both see and hear.
- One month before they died, 30 percent could walk, 63 percent could feed themselves; 78 percent knew who and where they were, and 77 percent could both see and hear.
- One year before they died, 59 percent could walk, 85 percent could feed themselves, 87 percent knew who and where they were, and 88 percent could both see and hear.

LIVING WILLS AND FINAL DECISIONS

If you become incapacitated and cannot speak for yourself and you want to direct the medical care you receive, it is important to prepare an advance medical directive. There are two types of advance medical directives: living wills, and written instructions that designate a health care surrogate of the person who will represent you when you can no longer speak for yourself.

To have the peace of mind of knowing that your intensely personal instructions will be honored, it is *absolutely vital* that you express your views clearly and completely in your living will and or that you discuss your views clearly and completely with your health care surrogate. The best time to prepare an advance medical directive is before you face admission to a hospital or nursing home, not when you are experiencing the anxiety and stress and disorientation that may accompany a severe illness.

Life-sustaining treatment in hospitals

A recent study publish in the *American Journal of Public Health* examined the views of physicians and nurses regarding life-sustaining treatments near the end of life (Solomon et al. 1993). The study surveyed 687 physicians and 759 nurses who worked in five hospitals located in Massachusetts, Georgia, Washington, D.C., and California.
- Almost half of the professionals surveyed reported that they "had acted against their conscience in providing care to terminally ill."
- Four times as many health professionals were concerned about over-treatment as those concerned about under-treatment (55 percent versus 12 percent)
- The treatments that were most frequently cited as being inappropriate for terminally ill patients were mechanical ventilation, cardiopulmonary resuscitation, artificial nutrition and hydration (food and water), and dialysis.
- A large majority (87 percent) of the health professionals believed that, "All competent patients, even if they are not considered terminally ill, have the right to refuse life support even if that refusal may lead to death."
- Eighty-seven percent also believed that "To allow patients to die by foregoing or stopping treatment is ethically different from assisting in their suicide."

The study concluded that "Many physicians and nurses were disturbed by the degree to which technological solutions influence care during the final days of a terminal illness and by the under-treatment of pain." An editorial accompanying the Soloman study contained an eloquent and poignant statement on the emotional, ethical, medical, and legal aspects of withdrawing life support (Dubler 1993):

> *"Removing life supports and permitting death is traumatic for some care-givers and alien to all. It demands a reexamination of the goals of care, an admission of the failure of medical science to forestall mortality, and an elevation of the patient's autonomy and legal right to refuse treatment over caregivers' notions of beneficence."*

Federal law—the patient self-determination act

The federal Patient Self-Determination Act took effect in 1991. The law requires hospitals, nursing homes, and certain other health care facilities to provide patients with written information regarding state law pertaining to living wills and advance directives at the time of enrollment or admission. Religious health care facilities may receive a "conscientious objection" exemption, although they are required to inform patients of their policies regarding advance medical directives.

Because neither state or federal law requires health care facilities to use a standard advance medical directive, many are in use. Thus, it is important to make sure that the advance medical directive you wish to use will be honored by your physician and the health care facility that you choose.

Florida law and the *Browning* decision

A state law was enacted in 1992 in response to the Florida Supreme Court's landmark *Guardianship of Estelle M. Browning* decision. The Browning decision can be found in *West's Florida Cases*, 567 So.2d on page 4. *West's Florida Cases* is a standard legal reference that is found in courthouse and other law libraries. The 1992 law, which is found in Chapter 765.1 through 765.4, *Florida Statutes*, states that:

- All adults have a fundamental right of self-determination regarding health care decisions, including the right to choose or refuse medical treatment;
- You may complete a Living Will to direct the provision, withholding, or with-drawal of life-prolonging procedures if you have a terminal illness or are in a permanent vegetative state; and
- You may designate another person—a health care "surrogate"—to make treatment decisions for you if you become incompetent and unable to make decisions for yourself.

The *Browning* decision states that every competent adult has the right to "choose or refuse medical treatment, and that right extends to all relevant decisions concerning one's health." According to *Browning*, this includes the right to refuse all types of medical treatment, both major and minor, and to refuse all types of life-sustaining or life-prolonging measures, including food and water.

The court said, "We are hopeful that this decision will encourage those who want their wishes to be followed to express their wishes clearly and completely." Preparing a living will is the best way to express your wishes "clearly and completely." The court also stated, however, that instructions regarding medical treatment can be verbal. If you make a verbal declaration, it should be witnessed. In addition, it also is important to discuss the content of your living will with your physician, with those close to you, and with a representative of the facility where you are likely to spend your final days.

If you leave a living will with instructions regarding life-sustaining treatment, these instructions must be followed by a health care surrogate. A surrogate may be a personal friend, family member, or legal guardian. In addition, it is important to designate an alternate health care surrogate, should your primary surrogate be unable to act in your behalf. *Browning* states that,

> *"The surrogate must make the medical choice that the patient, if competent, would have made, and not one that the surrogate might make for himself or herself, or that the surrogate might think is in the patient's best interest."*

The new Florida law does not mention artificial nutrition and hydration (food and water). The *Browning* decision, however, states that there is no legal distinction between supplying food and water through a feeding tube and other means of artificial life-support, such as being connected to a ventilator. If you do not want food and water, it is important to specifically state this in your living will and to state it verbally to your surrogate and your physician.

Copies of your living will should be given to family members, to your physician for placement in your medical record, and to your surrogate health care decision-maker. You can always modify your medical directive whenever you want, but remember to update all copies of the older version.

ADVANCE MEDICAL DIRECTIVE CHECKLIST

—Is your living will sufficiently detailed with regard to what life-prolonging procedures and other medical care you want, including nutrition and hydration (food and water)?

—Does your living will clearly describe the circumstances under which you want your directives to apply?

—Does your living will include a clear and complete personal statement?

—Did you discuss the content of your living will with your physician, medical surrogate, family, and medical facility?

—Was the living will properly witnessed? Florida requires that a both a Living Will and a document designating a health care surrogate be signed in the presence of two witnesses, one of whom can not be a spouse or blood relative.

—Did you give copies to your physician, surrogate, and to others important to you?

Sources of information on advance directives

A suggested form for a living will appears in Chapter 765.303, Florida Statues, as a "Suggested Form of a Living Will" for persons with a terminal condition. The chair of the Florida Bar's health law section stated that the statutory living will should "work in about 80 percent of the cases. It doesn't cover everybody every time," (Cutter, 1993). Unlike the Harvard Medical Directive, Florida's "suggested" living will is simply constructed.

The best advance directives are the most comprehensive and most detailed, such as the one published by the Harvard Medical School. The Harvard advance medical directive governs the extent of medical treatment in four different situations. In each of the four situations you indicate if you want medical treatment such as cardiopulmonary resuscitation, mechanical breathing, surgery, antibiotics, diagnostic testing, pain medications, and artificial nutrition and hydration (food and water). The Harvard directive is discussed in detail in "The Medical Directive" by Linda L. Emanuel and Ezekiel J. Emanuel, published in the *Journal of the American Medical Association*, Vol. 261, No. 22 (June 9, 1989).

The Harvard advance directive is easy to complete and includes provisions for a durable power of attorney, organ donation, and for a personal statement. Two copies of the advance directive are available for $5 from:

Advance Medical Directive
Harvard Medical School
Health Publications Group
164 Longwood Avenue, 4th Floor
Boston, MA 02115.

Single copies of the following publications on advance directives are available at no charge:

The Patient Self-Determination Directory and Resource Guide
National Health Lawyers Association, Development Office
1620 Eye Street, N.W., Suite 900,
Washington, D.C. 20006

A Matter of Choice: Planing Ahead for Health Care Decisions
Publication Number D12776
AARP Fulfillment Division
1909 K Street, N.W.
Washington, D.C. 20049.

Health Care Powers of Attorney
Publication Number D13895
AARP Fulfillment Division
1909 K Street, N.W.
Washington, D.C. 20049.

Advance Medical Directives for Patients
American Medical Association
Order #NC634492BN
(800) 621-8335

A national organization, Concern for Dying, publishes a newsletter and makes available publications on living wills and refusing life-sustaining treatment.

Concern for Dying
250 West 57th Street
New York, New York 10107
(212) 246-6962

Euthanasia and assisted suicide

The concept of euthanasia, or "mercy killing," is a very controversial and difficult subject. Numerous writers have written on its ethical and philosophical aspects (see Brody 1992; Quill 1993; and Caine and Conwell 1993). Others have proposed criteria for physician assisted suicide (Quill, Cassel and Meier 1992).

A report by the Council on Ethical and Judicial Affairs of the American Medical Association (AMA) defines euthanasia as, "The act of bringing about the death of a hopelessly ill and suffering person in a relatively quick and painless way for reasons of mercy" (Council on Ethical and Judicial Affairs 1992). The withholding or withdrawal of life-prolonging or life-sustaining treatment is not euthanasia.

Neither Florida nor any other state permits euthanasia or mercy killing. However, despite overwhelming legal and institutional opposition, public support for euthanasia has increased. A study conducted by Harvard University researchers and the *Boston*

Globe published in the *Journal of the American Medical Association* (Blendon, Szalay and Knox 1992) found that the percentage of Americans who "thought physicians should be allowed to end the lives of patients with incurable diseases if they and their families requested it" increased from 34 percent in 1950 to 63 percent in 1991. Despite this finding, voters in both Washington and California recently have defeated proposals to legalize euthanasia.

Assisted suicide, like euthanasia, is opposed by the American Medical Association (AMA) and numerous other organizations. According to the AMA, "Assisted suicide occurs when a physician facilitates a patient's death by providing the necessary means and/or information to enable the patient to perform the life-ending act." Florida law states that a person who deliberately assists in a suicide is guilty of manslaughter, a second degree felony.

The AMA report reflects concern in the medical profession over the issues of euthanasia and assisted suicide. The council states that,

> *"Physicians must not perform euthanasia or participate in assisted suicide. A more careful examination of the issue is necessary. Support, comfort, respect for patient autonomy, good communication, and adequate pain control may decrease dramatically the demand for euthanasia and assisted suicide. In certain carefully defined circumstances, it would be humane to recognize that death is certain and suffering is great. However, the societal risks of involving physicians in medical interventions to cause patients' deaths is too great in this culture to condone euthanasia or physician-assisted suicide at this time,"* (Council on Ethical and Judicial Affairs, 1992).

CHAPTER 10
Environmental health care problems

Florida's environment poses a unique mix of health hazards. Residents face hazards related to ocean creatures, reptiles, insects, heat and exposure to the sun's ultraviolet radiation. Florida's Poison Information Center and the National Cancer Institute are two excellent sources of information on the prevention and treatment of health care problems that result from environmental factors.

POISONS IN FLORIDA'S ENVIRONMENT AND THE FLORIDA POISON INFORMATION CENTER

Two Florida teaching hospitals, Tampa General Hospital in Tampa and University Medical Center in Jacksonville, jointly staff the Florida Poison Information Center. The center responds to telephone requests for information on poisons 24 hours a day, seven days a week. Both hospitals share the same (800) telephone number. Persons who live in the (904) area code are served by staff at the University Medical Center in Jacksonville and those who live in the (305), (407), and (813) area codes are served by staff at Tampa General Hospital.

The Florida Poison Information Center can provide life-saving medical advice in the event of insect, reptile, marine, plant, or other poisonings. It also provides information on poison prevention.

Florida Poison Information Center
Information and Medical Emergencies
24 hours a day, 7 days a week
(800) 282-3171

Marine life

Certain marine life can be very dangerous. The following information is from a publication prepared by the Florida Poison Information Center in Jacksonville.

- Portuguese man-of-war (jellyfish) skin eruptions should be soaked with vinegar until pain is relieved or baking soda (mixed with water to form a paste) should be rubbed over the affected area. Seek medical attention because allergic symptoms can develop quickly. Don't touch dead jelly fish on the beach, the poisons can remain active for weeks, even months if tentacles stay moist.
- Sea nettles are a smaller and less dangerous jelly fish that cause skin eruptions. If symptoms progress to nausea, aching muscles, or drowsiness, seek medical attention.
- If stung by a sting ray, irrigate the wound immediately with cold water to dilute the venom. Then soak the injured area in hot, but not scalding, water to relieve pain. Seek medical attention as soon as possible to reduce the risk of infection and to possibly remove remnants of the sting ray's barb.

- Catfish have poison in the skin and under the fins. Symptoms of catfish poisoning may include intense throbbing or scalding pain spreading upward from the wounds and lasting from 30 to 60 minutes. The affected area swells quickly and is easily infected. Muscle spasms usually follow and victims may also experience fainting, decreased heart rate, and slowed breathing. Immerse the wound immediately in hot, but not scalding, water for thirty minutes to an hour and a half.

SEABATHER'S ERUPTION

Jellyfish larvae are believed to be responsible for another marine hazard, seabather's eruption (SE), an intensely itchy skin eruption which is commonly (and inaccurately) believed to result from 'sea lice.' An article in the *Journal of the American Medical Association*, has attributed SE to the tiny larvae of the jellyfish, *Linuche unguiculata* (Tomchik et al. 1993).

Linuche unguiculata is also known as 'thimble jellyfish,' a cnidarian. Adults are brown in color and between 5 and 20 millimeters in length (about 3/16ths to slightly more than 3/4ths of an inch). According to the Tomchik article, the larvae are invisible, but have been reported to "cluster" in "clouds" by lifeguards who experience immediate stinging when they swim. It is believed that the susceptibility to SE varies among individuals, and that prior sensitization may be a factor in subsequent exposure.

The Tomchik article states that SE is characterized by intense itchiness and small lesions that begin to occur 4 to 24 hours after swimming in the ocean. However, some persons may experience a "prickling" sensation, and develop lesions, while in the water. The skin eruptions are most commonly found on the skin underneath the swimsuit. The larvae pass through the fabric of the swimsuit and sting when they become trapped against the skin. Other symptoms commonly include "headaches, malaise, weakness, perspiration, fever, chills, diarrhea, muscle spasms, and arthralgias." In addition, children have been reported to experience high fevers and vomiting. Cases of conjunctivitis and urethritis have also been reported.

In an interview, Tomchik stated that the severity of cases varies tremendously and a physician should treat unusual and severe cases. Some persons may only experience a few lesions, others may be covered from head to toe. The skin eruptions usually last about three to five days before the problem disappears on its own. Applying vinegar to the area may help.

According to the authors, cases of SE began appearing in South Florida in 1981 after an absence of 25 years, and a "conservative" estimate is that more that 10,000 people in South Florida had a case of SE during 1992. Cases of SE have been reported between Stuart and Key West and in the Caribbean. The authors report that the peak time of the year to encounter the jellyfish larvae is between March and August and that May is the worst month for thimble jellyfish because this is when swarming and spawning are the most intense. "High incidence" areas are Palm Beach County, northern Broward County, and the Keys. The authors suggest these precautions to minimize SE:

- Note if lifeguards have posted warnings.
- Avoid swimming in 'high incidence' areas between April and July.
- Avoid swimming if there are adult 'thimble jellyfish" on the beach.
- Strong offshore (Easterly) winds are associated with outbreaks.
- Men should not wear T-shirts while swimming, and women may want to wear two-piece swim suits.
- Remove the swim suit as soon as possible after leaving the water and remove the suit before showering.
- Discard affected swimsuits. There have been reports of persons contacting SE from previously worn garments.

- Surfers, snorkelers, and divers may "minimize symptoms by wearing wet suits with restrictive cuffs."
- Children, persons with allergies, autoimmune disease, or other immune-mediated conditions "may be at risk for unusual or sever reactions." The authors caution that although these reactions are rare, "such persons may wish to exercise extra caution when engaging in ocean activities, particularly during outbreaks."

SKIN CANCER

Because of its proximity to the equator, and because many people enjoy outdoor activities, Florida is a particularly dangerous environment for skin cancer. According to a research report published by the National Cancer Institute (NCI), approximately 30 percent of people who live in southern states will develop nonmelanoma skin cancer sometime during their lives.

Skin cancer is the most prevalent type of cancer. Fortunately, according to the NCI, nearly all cases can be successfully cured if identified early and treated promptly.

Although exposure to the sun's ultraviolet radiation is the main cause of skin cancer, there are genetic factors that increase susceptibility to skin cancer. NCI states that individuals at highest risk live in sunny climates, have red or blond hair, blue or light-colored eyes, fair skin that tends to freckle or burn rather than tan.

Reducing exposure to the sun is the easiest and most effective way of lowering the risk of developing nonmelanoma skin cancer. The sooner exposure is reduced the better. This is because the effect of exposure to ultraviolet radiation from the sun is cumulative over one's lifetime. It is estimated that up to half of a person's lifetime sun exposure occurs before age 18. Because of the cumulative effect of sun exposure, most skin cancers begin after age 50.

To minimize the risk of developing skin cancer, the best strategy is to protect yourself from the sun's ultraviolet radiation. The NCI recommends the following strategies:

- Wear hats with wide brims.
- Wear long sleeve shirts and pants made of tightly woven fabric.
- Use sunscreens with an SPF (sun protection factor) of 15 or higher to help protect exposed skin. Even on overcast days, about 80 percent of the sun's UV radiation can reach earth. Sand and concrete can reflect from 10 percent to more than 50 percent of the sun's damaging rays. The better sunscreens help protect against two types of UV radiation, UVA and UVB.
- Avoid exposure to the midday sun (from 10 a.m. to 2 p.m.).

Persons taking photosensitizing medications and immunosuppressive therapy should check with their physician before tanning. Be aware that all evidence indicates that both natural and artificial sun tanning is harmful to the skin.

The NCI produces free publications on all types of cancer. Publications on skin cancer include, "*Skin Cancers, Basal Cell and Squamous Cell Carcinomas Research Report*" and "*What You Need to Known About Skin Cancer.*" To obtain free copies, telephone (800) 4-CANCER. The National Institutes of Health publishes a consensus statement on skin cancer, "*Sunlight, Ultraviolet Radiation, and the Skin*" (consensus statement #74). To obtain a copy, consult the National Institutes of Health Consensus Statement section in Chapter 1.

Many medications and other substances can cause increased skin sensitivity to sunlight. The harmful reactions that may occur can range from skin burn, premature aging, allergic reactions, and cataracts to cancer. These effects can be caused by creams or ointments applied to the skin, oral or injectable medications, or prescription inhalers.

Persons using such medications should ask their physician or pharmacist about possible photosensitizing effects before they spend extended amounts of time in Florida's sunshine (or in tanning booths). The Food and Drug Administration has produced a very useful pamphlet titled "Medications That Increase Sensitivity to Light" which lists many such agents (FDA Publication No. FDA 91-8280).

PRECAUTIONS IN HOT WEATHER

As one ages, it is increasingly important to take extra precautions in hot weather. According to the National Institute on Aging, this is because the body becomes less effective in cooling itself. Sweat glands work less efficiently, producing less perspiration. Perspiration is the way our body cools itself.

Hot weather poses special health risks for older people, the most serious of which is hyperthermia. Hyperthermia includes heat stroke and heat exhaustion. Heat stroke is a medical emergency that requires treatment by a physician. Symptoms include nausea, dizziness, confusion, lethargy, and coma. The symptoms of heat exhaustion include weakness, heavy sweating, nausea, and giddiness. Both problems can be avoided by taking proper precautions.

Some older persons are at an increased risk for hyperthermia, including people with chronic health problems, such as diabetes mellitus; those with heart, lung, and kidney diseases and people who take diuretics, sedatives, antidepressants, tranquilizers, anticholinergic drugs, antihistamines, drugs for Parkinson's disease, and heart and blood pressure medication.

The National Institute on Aging recommends that older persons take the following precautions during hot weather:
- Drink plenty of water and juices and avoid alcohol;
- Eat light, avoid heavy meals;
- Wear light, loose fitting clothing;
- Wear a hat or use an umbrella if out in the sun;
- Maintain your exercise program, but work out in a cool, practical way; and
- Use fans and air conditioners liberally.

For more information, the National Institute on Aging can be contacted at (800) 222-2225.

CHAPTER 11
Health insurance, accreditation, information resources

PUBLIC AND PRIVATE HEALTH INSURANCE

Medicare

The Medicare program covers most people age 65 years of age and older and some disabled persons. Medicare enrollment is automatic when you apply for Social Security.

There are two "parts" to Medicare coverage. Part "A" covers most, but not all, of the costs for hospital inpatient care, nursing home care (with certain limitations), home health care, and hospice care. Part "B" covers other health care services, including physician care. Prescriptions are not covered at this time.

Most people do not have to pay a premium for Part A coverage because they worked for at least ten years under Social Security, worked as a government employee, or were covered under railroad retirement. Persons not eligible for premium free coverage can contact Social Security to learn if they can purchase coverage.

Part A will pay for home health care if: a physician determines that the patient needs home health care; skilled nursing care, physical therapy, or speech therapy is prescribed by the physician; the patient is "homebound;" and care is provided by a Medicare-certified home health agency. Medicare does not pay for custodial care when this is the only care needed. Custodial care is care that can be provided by persons without professional skills or training that helps people with daily living activities, such as taking medications, bathing, dressing, and eating. Help with the activities of daily living may be covered, however, if one is eligible to receive home health care or hospice services.

In 1993, the Part A hospital deductible was $676 for each benefit period. There can be more than one benefit period during a year. A benefit period begins upon entry into a hospital or skilled nursing facility and ends 60 days after discharge. The daily hospital copayment for hospital stays beyond 60 days was $169 for days 61 to 90 and $338 per day for days 91 to 150.

The copayment for skilled nursing facility care during 1993 was $84.50 per day for days 21 to 100 (there is a 100 day cap on Medicare covered skilled nursing facility care). There was no copayment for the first 20 days.

"Part B" covers doctors' services and outpatient services, such as diagnostic tests. If you are eligible for Part A, you also are eligible for Part B, which requires a monthly premium. In 1993, the monthly premium was $36.60. Usually, this is deducted from Social Security checks. The annual deductible was $100.

To avoid late enrollment penalties, most people must enroll in Part B during a seven-month enrollment period that begins three months before the month you first become eligible for Medicare. The enrollment period is different for persons who continue to work and are covered under an employer plan.

All physicians who treat Medicare patients must follow guidelines regarding how much they may charge Medicare for their services. Physicians who accept Medicare assignment bill Medicare directly and accept the Medicare fee as payment in full. During 1993, physicians who did not accept Medicare assignment could charge no more that 115 percent of what Medicare allowed for the service. This means that if the Medicare fee limit was $100, the physician could not charge more than $115.

The Medicare Part B Customer Service Line answers questions regarding Part B and provides information on the status of claims, copies of Explanations of Medicare Benefits (EOMBs), and directories (called the MEDPARD directory) that lists physicians and other providers who participate in Medicare and physicians who accept Medicare assignment.

Medicare Part A Customer Service
(904) 355-8899

Medicare Part B Customer Full Service
(800) 333-7586

Medicare Part B Short Order Express
(touch tone claims information)
(800) 666-7586

The Medicare Telephone Hotline answers questions on Medigap insurance and Medicare. Callers may request the *Guide to Health Insurance for People with Medicare*, Publication No. HCFA-02110, which discusses Medigap insurance and "The Medicare Handbook" Publication No. HCFA 10050, which is a comprehensive guide to Medicare eligibility and benefits. Additional pamphlets available include *Medicare and Coordinated Care Plans, Medicare Hospice Benefits, Medicare and Employer Health Plans, Medicare Coverage for Second Surgical Opinions, and Medicare Savings for Qualified Beneficiaries* (the QMB program).

The Medicare QMB program, administered by HRS in Florida, helps persons with low-incomes pay for some or all of their Medicare co-payments and deductibles. The hot line also will provide local telephone numbers for Medicaid offices where QMB benefits may be applied for.

Medicare Telephone Hotline
Health Care Financing Administration
U.S. Department of Health and Human Services
(800) 638-6833

Free guides on Social Security, Medicare, and Supplemental Security Income (SSI) are available. *Medicare*, Publication No. SSA 05-10043, summarizes Medicare in easy to understand language. *SSI,* Publication No. SSA 05-11000, discusses Supplemental Security Income eligibility and benefits.

Medicare and Supplemental Security Income
Social Security Administration
(800) 772-1213

By calling the telephone number above, information also can be obtained on the Social Security program, including obtaining Social Security cards and statements of Social Security earnings.

Private health insurance

Purchasing private health insurance requires comparative shopping. Generally, the higher the co-payments and deductibles, the lower the premium. Key points to consider are:

- What services are covered by the policy?
- Are there limitations on coverages, such as a maximum number of hospital or nursing home days?
- Are any medical problems excluded from coverage, such as preexisting conditions?
- What are the renewal provisions? Can you renew automatically?
- What is the premium cost?
- What is the maximum cost for "out-of-pocket" expenses?

An excellent booklet on health insurance choices is available from the federal Agency for Health Care Policy Research. The booklet is for persons who don't have health insurance or for those who want to reexamine their current policies. The booklet includes discussions of health maintenance organizations (HMOs) and traditional private insurance policies, shopping tips, a self-quiz, a checklist for important services, important questions to ask, and a work sheet for evaluating the best buy. The booklet, *Checkup on Health Insurance Choices* (AHCPR Publication Number 92-0091) is available at no charge from:

The Agency for Health Care Policy Research
Publications Clearinghouse
P.O. Box 8547
Silver Spring, MD 20907
(800) 358-9295

The Florida Department of Insurance publishes a guide on health insurance that provides tips on how to select health insurance policies. The department also publishes a guide on "Medigap" policies. Comparative shopping is important in this area as well. Contact the Florida Department of Insurance at:

Florida Department of Insurance Help-Line
(800) 342-2762

The National Insurance Consumer Helpline is sponsored by private health insurance companies and helps consumers with questions on health, life and auto insurance. The National Insurance Consumer Helpline can be reached at:

National Insurance Consumer Helpline
(800) 942-4242

Brochures and general information on health insurance also are available from the Health Insurance Association of America (HIAA). The association represents private health insurance companies. Publications available from the HIAA include *The Consumer's Guide to Medicare Supplement Insurance*, *The Consumer's Guide to Disability Insurance*, and *The Consumer's Guide to Long-Term Care Insurance*.

Health Insurance Association of America
PO Box 41455
Washington, D.C. 20018
(800) 635-1271

Long-term care insurance

The United Seniors Health Cooperative publishes "Long Term Care: A Dollar and Sense Guide," available for $10. The guide contains descriptions of what Medicare and Medicaid will pay for and suggestions on how to determine if the purchase of long-term care insurance makes financial sense. A more comprehensive publication, "Long-Term Care Insurance: Professional's Guide to Selecting Policies," is available for $36.50, including postage.

United Seniors Health Cooperative
1331 H Street, N.W., Suite 500
Washington, D.C. 20005

A copy of, *Before You Buy—A Guide to Long-Term Care Insurance*, is available for free from the American Association of Retired Persons (AARP). The AARP also will send a copy of *Resources to Go*, a free listing of consumer publications.

AARP Program Department
601 E Street, N.W.
Washington, D.C. 20049
(800) 523-5800
(202) 434-2277

Consumer Reports published an article in June 1991 on long-term care insurance, "An Empty Promise to the Elderly?" This article is available in many public libraries or can be ordered for $3 from:

Consumer Reports Reprints
101 Truman Avenue
Yonkers, New York 10703-1057

To obtain a survey that compares long-term care policies offered by several large insurance companies, send a large self-addressed envelope stamped with 75 cents postage to:

The National Association of Life Underwriters
Dept. PR-SP
1922 F Street, N.W.
Washington, D.C. 20006

The Florida Department of Insurance publishes an excellent consumer guide that describes long-term care insurance in detail. The guide contains a series of questions you should ask in selecting a policy and lists companies licensed to sell long-term care insurance in Florida. The department also maintains a toll-free Insurance Consumer Hotline to answer questions about health insurance, long-term care insurance, and other types of insurance. To request a free copy of the Long-Term Care Insurance Consumers' Guide, contact:

Long-Term Care Insurance Consumers' Guide
Florida Department of Insurance
The Capitol, LL25
Tallahassee, FL 32399-0300
Hotline: (800) 342-2762

Medigap insurance

"Medigap" insurance pays for health care services that are not covered by Medicare—it fills the "gaps" in Medicare coverage. Medigap policies pay for deductibles and coinsurance, medically necessary emergency care in foreign countries, prescription drugs, preventive care, and other services.

In 1992 a federal law became effective that standardized and simplified Medigap insurance. Insurance companies can offer up to ten different types of standardized Medigap policies. The law also guarantees that you can purchase Medigap insurance, regardless of any health problems you may have, provided you purchase it within certain time periods.

After enrollment in Part B of Medicare, there is a six-month period to purchase Medigap supplemental coverage. Most people enroll in Medicare Part B when they turn 65 or during a seven-month enrollment period that begins three months before they turn 65. If you delay enrollment until after you reach 65 because you continue to work and are covered under an employer plan, your six-month Medigap enrollment period begins whenever your Part B coverage starts.

According to Medicare, if you are a member of a health maintenance organization (HMO) or other managed care plan that has a contract with Medicare, it is likely that you do not need Medigap insurance.

- The federal government publishes an excellent booklet that answers scores of questions on Medicare and Medigap. The *Guide to Health Insurance for People with Medicare*, Publication No. HCFA-02110, is free and can be ordered by calling the Medicare Hotline (discussed in the previous section on Medicare).
- The United Seniors Health Cooperative (see previous section on long-term care insurance) publishes a guide, *Managing Your Health Care Finances: Getting the Most Out of Medicare and "Medigap Insurance*, for $10.
- The Florida Department of Insurance Help-Line (see previous section on private health insurance) publishes a guide on Medigap insurance.
- The Health Insurance Association of America publishes the *Consumer's Guide to Medicare Supplement Insurance* (see previous section on Medigap).

Medicaid

Medicaid pays for health care services for certain low-income individuals. Coverage depends on:

- Eligibility for Aid to Families with Dependent Children and Supplemental Security Income; and
- Age and financial status of the elderly, pregnant women, children and certain persons with high out-of-pocket medical expenses whose families include children.

Specific information on Medicaid eligibility can be obtained from the Florida Department of Health and Rehabilitative Services. Consult the "government pages" of your local telephone directory. Look under "state government," then "Florida Department of Health and Rehabilitative Services," then "Economic Services," then "Medicaid" or "eligibility."

The federal Health Care Financing Administration (HCFA) publishes the *Medicaid Fact Sheet* a general information publication on the Medicaid program. For a free copy, write to:

Health Care Financing Administration
Office of Public Affairs
Room 403B Hubert H. Humphrey Building
200 Independence Avenue, S.W.
Washington, D.C.

ACCREDITATION ORGANIZATIONS

Although the authors of this book are unaware of any research that has shown that accredited health care facilities provide better care than those that are not accredited, accreditation does indicate that the provider has sought verification from independent, impartial experts that it meets staffing and other standards. The federal Office of Technology Assessment (OTA), an agency of the U.S. Congress, states that accredited facilities have been recognized by independent experts as having, "the appropriate resources to provide care, either overall or for specific conditions." Some health care experts believe, however, that accreditation is not a useful indicator of quality care. The inclusion of an accredited facility in this book does not constitute an endorsement of that facility either by the author or the publisher.

The Joint Commission on the Accreditation of Healthcare Organizations (JCAHO), the nation's largest health care accreditation organization, accredits hospitals, ambulatory care facilities, long-term care facilities, home health agencies, and mental health and substance abuse treatment facilities. JCAHO was founded in 1917 when a hospital standards program was created by the American College of Surgeons. In 1951, the hospital standards program became the Joint Commission on Accreditation of Hospitals, an independent nonprofit organization. In 1988, the organization changed its name to the Joint Commission on Accreditation of Healthcare Organizations.

According to the JCAHO, their mission is to "Improve the quality of health care provided to the public." Information from the JCAHO is available to anyone, including the accreditation history of a facility from the mid-1970s. Also available is the accreditation status of a facility which indicates if the facility is "Accredited with Commendation," "Accredited," or has a "Conditional" accreditation status. In addition, some facilities are denied accreditation.

The JCAHO also publishes a catalog that includes numerous publications that concern quality of care in hospitals and long-term care, ambulatory care, mental health services home care, and laboratory service providers.

The information in this book on the JCAHO accredited facilities was obtained from the JCAHO over a period of several months through several communications. Some facilities have incomplete data. It is the experience of the authors that large data bases are seldom free of errors. To obtain accreditation information, or to verify accreditation information, the JCAHO can be contacted at:

The Joint Commission on Accreditation of
Healthcare Organizations
One Renaissance Boulevard
Oakbrook Terrace, Illinois 60181
(708) 916-5800
(ask for the "Customer Service Center")

The Commission on Accreditation of Rehabilitation Facilities (CARF) accredits hospital comprehensive inpatient rehabilitation programs, spinal cord injury programs, chronic pain management programs, brain injury programs, outpatient medical rehabilitation programs, infant and early childhood developmental programs, residential services programs (supervised living, supported independent living, and family living programs), respite programs, independent living programs, alcoholism and other drug dependency rehabilitation programs, community mental health organizations, and psychosocial programs.

Commission on Accreditation of
Rehabilitation Facilities
101 North Wilmot Road, Suite 500
Tucson, Arizona 85711
(602) 748-1212

The Community Health Accreditation Program (CHAP) accredits home care agencies. CHAP has received financial assistance from the W.K. Kellogg Foundation to develop the first-ever consumer- oriented quality standards for home care. In addition, CHAP accredited home care agencies are deemed to be in compliance with Medicare standards.

Community Health Accreditation Program
350 Hudson Street
New York, New York 10014
(212) 989-9393

The Continuing Care Accreditation Commission is an independent accrediting commission sponsored by the American Association of Homes for the Aging. Accredited facilities must meet financial, health care, and other standards. To obtain a list of accredited continuing care communities, send a self-addressed stamped legal envelope to:

Continuing Care Accreditation Commission
901 E Street N.W., Suite 500
Washington, DC 20004-2037
(202) 783-7286

The Accreditation Association for Ambulatory Health Care accredits ambulatory and outpatient surgical centers (including eye surgery centers), physician offices, health maintenance organizations (HMOs), health clinics, and ambulatory health care programs.

Accreditation Association for
Ambulatory Health Care
9933 Lawler Avenue
Skokie, Illinois 60077-3702
(708) 676-9601

The National Committee for Quality Assurance (NCQA) was founded in 1979 as a nonprofit organization by the Group Health Association of America and the American Managed Care and Review Association. In 1990, NCQA became an independent organization, in part because of assistance provided by the Robert Wood Johnson Foundation. NCQA accredits managed care plans such as health maintenance organizations and independent practice associations. The mission statement of the NCQA states that, "NCQA's primary function is to develop and apply oversight processes and measures of performance for health plans. NCQA is committed to providing information on quality to the public, consumers, purchasers, health plans and other relevant parties."

NCQA has five categories of accreditation: full accreditation; accreditation with recommendations; provisional accreditation; denial/revocation of accreditation status; and deferral of accreditation review.

National Committee for Quality Assurance
1350 New York Ave, N.W., Suite 700
Washington, D.C. 20005
(202) 628-7788

The American Osteopathic Association accredits physicians and hospitals that practice osteopathy. See the "Osteopathic Hospital" section of Chapter 3 for a discussion of osteopathy.

American Osteopathic Association
142 East Ontario Street
Chicago, Il 60611
(800) 621-1773

LEGAL ADVICE

The Florida Bar's "Lawyer Referral Service" can be contacted to obtain the names of attorneys who specialize in continuing care contracts, advance medical directives, Medicare, social security, and other legal matters. The referral service gives the name of one attorney at time. However, persons can call back for the name of another attorney if they wish.

The Florida Bar
Lawyer Referral Service
(800) 342-8011

The American Association of Retired Persons, Legal Council for the Elderly, and Legal Services of Greater Miami have a toll free legal help line. Although there is a limit of one question per telephone call, persons may call again with a different question.

Elder Legal Hotline
(800) 252-5997

LOCAL HEALTH COUNCILS

Local health councils can be an excellent source of information on nursing homes, hospitals, adult congregate living facilities, and other health care providers. Florida has eleven local health councils which have nine staffs. One staff serves Districts 1 and 2 and another staff serves Districts 5 and 6. Hospitals, nursing homes, and other health care providers pay an annual assessment to support the councils. The councils are independent. Some local health councils publish nursing home and adult congregate living facility (ACLF) directories for their areas.

District 1—Escambia, Okaloosa, Santa Rosa, and Walton
District 2—Bay, Calhoun, Franklin, Gadsden, Gulf, Holmes, Jackson, Jefferson, Leon, Liberty, Madison, Taylor, Wakulla, and Washington

N.W. Florida and Big Bend Health Councils
2629 West Tenth Street
Panama City, FL 32401
(904) 872-4128

District 3—Alachua, Bradford, Citrus, Columbia, Dixie, Gilchrist, Hernando, Hamilton, Lafayette, Lake, Levy, Marion, Putnam, Sumter, Suwannee, and Union

North Central Florida Health Planning Council
11 West University Avenue, Suite 7
Gainesville, FL 32601
(904) 377-4404

District 4—Baker, Clay, Duval, Flagler, Nassau, St. Johns, and Volusia

Health Planning Council of Northeast Florida
2236 St. Johns Avenue
Jacksonville, FL 32204
(904) 381-6035

District 5—Pasco and Pinellas
District 6—Hardee, Highlands, Hillsborough, Manatee, and Polk

Health Council of Pasco-Pinellas/West Central Florida
9887 North Gandy Blvd., Suite 200
St. Petersburg, FL 33702-2451
(813) 576-7772

District 7—Brevard, Orange, Osceola, and Seminole

Local Health Council of East Central Florida
1155 S. Semoran Blvd., Suite 1137
Winter Park, FL 32792
(407) 671-2005

District 8—Charlotte, Collier, Glades, Desoto, Hendry, Lee, and Sarasota.

District Eight Health Council
12811 Kenwood Lane, Suite 203
Ft. Myers, FL 33907
(813) 278-7160

District 9—Indian River, Martin, Okeechobee, Palm Beach, and St. Lucie

District Nine Health Council
8895 N. Military Trail, Suite 300E
Palm Beach Gardens, FL 33401
(407) 624-1100

District 10—Broward

Broward Regional Health Planning Council
915 Middle River Drive, Suite 309
Fort Lauderdale, FL 33304
(305) 561-9681

District 11—Dade and Monroe

Health Council of South Florida
5757 Blue Lagoon Drive, Suite 170
Miami, FL 33126
(305) 263-9020

AREA OFFICES OF HEALTH FACILITY REGULATION

These offices inspect and license health care facilities. They can be contacted to: verify the status of a hospital, nursing home, ACLF, home health care agency, birth center, hospice, ambulatory surgical center, or certain other health care facility license; or to file a complaint against a health care facility.

Area 1—Escambia, Okaloosa, Santa Rosa, Walton
Area Office 1
4900 Bayou Blvd., Suite 106
Pensacola, FL 32503
(904) 484-5120

Area 2—Bay, Calhoun, Franklin, Gadsden, Gulf, Holmes, Jackson, Jefferson, Leon, Liberty, Madison, Taylor, Wakulla, and Washington
Area Office 2
2727 Mahan Drive, Room 108
Tallahassee, FL 32308
(904) 922-6463

Area 3—Alachua, Bradford, Citrus, Columbia, Dixie, Gilchrist, Hernando, Hamilton, Lafayette, Lake, Levy, Marion, Putnam, Sumter, Suwannee, and Union
Area Office 3
5700 S.W. 34th Street, Suite 1120
Gainesville, FL 32608
(904) 336-3070

Area 4—Baker, Clay, Duval, Flagler, Nassau, St. Johns, and Volusia
Area Office 4
111 East Coastline Drive, Room 468
Jacksonville, FL 32231
(904) 359-6046

Area 5—Pasco and Pinellas
Area Office 5
877 Executive Center Drive, West
The Glades Building, Suite 201
St. Petersburg, FL 33702
(813) 570-5181

Area 6—Hardee, Highlands, Hillsborough, Manatee, and Polk
Area Office 6
7827 N. Dale Mabry Highway, Suite 100
Tampa, FL 33614
(813) 272-3440

Area 7—Brevard, Orange, Osceola, and Seminole
Area Office 7
400 West Robinson, Suite 309
Orlando, FL 32801
(407) 423-6830

Area 8—Charlotte, Collier, Glades, Desoto, Hendry, Lee, and Sarasota
Area Office 8
12381 S. Cleveland Avenue, Room 110
Ft. Myers, FL 33907
(813) 278-7221

Area 9—Indian River, Martin, Okeechobee, Palm Beach, and St. Lucie
Area Office 9
1199 W. Lantana Road, Room 201
Lantana, FL 33465
(407) 586-3071

Area 10—Broward
Area Office 10
3800 Inverrary Blvd., Suite 101
Lauderhill, FL 33319
(305) 497-3395

Area 11—Dade and Monroe
Area Office 11
401 N.W. 2nd Avenue, 526 North Tower
Miami, FL 33128
(305) 377-7100

NURSING HOME AND LONG-TERM CARE FACILITY OMBUDSMAN COUNCILS

The Statewide Nursing Home and Long-Term Care Facility Ombudsman Council receives, investigates, and resolves complaints made by or on behalf of persons who live in nursing homes and ACLFs.

The district councils may be contact to learn about complaints filed against nursing homes and ACLFs. Ask to speak with the District Ombudsman Council Coordinator. The District Ombudsman Council Coordinator will be able to tell you how many complaints they have received against a particular nursing home or ACLF, the types of complaints, and if the complaints were minor or serious.

The ombudsman program also acts as an advocacy program for persons who live in these facilities and recommends needed changes to the Florida Legislature.

District 1—Escambia, Okaloosa, Santa Rosa, Walton
District 1 Ombudsman Council
160 Government Center
Pensacola, FL 32505-8420
(904) 436-8243

District 2—Bay, Calhoun, Franklin, Gadsden, Gulf, Holmes, Jackson, Jefferson, Leon, Liberty, Madison, Taylor, Wakulla, and Washington
District 2 Ombudsman Council
2639 North Monroe Street, Suite 200-A
Tallahassee, FL 32303
(904) 488-9875

District 3-A—Alachua, Bradford, Columbia, Dixie, Gilchrist, Hamilton, Lafayette, Levy, Putnam, Suwannee, and Union
District 3-A Ombudsman Council
1000 N.E. 16th Avenue, Bldg. H.
Gainesville, FL 32609
(904) 336-5015

District 3-B—Citrus, Hernando, Lake, Marion, and Sumter
District 3-B Ombudsman Council
3001 W. Silver Springs Blvd., B-13
Ocala, Florida 34475
(904) 620-3088

District 4—Baker, Clay, Duval, Flagler, Nassau, St. Johns, and Volusia
District 4 Ombudsman Council
5920 Arlington Expressway
Jacksonville, FL 32231
(904) 723-2058 or (800) 342-9685

District 5—Pasco and Pinellas
District 5 Ombudsman Council
11351 Ulmerton Road, Suite 100
Largo, Florida 34648-1630
(813) 588-6912

District 6—Hardee, Highlands, Hillsborough, Manatee, and Polk
District 6 Ombudsman Council
8900 North Armenia Street, Suite 1
Tampa, FL 33604
(813) 935-7084

District 7—Brevard, Orange, Osceola, and Seminole counties.
District 7 Ombudsman Council
400 West Robinson Street, Suite 1129
Orlando, FL 32801
(407) 423-6114

District 8—Charlotte, Collier, Glades, Desoto, Hendry, Lee, and Sarasota
District 8 Ombudsman Council
PO Box 6085
Ft. Myers, FL 33906
(813) 338-1493

District 9—Indian River, Martin, Okeechobee, Palm Beach, and St. Lucie
District 9 Ombudsman Council
111 Georgia Avenue
West Palm Beach, FL 33401
(407) 837-5038

District 10—Broward
District 10 Ombudsman Council
3800 Inverrary Blvd., Suite 306, Room 24
Lauderhill, FL 33319
(305) 467-4223

District 11—Dade and Monroe
District 11 Ombudsman Council
1320 South Dixie Highway, 3rd Floor
Coral Gables, FL 33146
(305) 663-2085

Statewide Ombudsman
(800) 352-3463

SOURCES OF INFORMATION ON SERVICES FOR THE ELDERLY

Area Agencies on Aging are located in communities throughout the United States. These organizations either provide or contract for a wide range of services to the elderly. In Florida, each Area Agency on Aging has a local "Elder Helpline." In addition, there is also a national Eldercare Locator which can be called to obtain the telephone numbers of local agencies in other states.

Area Agencies on Aging

Each county in Florida is served by a regional Area Agency on Aging. These publicly supported agencies have an "Elder Helpline" in each county which can be called for help with home delivered meals, transportation, legal assistance, housing options, recreation and social activities, adult day care, senior center programs, and home health services.

In addition, the Elder Helplines can also be valuable sources of information on local health care providers, consumer protection matters, social security, Medicare, Medicaid, charitable organizations, employment, recreation, insurance, and other matters.

Florida Elder Helplines
Voice/TDD lines are marked with an asterisk (*)

Northwest Florida
Northwest Florida AAA
Gaslight Square
6706 N. 9th Avenue, Bldg. A, Suite 1
Pensacola, FL 32504-7398
(904) 484-5150

Escambia ....(904) 432-1475
Voice/TDD ....(904) 432-0891*
Okaloosa ....(904) 833-9165
Santa Rosa ....(904) 623-0467
Walton ....(904) 892-8168

North Florida
AAA of North Florida, Inc.
2639 N. Monroe St., Suite 145-B
Tallahassee, FL 32303
(904) 488-0055

Bay ....(904) 769-3468
Calhoun..............................(904) 674-4163
Franklin..............................(904) 697-3760
Gadsden ....(904) 627-2223
Gulf ....(904) 229-8466
Holmes ....(904) 547-2345
Jackson ....(904) 482-5028
Jefferson ....(904) 997-3418
Leon ....(904) 575-9694
Liberty ....(904) 643-5613
Madison ....(904) 973-2006
Taylor ....(904) 584-4924
Wakulla..............................(904)926-7145
Washington ....(904) 638-6216

Mid-Florida
Mid Florida AAA
5700 S.W. 34th Street, Suite 222
Gainesville, FL 32608
(904) 378-6649

The mid-Florida region has a separate helpline operated by the Center for Aging Resources; (800) 262-2243 (Florida) and (904) 375-1155 (out of state).

Alachua ....(904) 336-3822
Bradford ....(904) 964-3837
Citrus ....(904) 746-1844
Columbia ....(904) 752-8235
Dixie ....(904) 498-7910
Gilchrist ....(904) 463-7681
Hamilton ....(904) 792-2136
Hernando ....(904) 796-0485
Lafayette ....(904) 294-1172
Lake ....(904) 326-5304
Levy ....(904) 493-7546
Marion ....(904) 629-7407
Putnam ....(904) 329-8963
Sumter................................(904) 793-5234
Suwannee...........................(904) 364-5673
Union ....(904) 496-2342

Northeast Florida
Northeast Florida AAA
2257 Riverside Avenue
Jacksonville, FL 32203
(904) 388-6495

Baker .... (904) 259-2223
Clay
   Key Stone Heights .... (904) 473-2112
   Middleburg .... (904) 259-2223
Duval .... (904) 798-9503*
Flagler .... (904) 437-7300*
Nassau
   Fernandina Beach .... (904) 261-0701
   Hilliard .... (904) 845-3331
St. Johns .... (904) 824-1648
Volusia .... (904) 253-4700
   also .... (800) 544-8127

Tampa Bay
Tampa Bay Regional Planning Council
9455 Koger Blvd, Hendry Bldg.
St. Petersburg, FL 33702
(813) 577-5151 (St. Petersburg)
(813) 224-9380 (Tampa)

Pasco
   East .... (904) 567-1111*
   Central .... (813) 228-8686*
   West .... (813) 848-5555*
Pinellas .... (813) 531-4664*

West Central Florida
West Central Florida AAA
1419 W. Waters Avenue, Suite 114
Tampa, FL 33604
(800) 336-2226
(813) 933-5945

Hillsborough .... (813) 653-7709*
Highlands
   Avon Park .... (813) 452-1288
   Lake Placid .... (813) 465-1199
   Sebring .... (813) 382-1288
Hardee .... (813) 773-6880
Manatee .... (813) 749-7127
Polk .... (813) 533-0741

East Central Florida
East Central Florida Regional Planning
   Council
1011 Wymore Road, Suite 207
Winter Park, FL 32789
(407) 623-1075

Brevard .... (407) 631-2747
Osceola .... (407) 847-4357
Orange .... (407) 648-4357
Seminole .... (407) 831-4357

South Central Florida
South Central Florida AAA
1402 Jackson Street
Fort Myers, FL 33901
(813) 332-4233

Charlotte .... (813) 637-2288
Collier .... (813) 774-8443
DeSoto .... (813) 494-5965
Glades .... (813) 946-1821*
Hendry-East .... (813) 893-7088*
Hendry-West .... (813) 675-1446
Lee .... (813) 433-3900
Sarasota
   North .... (813) 955-2122*
   Englewood/N. Port .... (813) 475-4056

Palm Beach/Treasure Coast
Palm Beach/Treasure Coast AAA
8895 N. Military Trail, Suite 201-C
Palm Beach Gardens, FL 33410
(407) 694-7601

Indian River .... (407) 569-0764
Martin .... (407) 283-2242
Okeechobee .... (813) 763-9444
Palm Beach .... (407) 930-5040
St. Lucie .... (407) 465-1485*

South Florida
AAA of Broward County
5345 N.W. 35th Avenue
Fort Lauderdale, FL 33309
(305) 670-6500

Alliance for Aging
9500 S. Dadeland Blvd, Suite 400
Miami, FL 33156
(305) 670-6500

Broward .... (305) 484-4357*
Dade .... (305) 358-6060
   also .... (800) 273-2044
Monroe .... (305) 296-3110
   also .... (800) 273-2044

Note: telephone numbers change frequently. Call the regional Area Agency on Aging or the Eldercare Locator (discussed in the next section) if a non-working telephone number is reached.

Nationwide Eldercare Locator

The Eldercare Locator is a nationwide service that helps people find information about community services for elders anywhere in the United States and its territories. Eldercare Locator will put you in touch with Area Agencies on Aging anywhere in Florida or the other 49 states. The Area Agencies on Aging in Florida were listed previously.

The Eldercare Locator accepts calls between 8 a.m and 6 p.m. Eastern Standard Time. When you call, Eldercare Locator recommends that you have the name and address of the older person you are helping, including the ZIP code; and a brief general description of the problem or type of assistance that is being sought.

Eldercare Locator
(800) 677-1116

NEWSLETTERS, RESEARCH SERVICES, AND ASSOCIATIONS

Newsletters and research services

Corecare Associates specializes in developing marketing programs for long-term care providers and publishes a newsletter for nursing homes, adult congregate living facilities, home health agencies, adult day care centers and other providers in the continuum of elder care services. The Corecare Registry newsletter, published by Corecare Associates, features articles on the regulatory aspects of health care, the individuals who shape health care policy, and other topics of interest to health care providers. For information contact:

Corecare Associates
701 S.E. 6th Avenue, Suite 201
Delray Beach, FL 33483-9929
(407) 274-9823

HealthTrac is a newsletter for health care providers who have an interest in state legislation and regulation. *HealthTrac* specializes in analyzing and tracking all health care bills in the Florida Legislature and providing "insider" views of major health care program and policy issues. HealthTrac has also published an excellent book on caregiving, the *Florida Caregivers Handbook*. For information contact:

HealthTrac
PO Box 13552
Tallahassee, FL 32317
(904) 222-8180

Health Planning and Development conducts health care research and analyses health care data. They developed computer software that produces analytical reports on the characteristics of patients discharged from hospitals. They are also engaged in health planning for hospitals and other health care providers, and they conduct research on health care topics. For information contact:

Jay Cushman
Health Planning and Development
12721 S.W. Edgecliff Road
Portland, Oregon 97219
(503) 636-3920

Healthcare Research Systems develops patient satisfaction measurement systems for hospitals, continuing care retirement communities, nursing homes, assisted living facilities, hospices, home care agencies, and other health care providers. Employee and physician satisfaction measurement surveys are also conducted.

Healthcare Research Systems
College of Medicine
Ohio State University
941 Chatham Lane, 201
Columbus, OH 43221
(614) 293-3630

Florida Associations of Medical Professionals

Florida Academy of Family Practitioners
1627 Rogero Road
Jacksonville, FL 32211-4866
(904) 743-6304

Florida Chiropractic Association
2851 Remington Green Circle, Suite C
Tallahassee, FL 32308-3729
(904) 385-9393

Florida College of Emergency Physicians
3717 S. Conway Road
Orlando, FL 32812-7607
(407) 281-7396

Florida Medical Association
PO Box 2411
Jacksonville, FL 32203
(904) 356-1571

Florida Nurses Association
PO Box 536985
Orlando, FL 32853-6985
(407) 896-3261

Florida Optometric Association
PO Box 13429
Tallahassee, FL 32317
(904) 877-4697

Florida Osteopathic Medical Association
2007 Apalachee Parkway
Tallahassee, FL 32301
(904) 878-7364

Florida Physical Therapy Association
PO Box 4283
Tallahassee, FL 32315
(904) 222-1243

Florida Society for Clinical Social Work
PO Box 3061
Tallahassee, FL 32315

Florida Society of Psychotherapists
PO Box 155
Fernandina Beach, FL 32034

Licensed Practical Nurse's Association of
Florida
PO Box 2304
Panama City, FL 32402-2304
(904) 265-2702

Mental Health Association of Florida
2337 Wednesday
Tallahassee, FL 32308
(904) 385-7527

National Association of Social Workers
Florida Chapter
345 S. Magnolia Drive, Suite B-14
Tallahassee, FL 32301-2971
(904) 224-2971

Florida Health Care Facility Associations

Associated Home Health Industries
1406 Hays
Tallahassee, FL 32301
(904) 942-0895

Association of Voluntary Hospitals of
Florida
Barnett Bank Building, Suite 808
315 South Calhoun Street
Tallahassee, FL 32301
(904) 222-9800

Florida Alliance of Birth Centers
260 East 6th Avenue
Tallahassee, FL 32303
(904) 224-0490

Florida Alcohol and Drug Abuse
  Association
1030 E. Lafayette St, Suite 100
Tallahassee, FL 32301
(904) 878-2196

Florida Assisted Living Association
PO Box 3706
West Palm Beach, FL 33402
(800) 785-3252 or (407) 844-8800

Florida Association of Health
  Maintenance Organizations
PO Box 13645
Tallahassee, FL 32317-3645
(904) 386-2904

Florida Association of Homes for the
  Aging
1018 Thomasville Road, Suite 200Y
Tallahassee, FL 32303
(904) 222-3562

Florida Council for Community Mental
  Health
111 N. Gadsden Street
Tallahassee, FL 32301
(904) 224-6048

Florida Health Care Association
(nursing homes and retirement facilities)
PO Box 1459
Tallahassee, FL 32301
(904) 224-3907

Florida Hospices, Inc.
317 East Park Avenue
Tallahassee, FL 32301
(904) 222-4239

Florida Hospital Association
PO Box 531107
Orlando, FL 32853-1107
(407) 841-6230

Florida League of Hospitals
215 South Monroe Street
Tallahassee, FL 32301
(904) 224-9407

Florida Society of Ambulatory Surgical
  Centers
4965 Palm Avenue
Winter Park, FL 32792
(407) 679-5252

Retirement Housing Council
(ACLFs and continuing care facilities)
PO Box 12934
Tallahassee, FL 32317-2934
(904) 561-9162

Other Florida health care organizations

The Florida Council on Aging, established in 1955, has over 750 members. The council provides a professional forum for health care providers, health care professionals, businesses, and numerous organizations that have an interest in aging and the elderly. The Council sponsors an annual educational conference, publishes a newsletter, sponsors a statewide awards program for older persons, supports a gerontology scholarship at Florida State University, and advocates for services for the elderly.

The Florida Council on Aging
1018 Thomasville Road, Box C-2, Suite 110
Tallahassee, Florida 32303-6236
(904) 222-8877

Located in the same offices is the Florida Foundation on Active Aging, which was chartered in 1990 to "develop and disseminate positive role models of active living for older adults, with a focus on health, work, contributions to community, education, social interactions and high self esteem." The Foundation has a distinguished Board of Trustees that includes some of Florida's most distinguished health care, academic, and aging professionals.

Florida Foundation on Active Aging
1018 Thomasville Road, Box C-2, Suite 110
Tallahassee, Florida 32303
(904) 222-4664

National Professional Organizations
(see individual chapters for listings of other associations)

American Association of Homes
for the Aging
901 E Street NW, Suite 500
Washington, D.C. 20004-2037
(202) 783-2242
Publications catalog available

American College of Healthcare Executives
840 North Lake Shore Drive
Chicago, IL 60611
(312) 943-0544
Publications catalog available
Ask for extension 3000 and mention catalog

American Hospital Association
840 North Lake Shore Drive
Chicago, Illinois 60611
(800) AHA-2626
Publications and products catalog available

National Association for Healthcare
Quality
5700 Old Orchard Road, First Floor
Skokie, Il 60077-1057
(708) 966-9392
Publications catalog available
Publishes *Journal for Healthcare Quality*
Certifies professionals in healthcare
quality

American Society for Quality Control
611 East Wisconsin Avenue
PO Box 3005
Milwaukee, Wisconsin 53201-3005
(800) 248-1946
Publications catalog available.

CHAPTER 12
Reform, malpractice, fraud, billing errors, complaints

HEALTH CARE REFORM

Although many researchers have concluded that the U.S. offers the most advanced health care in the world, our system is expensive, wasteful, and far too many people lack health insurance. Over the past few years, rising health care costs, increasing numbers of people without insurance, and other factors, have caused health care reform to emerge as a major concern.

Patients are concerned about high costs, while physicians, nurses and other health care professionals are distraught over increasingly burdensome "red tape." Businesses increasingly cannot afford to purchase coverage for their employees, and government budgets have less money for criminal justice, education, and other needed programs.

A large underserved population also exists that cannot access health care services for reasons that are more within the realm of sociology than the simple absence of health insurance coverage. In fact, many practitioners are reluctant to see Medicaid patients; thus coverage and access are not synonymous.

The potential for significant financial rewards stimulates a large research and development effort to invent new medical technologies and develop new pharmaceuticals. Despite the advantages of a market-driven free enterprise health care system, the business nature of health care has made many uncomfortable. According to a physician writing in the *New England Journal of Medicine* (Alper 1987),

> *"This rush toward what some have termed the 'commercialization' of medicine and others have called the 'industrialization' of medicine has bewildered physicians, perhaps because we instinctively sense that although there have always been some business aspects to medical practice, medicine, in the most fundamental sense, is not a business."*

Among developed industrialized countries, only the U.S. and the Republic of South Africa do not make health care available to all citizens. Why is it that the U.S. does not have a national health care program? There are at least three major inter-related reasons.

First, public opinion in the U.S. is very different from European countries with regard to the fundamental role of government in society. To clarify this point, consider the results of polls contained in an article in the *New England Journal of Medicine* on the subject of health care reform (Blendon and Donelan 1990). These polls compared public opinion in the U.S. with five European countries. In 1985, the question was asked if it was the responsibility of government to provide medical care. In the United States, approximately 40 percent said yes. In Italy, the "yes" response was nearly 80 percent; in the United Kingdom, 75 percent; in West Germany and Austria, 60 percent; and in the Netherlands, 55 percent.

Another question asked is whether it is the responsibility of government to reduce income differences between the rich and the poor. In the United States, approximately

30 percent said yes, in contrast to more than 80 percent in Italy and Austria.

The authors commented that "These views are somewhat surprising, given that the United States currently has one of the lowest levels of taxation among the 18 wealthiest industrialized countries. Only Japan raises less tax revenue."

The second reason is given by George D. Lundberg, M.D., editor of the *Journal of the American Medical Association* (Lundberg 1991). According to Dr. Lundberg, one of the reasons that all Americans do not have sufficient access to medical care is because of "long-standing, systematic, institutionalized racial discrimination." Dr. Lundberg adds, "It is not a coincidence that the United States of America and the Republic of South Africa—the only two developed industrialized countries that do not have a national health policy ensuring that all citizen have access to basic health care—are also the only two such countries that have within their borders substantial numbers of underserved people who are different ethnically from the controlling group."

The final reason is that the powerful influence and divergent views of the health care special interest groups—insurance companies, physicians, hospitals, and others—makes forming a political consensus for meaningful health care reform very difficult. There is simply too much at stake financially.

Making substantial improvements in America's health care system may well await the emergence of a national consciousness that embraces ethics and values that are similar to those in European countries. According to C. Everett Koop, M.D., the former Surgeon General of the United States, (*St. Petersburg Times*, September 6, 1992):

> *"It would be easier to enact the sweeping reforms we need in health care if we, as Americans, could agree on the basic values and ethics upon which our health care system—and our society—is based and from which it derives its moral power. If we could reach an ethical consensus, many of the economic and political problems of health care reform would be easily solved."*

Unfortunately, fraud is now a major factor in the cost of health care. A widely used estimate is that fraud comprises 10 percent of health care expenditures. We all pay for this illegal behavior. Health care fraud represents a staggering amount of money: almost $4 billion annually in Florida and over $90 billion annually nationally. Although a system free of fraud would not necessarily improve access to health care to people who do not have insurance, this represents enough money to provide health care to all who currently lack health insurance.

The underlying cause of our huge health care fraud problem lies in the change in the ethics and values of a minority of persons that, unfortunately, has an impact far greater than their numbers. The same problems that plague our health care system caused havoc in the savings and loan industry, in our financial markets with insider trading, in defense contracts, and in many other areas.

Meaningful health care reform likely will require us, as Dr. Koop stated, to agree on the basic values and ethics upon which our society is based. If the traditional values of honesty, service, and fairness were practiced by all health care insurers, manufactures, and providers a large part of our health care crisis would disappear.

PERSONAL HEALTH CARE STRATEGIES

Everyone can take steps to use our health care system appropriately, and to contain health care costs, by taking "personal responsibility" to help our health care system function more effectively. This is the same concept as "thinking globally and acting locally." Here are some personal strategies that have emerged from medical literature.

- Live a healthy lifestyle. Many researchers have concluded that proper diet, exercise, avoiding harmful substances such as tobacco, and maintaining a happy and inquisitive attitude towards life promotes good health, enhances longevity, and helps maintain independence in later years.
- Do not use more medical services than you need.
- Participate in making health care decisions. When necessary, particularly if there is a severe or rare problem, ask questions about medical effectiveness, conduct research such as obtaining practice guidelines, and seek a second opinion. Advances in medical diagnosis and treatment are occurring at a rapid rate.
- State-of-the art medical information is becoming increasingly available from many sources as is information on clinical trials. The MEDLINE medical research system, the most comprehensive medical data base in existence, is readily available to the public in many large Florida cities.
- Be cost conscious. Ask questions about costs for laboratory, radiology, prescription drugs, and other medical ancillaries. Can the same service or item be obtained at a lower cost elsewhere? Does the physician accept Medicare assignment?
- Identify and report fraud. Fraud is estimated to comprise up to 10 percent of all health care expenditures. We all end up paying for those who are dishonest, and dishonest and illegal behavior is something we cannot afford.
- Consider alternatives to nursing home care whenever medically appropriate. Discuss options with your physician (see Chapter 9 for a discussion of options) such as arranging for home health care (Chapter 6) or living in an adult congregate living facility (Chapter 5).
- Prepare a living will and designate a health care surrogate (Chapter 9) to direct your medical care should you become incompetent. A clearly written advance medical directive helps ensure that your wishes will be followed.

MEDICAL MALPRACTICE

How often does medical malpractice occur in hospitals? Do certain types of hospitals have higher rates? Are elderly persons at greater risk? What proportion of physicians are sued and what proportion of malpractice cases go to court? Who usually wins, the patient or the doctor? Recent studies have provided some answers to these questions.

Although medical malpractice lawsuits have increased in recent years, malpractice litigation also has increased in other professions such as accounting, engineering, and even funeral direction. According to experts, medical malpractice lawsuits have increased because of riskier medical procedures and an increase in "consumerism." Although an increase in the number of lawyers is sometimes mentioned as a factor, a RAND study found no evidence that a high density of lawyers had any systematic effect on the frequency of malpractice claims (Danzon, 1986).

An unrealistic view of our advanced science and technology is also a large factor. Our rapid technological advances have increased expectations that technology will solve many of our problems. Despite our achievements in technology, medicine is far from being an exact science. Rather it is an "art" in many respects. Some medical problems are difficult to diagnose, many others have no cure, and treatment is not always clear cut. Medical science cannot cure the common cold, nor can it cure AIDS.

Although advances in medical science have made tremendous improvements in the quality of medical care, some high-tech medical procedures carry risk. Writing in the *Journal of the American Medical Association*, Harvard Medical Practice Study researchers stated that,

> *"Advances in medical science have made possible bolder interventions (and more favorable outcomes), often in more fragile patients. Therefore, the consequences of errors are likely to be far more serious"* (Weiler, Newhouse and Hiatt 1992).

A 1989 Institute of Medicine study indicated that unrealistic patient expectation is a factor which has caused medical malpractice law suits to increase. The study stated, "Behind many medical malpractice claims is a disappointed consumer who believed he or she was purchasing a cure, is disappointed with the results, and, often without any other avenue of compensation, is seeking relief through the legal system."

Another problem is the practice of "defensive medicine." The fear of a malpractice lawsuit may cause physicians to order diagnostic tests, and to make other decisions, to reduce the threat of litigation. These practices increase costs unnecessarily.

Despite all of these problems, there is a silver lining—malpractice litigation has improved the quality of health care. Researchers cite more detailed medical record keeping, the creation of incident reports and medication control systems, and physicians spending more time with patients as positive benefits from malpractice litigation. In addition, "defensive medicine" sometimes can identify medical problems that might have been overlooked.

The extent of medical malpractice

The most detailed study ever undertaken of medical malpractice examined 30,195 patients who were treated in 51 urban and rural hospitals in New York state during 1984. The study was conducted by the Harvard Medical Practice Study team (see Brennan et al. 1991; Leape et al. 1991 and Localio et al. 1991). One of the sponsors of the study, the Robert Wood Johnson Foundation (see *Abridge*, Spring 1991), also reported findings.

The study reviewed patient medical records to determine the number of patients who experienced "adverse events" and "negligent adverse events." Adverse events are medical injuries that prolong a hospital stay or cause a disability. Most adverse events are not, however, caused by negligence. On the other hand, a "negligent adverse event" results from substandard medical care. An unforeseeable adverse drug reaction is an example of an adverse event, while a surgical error is an example of a negligent adverse event.

The Harvard researchers found that 1,133 (3.8 percent) of the 30,195 patients studied experienced adverse events and 280 (1 percent) experienced negligent adverse events. Breaking down the 1 percent who experienced negligent adverse events:

- 45.7 percent had injuries resulting in "minimal impairment" with recovery in one month or less;
- 12.1 percent had "moderate impairment" causing one to six months disability;
- 3.0 percent had moderate impairment for more than six months;
- 6.4 percent were permanently impaired;
- 25.4 percent had injuries that caused death; and,
- 7.3 percent of the cases could not be judged.

Although one-fourth (25.4 percent) of the negligent injuries resulted in death, one of the authors of the study, Howard H. Hiatt, M.D., stated that "Most of these patients were very ill. A patient in shock following a severe heart attack, for example, was given an overdose of a drug and died immediately as a result of that overdose. Even though the patient might well have died within a day or two even without the drug overdose, the death was considered to have been a result of negligence" (Grady and Siegel 1992).

Medical injury risk factors

The Harvard study also examined factors that influence adverse events and negligent adverse events. The study found that:
- Vascular surgery had the highest adverse event rate (16.1 percent of patients were judged to have experienced an adverse event) followed by thoracic and cardiac surgery (10.8 percent).
- Both adverse events and negligent adverse events increase as the age of the patient increases. Persons over age 65 had twice the rate of adverse events (5.9 percent) than persons ages 16 to 44 (2.6 percent).
- Obstetrics has a "very low" adverse event rate (1.5 percent). Claims can, however, be very large because of lifetime medical and other costs when there are severe injuries to newborns.
- The rate of negligent adverse events in teaching hospitals was one-half the rate in non-teaching hospitals.
- Hospitals with financial difficulties had "significantly higher" negligence rates.

Malpractice litigation

The table below shows data from the Harvard study on the incidence of adverse events, negligent adverse events, and medical malpractice claims per 10,000 hospitalized patients. The Harvard study found that about 1 in 10,000 hospitalized patients received compensation (a paid claim) as a result of a medical malpractice lawsuit.

Medical Injuries and Medical Malpractice Claims per 10,000 Hospitalized Patients Harvard Medical Practice Study III

	Patients	Percent
No adverse event	9,630	96.3
Adverse event, no negligence	270	2.7
Negligent adverse event, no claim	98	1.0
Negligent adverse event, claim, not paid	1	.01
Negligent adverse event, claim, paid	1	.01
	10,000	100

Source: Robert Wood Johnson Foundation, 1991.

The Harvard researchers found that only one in eight claims was litigated in court, and that there was only one claim for every 50 negligent injuries. The study concluded, "Medical-malpractice litigation infrequently compensates patients injured by medical negligence and rarely identifies, and holds providers accountable for, substandard care."

Researchers have found that the vast majority of malpractice claims are settled either before trial, or after trial has begun but before there is a jury verdict. A major study, published in 1991 in *Law and Contemporary Problems*, (Metzloff 1991 also see *Abridge*,

Spring 1991) examined all medical malpractice lawsuits litigated during a three-year period in North Carolina. The study found that:
- 25 percent of cases were dropped before trial without a payment;
- 60 percent of cases were settled with a payment;
- 15 percent of cases went to trial; and,
- 80 percent of medical malpractice cases that went to court were won by doctors.

A RAND study found that when the total costs of medical liability litigation are considered, injured patients receive 43 percent, while 57 percent is spent on litigation expenses, including attorney fees, and costs incurred by insurance companies (Hensler 1987).

A 1992 U.S. General Accounting Office (GAO) study examined alternatives to medical malpractice litigation. The study cited research that found that claims take a long time to be resolved, the court system has high legal costs, settlements and awards are unpredictable, and that many claims that have merit never reach the courts.

Research studies have concluded that our court system does a poor job in compensating persons for medical injuries resulting from substandard care. Although this may be so, many argue that the protections and fairness assured by our court system outweigh this disadvantage. In addition, many experts believe that because medical liability litigation is very technical and complex, law firms that specialize in medical liability are usually the most capable in handling such lawsuits.

Malpractice and Florida physicians

A collaborative study involving Vanderbilt University, the American Medical Association, and the Urban Institute analyzed medical malpractice insurance claims in Florida between 1975 and 1988 (Sloan et al. 1989). This study confirmed other research that had found that a small minority of physicians are responsible for the great majority of medical malpractice legal costs and awards. The principal findings of the study were:
- Three percent of Florida physicians practicing internal medicine and pediatrics accounted for 85 percent of insurers' losses for their specialties. Over a six-year period, 15 percent of these physicians were sued.
- Six percent of Florida OB/GYNs and anesthesiologists accounted for 85 percent of insurers' losses for their specialities. One-third of these physicians were sued over a six-year period.
- Eight percent of Florida's orthopedic surgeons, plastic surgeons, and neurosurgeons accounted for three-quarters of insurers' losses for their specialities. Approximately one-half of these surgeons were sued over a six-year period.
- A good predictor of future problems is prior malpractice claims experience. Contrary to expectations, physicians with adverse claims experiences were found to be less likely to leave Florida than physicians who had lawsuits that did not result in payments. Physicians with unfavorable claims experiences also were less likely to retire or to practice another area of medicine than physicians with favorable claims experiences.
- A "handful" of physicians were responsible for the vast majority of payments for compensation and associated costs.

HEALTH CARE FRAUD

Although government agencies and insurance companies are actively trying to reduce fraud, health care consumers can play a key role. The most common types of consumer health care fraud include:

- Billing for services not performed;
- Fraudulent diagnosis, including mischaracterizing services and billing for a more costly procedure than was performed;
- Prescribing unnecessary or inappropriate laboratory tests, surgeries, x-rays, medical supplies, and medical equipment; and
- Charging for brand name drugs when generic drugs are dispensed.

Although the vast majority of physicians and other health care providers are honest, there are exceptions. Below are strategies individuals can use to help prevent fraud and abuse.

- If you don't understand why a procedure is necessary, ask for an explanation.
- Check your Medicare Explanation of Medicare Benefits (EOMB) form, bill, or insurance company notice to be sure that you received the services shown. If you have questions, ask the provider for an explanation.
- Date and sign only one claim form for each visit and never sign a blank claim form.
- Although free medical screenings and tests are offered as a public service by reputable providers, beware of free medical checkups offered to you over the telephone, and beware of any free checkup where you are asked to sign an insurance claim form.
- Most insurers require that copayments and deductibles be paid. In such cases, it is fraudulent to waive them.
- Ask what services are covered by Medicare or other insurance and what you have to pay out of pocket.
- Make sure you receive a receipt that includes the services that were provided and the charges for them.

Reporting health care fraud

Medicare Fraud Branch
P.O. Box 45087
Jacksonville, FL 32231-5087
(800) 333-7586

Florida Blue Cross/Blue Shield
(members of Blue Cross/Blue Shield plans)
Fraud Hot Line
(800) 678-8355

Medicaid Program
Fraud Hot Line
Office of the Auditor General
(800) 892-0375

The National Insurance Fraud Hotline
(possible fraud in any commercial,
state,
or federal health insurance program)
(800) 835-6422

The Florida Department of Insurance, Division of Fraud investigates health insurance fraud. The Division of Fraud has regional field offices in Fort Myers, Jacksonville, Miami, Ocala, Orlando, Pensacola, Tallahassee, and Tampa.

Pensacola Office
315-B South Palafox Street
Pensacola, Florida 32501
(904) 444-2394

Orlando Office
400 West Robinson Street, Suite N-511
Orlando, FL 32801
(407) 423-6348

Tallahassee Office
645 Fletcher Building
Tallahassee, FL 32399
(904) 922-3115

Tampa Office
1313 North Tampa Street, Suite 805
Tampa, Florida 33602
(813) 272-3565

Jacksonville Office
4151 Woodcock Drive, Suite 117
Jacksonville, FL 32207
(904) 348-2740

Fort Myers Office
2295 Victoria Avenue
Fort Myers, FL 33901
(813) 338-2323

Ocala Office
11655 N.W. Gainesville Hwy., Bldg. 8
Ocala, FL 32675
(904) 732-1746

Miami Office
401 N.W. 2nd Avenue, Suite N-321
Miami, FL 33128
(305) 377-5957

HOSPITAL BILLING ERRORS

The state Agency for Health Care Administration (AHCA) has a "Hospital Bill Program" to help resolve billing misunderstandings. If you have questions or complaints about your hospital bill, and your hospital has not provided you with a satisfactory response, contact the Hospital Bill Program. If necessary, AHCA will contact the hospital on your behalf and the hospital must respond within 30 days. AHCA suggests that you check your bill for the following:

- Were there repeat billings for identical services on the same day?
- Were all laboratory tests ordered by your physician?
- If you were discharged early in the morning, were you charged room and board for the entire day?
- Did you have all the X-rays for which you were billed?
- Were you charged for medications that were ordered but discontinued?
- Does the bill have the correct number of days spent in a special unit, such as intensive care?
- Were you billed for items you never received or that you were not allowed to take home?

AHCA also publishes regional information brochures on hospital and physician charges. To obtain information about the Hospital Bill Program, hospital charges, or physician charges, write or telephone:

Agency for Health Care Administration
301 Atrium Building
325 John Knox Road
Tallahassee, FL 32303
(Hospital Bill Program)
(904) 487-3183
(Publications)
(800) 342-0828

Because AHCA receives a large number of requests for information and assistance, you may reach a recording. Leave a message, speak slowly and carefully, include your name and address, and indicate if you want information about the Hospital Bill Program, the hospital charges brochure, or the physician charges brochure. You will receive the requested information in the mail within a few days.

The Department of Insurance also has a program to resolve billing disputes between patients and health care providers. Contact the Department of Insurance at (800) 435-7352.

AGENCIES THAT INVESTIGATE AND RESOLVE HEALTH CARE COMPLAINTS

HEALTH CARE PROFESSIONALS
PHYSICIANS, NURSES, AND OTHERS
Florida Department of Professional Regulation
(800) 342-7940 or (904) 488-6602
(to file a complaint or to inquire about
the status of the license of a health care professional)

HEALTH INSURANCE COVERAGE
Florida Department of Insurance
Help Line
(800) 342-2762

HEALTH INSURANCE FRAUD
(see listings earlier in this chapter)

HEALTH MAINTENANCE ORGANIZATIONS (HMOS)
Agency for Health Care Administration
(800) 342-7940

HOME HEALTH AGENCY HOT LINE
Agency for Health Care Administration
(800) 962-6014

HOSPITAL CHARGES OR BILLING PROBLEMS
(see listings earlier in this chapter)

HOSPITAL PATIENT CARE & CONDITION OF FACILITY
Agency for Health Care Administration
(904) 487-2527 (State Headquarters)
(see Chapter 11 for a list of Health
Facility Regulation Area Offices)

MEDICAL DEVICES
Food and Drug Administration
(800) 638-6725
(301) 881-0256 (in Maryland)

NURSING HOMES
Nursing Home Complaints
(see complaint section in Chapter 4)
(see list of Ombudsman Councils in Chapter 11)

PATIENT ABUSE
Abuse Hotline
(800) 342-9152

RETIREMENT FACILITIES (ACLFS AND CONTINUING CARE FACILITIES)
(see complaint section in Chapter 5)
(see Chapter 11 for a list of Health
Facility Regulation Area Offices)
(see list of Ombudsman Councils in Chapter 11)

Bibliography

_____. "A Special Edition on Medical Malpractice," ABridge. Princeton, N.J.: Robert Wood Johnson Foundation (Spring, 1991).

_____. "Brightening the Days of Nursing Home Residents." Aging. Washington D.C.: U.S. Department of Health and Human Services. Number 365 (1993).

_____. "In Search of the Secrets of Aging." National Institutes of Health, NIH Publication No. 93-2756 (May 1993).

Agency for Health Care Administration. "Cesarean Section Rates in Florida Hospitals, 1991." Tallahassee, FL: Author (January 1, 1993).

Alper, Philip R. "Medical Practice in the Competitive Market." *New England Journal of Medicine*, Vol. 316, No. 6 (February 5, 1987).

American Academy of Pediatrics and American College of Obstetricians and Gynecologists. "Guidelines for Perinatal Care," Second Edition. Elk Grove Village, IL: American Academy of Pediatrics; 1988.

Banta, David H. and Stephen B. Thacker. "The Case for Reassessment of Health Care Technology." *Journal of the American Medical Association*. Vol. 264, No. 2 (July 11, 1990).

Bernstein, Steven J., Lee H. Hilborne, Lucian L. Leape, et al. "The Appropriateness of Use of Coronary Angiography in New York State." *Journal of the American Medical Association*. Vol. 269, No. 6 (February 10, 1993).

Bernstein, Steven J., Elizabeth A. McGlynn, Albert L. Siu, et al. "The Appropriateness of Hysterectomy." *Journal of the American Medical Association*. Vol. 269, No. 18 (May 12, 1993).

Blendon, Robert J., Ulrike S. Szalay, and Richard A. Knox, "Should Physicians Aid Their Patients in Dying." *Journal of the American Medical Association*. Vol. 267, No. 19 (May 20, 1992).

Blendon, Robert J. and Karen Donelan. "The Public and the Emerging Debate Over National Health Insurance." *The New England Journal of Medicine*. Vol. 323, No. 3 (July 19, 1990).

Blue Cross and Blue Shield Association. "National Health Care Reform: Organizing the Solutions" (1991).

Bower, B. "Mental Disorder Numbers Outpace Treatment." *Science News*. Vol. 143, No 9 (February 27, 1993).

Brennan, Troyen A., Lucian L. Leape, Nan M. Laird, et al. "Incidence of Adverse Events and Negligence in Hospitalized Patients—Results of the Harvard Medical Practice Study I." *New England Journal of Medicine*. Vol. 324, No. 6. (February 7, 1991).

Brennan, Troyen A., Liesi E. Hebert, Nan M. Laird, et al. "Hospital Characteristics Associated with Adverse Events and Substandard Care." *Journal of the American Medical Association*. Vol. 265. No 24 (June 26, 1991).

Brock, Dwight B. and Daniel J. Foley. "A Survey of the Last Days of Life: Methodology Considerations and Pretest Results." Social Statistics Section, Proceedings of the American Statistical Association (1985).

Brock, Dwight B. and Daniel J. Foley. "Health Status Trends in the Last Year of Life." Proceedings of the Social Statistics Section of the American Statistical Association (1988).

Brody, Howard. "Assisted Death—A Compassionate Response to a Medical Failure." *The New England Journal of Medicine*. 1992; Vol. 327, No. 19 (November 5, 1992).

Brook, Robert H. "Practice Guidelines and Practicing Medicine." Journal of the American Medical Association. Vol. 262, No. 21 (December 1, 1989).

Brook, Robert H., Rolla Edward Park, Mark R. Chassin, et al. "Predicting the Appropriate Use of Carotid Endarterectomy, Upper Gastrointestinal Endoscopy, and Coronary Angiography." *The New England Journal of Medicine*. Vol. 323, No. 17 (October 25, 1990).

Brook, Robert H. "Maintaining Hospital Quality." *Journal of the American Medical Association*. Vol. 270, No. 8 (August 25, 1993).

Bulkin, Wilma and Herbert Lukashok. "Rx for Dying: The Case for Hospice." *New England Journal of Medicine*. Vol. 318, No. 6 (February 11, 1988).

Burns, Lawton R. and Douglas R. Wholey. "The Effects of Patient, Hospital, and Physician Characteristics on Length of Stay and Mortality." *Medical Care*. Vol. 29., No. 3 (March, 1991).

Burstin, Helen R., Stuart R. Lipsitz, Steven Udvarhelyi and Troyen A. Brennan. "The Effect of Hospital Financial Characteristics on Quality of Care." *Journal of the American Medical Association*. Vol. 270, No. 7. (August 18, 1993).

Caine, Eric D. and Yeates C. Conwell. "Self-determined Death, the Physician, and Medical Priorities." *Journal of the American Medical Association*. Vol. 270, No. 7 (August 18, 1993).

Catalan-Fernandez, J.G., O. Pons-Sureda, A. Recober-Martinez, et al. "Dying of Cancer, The Place of Death and Family Circumstances." *Medical Care*. Vol. 29, No. 9 (September 1991).

Chassin M.R., Jacqueline Kosecoff, R.E. Park, et al. "Does Inappropriate Use Explain Geographic Variations in the Use of Health Care Services? A Study of Three Procedures." *Journal of the American Medical Association*. Vol. 258, No. 18 (November 13, 1987).

Chassin, Mark R. "The Missing Ingredient in Health Reform—Quality of Care." *Journal of the American Medical Association*. Vol. 270, No. 3 (July 21, 1993).

Clinton, Jarrett. J. "Improving Clinical Practice." *Journal of the American Medical Association*. Vol. 267, No. 19 (May 20, 1992).

Congressional Budget Office, Congress of the United States. "Rising Health Care Costs: Causes, Implications, and Strategies." Washington, D.C.: U.S. Government Printing Office; April, 1991.

Council on Ethical and Judicial Affairs, American Medical Association. "Council Report: Decisions Near the End of Life." *Journal of the American Medical Association.* Vol. 267, No. 16 (April 22/29 1992).

Council on Ethical and Judicial Affairs, American Medical Association. "Conflicts of Interest: Physician Ownership of Medical Facilities." *Journal of the American Medical Association.* Vol. 267, No. 17 (May 6, 1992).

Crenshaw, Albert B. "Diagnosing Medical Fraud." *The Washington Post* (June 16, 1991).

Cutter, John A. "Be Sure it's Your Decision." *St. Petersburg Times, Seniority* (June 29, 1993) p. 10.

Danzon, Patricia M. "New Evidence on the Frequency and Severity of Medical Malpractice Claims." Institute for Civil Justice, RAND Corporation. R-3410-ICJ. (1986).

Department of Veterans Affairs. "Federal Benefits for Veterans and Dependents," Washington, DC: U.S. Government Printing Office; March 15, 1989.

DesHarnais, Susan I., Laurence F. McMahon, Roger T. Wroblewski and Andrew J. Hogan. "Measuring Hospital Performance." *Medical Care.* Vol. 28, No. 12 (December 1990).

Dubler, Nancy Neveloff. "Commentary: Balancing Life and Death—Proceed with Caution." *American Journal of Public Health.* Vol. 83, No. 1 (January, 1993)

Emanuel, Ezekiel J. and Linda L. Emanuel. "Four Models of the Physician-Patient Relationship." *Journal of the American Medical Association.* Vol. 267, No. 16. (April 22/29, 1992).

Evans, Denis A., H. Harris Funkenstein, Marilyn S. Albert et al. "Prevalence of Alzheimer's Disease in a Community Population of Older Persons." *Journal of the American Medical Association.* Vol. 262, No. 18 (November 10, 1989).

Farley, Dean E. and Ronald J. Ozmikowski "Volume-Outcome Relationships and Inhospital Mortality: The Effect of Changes in Volume Over Time." *Medical Care.* Vol. 30, No. 1 (January, 1992).

Feinstein, Jonathan S. "The Relationship between Socioeconomic Status and Health: A Review of the Literature." *The Milbank Quarterly.* Vol. 71, No. 2 (1993).

Finkel, Madelon Lubin and David J. Finkel. "The Effect of a Second Opinion Program on Hysterectomy Performance." *Medical Care.* Vol. 28, No. 9 (September 1990).

Florida Department of Health and Rehabilitative Services. "A Comparative Analysis of Florida's Teaching and Research Hospitals," (March, 1988).

Florida Health Care Cost Containment Board. "Study of Cesarean Section Rates in Florida Hospitals Using Small Area Analysis," (March, 1990).

Florida Health Care Cost Containment Board. "1989 Annual Report," (March, 1990).

Florida Health Care Cost Containment Board. "Nursing Home Reporting System, 1987 Annual Report," (December, 1987).

Florida Health Care Cost Containment Board. "Neonatal Intensive Care Study," (January, 1987).

Frieden, Joyce. "Fraud Squad Target Suspect Claims," *Business and Health*. Vol. 9, No. 4 (April 1991).

Friedman, Emily, "Policy Perspectives: Changing the System. *Journal of the American Medical Association*. Vol. 269, pages 2437–2442 (1993)

Friedman, Robert M. and Krista Kutash. "Mad, Bad, Sad, Can't Add? Florida Adolescent and Child Treatment Study," Department of Epidemiology and Policy Analysis, Florida Mental Health Institute, University of South Florida; September, 1986.

Fuchs, Victor R. "No Pain, No Gain: Perspectives on Cost Containment." *Journal of the American Medical Association*. Vol. 269, No. 5 (February 3, 1993).

General Accounting Office. "VA Health Care: Variabilities in Outpatient Care Eligibility and Rationing Decisions." GAO-HRD-93-106 Gaithersburg, MD: General Accounting Office (July, 1993)

Gentry, Carol. "Intensive Care Not Always Best for Cancer Patients." *St. Petersburg Times*. P. 1A (February 10, 1993).

Goldsmith, J. "Commentary: Hospital/Physician Relationships. *Health Affairs*. Vol. 12, No. 3 (1993).

Graduate Medical Education National Advisory Committee. "Physician Requirements, 1990, for Psychiatry," Washington, DC: Public Health Service; 1981.

Grady, Mary L. and Randie A. Siegel, editors. "Summary Report: Issues in Medical Liability: A Working Conference" AHCPR 92-0011. Washington, D.C.: U.S. Department of Health and Human Services, Agency for Health Care Policy and Research; 1992.

Green, Jesse and Neil Wintfeld. "How Accurate are Hospital Discharge Data for Evaluating Effectiveness of Care?" *Medical Care*. Vol. 31, No. 8, (1993).

Greenfield, Sheldon, Eugene C. Nelson, Michael Zubkoff, et al. "Variations in Resource Utilization Among Medical Specialties and Systems of Care—Results from the Medical Outcomes Study." *Journal of the American Medical Association*. Vol. 267, No. 12 (March 25, 1992).

Grimes, David A. "Technology Follies—The Uncritical Acceptance of Medical Innovation." *Journal of the American Medical Association*. Vol. 269, No. 23 (June 16, 1993).

Guralnik, Jack M. and George A. Kaplan. "Predictors of Healthy Aging: Prospective Evidence from the Almeda County Study." *American Journal of Public Health*. Vol. 79, No. 6 (June 1989).

Hand R., Stephen Sener, Joseph Imperato, et al. "Hospital Variables Associated with Quality of Care for Breast Cancer Patients." *Journal of the American Medical Association*. Vol. 266, No. 24 (December 25, 1991).

Hannan, Edward L., Joseph F. O'Donnell, Harold Kilburn, et al. "Investigation of the Relationship Between Volume and Mortality for Surgical Procedures Performed in New York State Hospitals." *Journal of the American Medical Association*. Vol. 262, No. 4 (July 28, 1989).

Hannan, Edward L., Harold Kilburn, Harvey Bernard, et al. Coronary Artery Bypass Surgery: The Relationship Between Inhospital Mortality Rate and Surgical Volume After Controlling for Clinical Risk Factors." *Medical Care*. Vol. 29, No. 11 (November, 1991).

Hartz A.J., Henry Krakaueret, Evelyn M. Kuhn, et al. "Hospital Characteristics and Mortality Rates." *The New England Journal of Medicine*. Vol. 321 No. 25 (December 21, 1989).

Haas, J.S., S. Udvarhelyi, and A.M. Epstein. "The Effect of Health Coverage for Uninsured Pregnant Women on Maternal Health and the Use of Cesarean Section." *Journal of the American Medical Association*. Vol. 270, No. 1, pp 61–64 (1993).

Hensler, D.R. et al. "Trends in Tort Litigation, The Story Behind the Statistics." The RAND Corporation, No. R-3583-ICJ (1987).

Hilborne, Lee H., Lucian L. Leape, Steven J. Bernstein, et al. "The Appropriateness of Use of Percutaneous Transluminal Coronary Angioplasty in New York State *Journal of the American Medical Association*. Vol. 269, No. 6 (February 10, 1993).

Hinton, John. "Comparison of Places and Policies for Terminal Care." *The Lancet*. Vol. 1 for 1979, No. 8106 (January 6, 1979).

Holahan, J., M. Moon, W.P. Welch, and S. Zuckerman. "Balancing Access, Costs, & Politics." Urban Institute Report 91-6. 79 pp. Washington, D.C. Urban Institute Press, 1991. ISBN 0-87766-518-4.

Institute of Medicine. (1989). Summary Medical Professional Liability and the Delivery of Obstetrical Care Volume 1. Washington, D.C.: National Academy Press.

Johnson, Mary Ann, Maureen A. Brown, Leonard W. Poon, et al. "Nutritional Patterns of Centenarians." *International Journal of Aging and Human Development*. Vol. 34, No. 1 (1992).

Johnson, William G., Troyen A. Brennan, Joseph P. Newhouse, et al. "The Economic Consequences of Medical Injuries, Implications for a No-fault Insurance Plan." *Journal of the American Medical Association*. Vol. 267. No. 18 (May 13, 1992).

Jonas, Harry S. and Sharon L. Dooley. "The Search for a Lower Cesarean Rate Goes On," *Journal of the American Medical Association*. Vol. 262, No. 11 (September 15, 1989).

Kahn, Katherine L., William H. Rogers, Lisa V. Rubenstein, et al. "Measuring Quality of Care with Explicit Process Criteria Before and After Implementation of the DRG-Based Prospective Payment System." *Journal of the American Medical Association*. Vol. 264, No. 15 (October 17, 1990).

Keeler, Emmett B., Lisa V. Rubenstein, Katherine L. Kahn, et al. "Hospital Characteristics and Quality of Care." *Journal of the American Medical Association*. Vol. 268, No. 13 (October 7, 1992).

Kelly, Joyce V. and Fred J. Hellinger. "Heart Disease and Hospital Deaths: An Empirical Study," *Health Services Research*. Vol. 22, No. 3 (August, 1987).

Kelly, Joyce V. and Fred J. Hellinger. "Physician and Hospital Factors Associated With Mortality of Surgical Patients," *Medical Care*. Vol. 24, No. 9 (September, 1986).

Kemper, Peter and Christopher M. Murtaugh. "Lifetime Use of Nursing Home Care." *The New England Journal of Medicine*. Vol. 324, No. 9 (February 28, 1991).

Kemper, P., C.M. Murtaugh, and B.C. Spillman. "Nursing Home Use After Age 65 in the United States: Differences in Remaining Lifetime Use Among Subgroups and States." Agency Rockville, MD: Agency for Health Care Policy and Research (1991, June).

Kirklin, John W., Charles Fisch, George A. Beller, et al. "ACC/AHA Task Force Report—Guidelines and Indications for Coronary Artery Bypass Graft Surgery." *Journal of the American College of Cardiology*. Vol. 17, No. 3 (March 1, 1991)

Laffel, Glenn L., Arnold I. Barnett, Stan Finkelstein, et al. "The Relation Between Experience and Outcome in Heart Transplantation." *The New England Journal of Medicine*. Vol. 327, No. 17 (October 22, 1992).

Laffel, Glenn L. and Donald M. Berwick. "Quality Health Care." *Journal of the American Medical Association*. Vol. 270, No. 2 (July 14, 1993).

Lair, T. and D. Lefkowitz. "Mental Health and Functional Status of Residents of Nursing and Personal Care Homes." (DHHS-PHS Publication No. 90-3470). *National Medical Expenditure Survey Research Findings 7*. Rockville, MD: Agency for Health Care Policy and Research, Public Health Service.

Larson, Eric B. "Illnesses Causing Dementia in the Very Elderly." *The New England Journal of Medicine*. Vol. 328, No. 3 (January 21, 1993).

Leape, Lucian L., Troyen A. Brennan, Nan Laird, et al. "The Nature of Adverse Events in Hospitalized Patients—Results of the Harvard Medical Practice Study II." *New England Journal of Medicine*. Vol. 324, No. 6. (February 7, 1991).

Leape, Lucian L., Lee H. Hilborne, Rolla Edward Park, et al. "The Appropriateness of Use of Coronary Artery Bypass Graft Surgery in New York State." *Journal of the American Medical Association*. Vol. 269, No. 6 (February 10, 1993).

Lentzner, Harold R., Elsie R. Pamuk, Elaine P. Rhodenshiser, et al. "The Quality of Life in the Year before Death." *American Journal of Public Health*. Vol. 82, No. 8 (August, 1992).

Libow, Leslie S., and Perry Starer. "Care of the Nursing Home Patient." *New England Journal of Medicine*. Vol. 321, No. 2 (July 13, 1989).

Lindberg, Donald A., Elliot R. Siegel, Barbara A. Rapp, et al. "Use of MEDLINE by Physicians for Clinical Problem Solving." *Journal of the American Medical Association*. Vol. 269, No. 24 (June 23/30, 1993).

Liu, K., Kenneth G. Manton, and Barbara M. Liu. "Morbidity, Disability, and Long-term Care of the Elderly: Implications for Insurance Financing." *The Milbank Quarterly*. Vol. 68, No. 3, 1990.

Localio, A. Russell, Ann G. Lawthers, Troyen A. Brennan, et al. "Relation Between Malpractice Claims and Adverse Events Due to Negligence: Results of the Harvard Medical Practice Study III." *The New England Journal of Medicine*. Vol. 325, No. 4. (July 25, 1991).

Localio, A. Russell, Ann G. Lawthers, Joan M. Bengtson, et al. "Relationship Between Malpractice Claims and Cesarean Delivery." *Journal of the American Medial Association*. Vol. 269, No. 3 (January 20, 1993).

Lomas, Jonathan, et al. "Do Practice Guidelines Guide Practice? The Effect of a Consensus Statement on the Practice of Physicians," *The New England Journal of Medicine*. Vol. 321, No. 19 (November 9, 1989).

Lomas, Jonathan, Murray Enkin, Geoffrey M. Anderson, et al. "Opinion Leaders vs Audit and Feedback to Implement Practice Guidelines." *Journal of the American Medical Association*. Vol. 265, No 17. (May 1, 1991).

Luft, Harold S. and Patrick S. Romano. "Chance, Continuity, and Change in Hospital Mortality Rates." *Journal of the American Medical Association*. Vol. 270, No. 3 (July 21, 1993).

Lumsdon, Kevin. "Interview—Health Policy Researcher John E. Wennberg." *Hospitals and Health Networks*. (August 5, 1993).

Lundberg, George D. "National Health Care Reform, An Aura of Inevitability is Upon Us." *Journal of the American Medical Association*. Vol. 265, No. 19 (May 15, 1991).

Margo, Geoffrey M. and John M. Manring. "The Current Literature on Inpatient Psychotherapy," *Hospital and Community Psychiatry*. Vol. 40, No. 9 (September, 1989).

Martin, Peter, Leonard W. Poon, Gloria M. Clayton, et al. "Personality, Life Events and Coping in the Oldest-Old" *International Journal of Aging and Human Development*. Vol. 34, No. 1 (1992).

Metzloff, Thomas B. "Resolving Malpractice Disputes: Imaging the Jury's Shadow." *Law and Contemporary Problems*. Vol. 54, No. 1. (Winter, 1991).

Michels, Robert and Peter M. Marzuk. "Progress in Psychiatry." *The New England Journal of Medicine*. Part I. Vol. 329, No. 8 (August 19, 1993a).

Michels, Robert and Peter M. Marzuk. "Progress in Psychiatry." *The New England Journal of Medicine*. Part II. Vol. 329, No. 9 (August 26, 1993b).

Millman, M. (editor). "Access to Health Care in America. Institute of Medicine. 240 pp. Washington, D.C., National Academy Press, (1993). ISBN 0-309-04742-0.

Myers, Stephen A. and Norbert Gleicher. "A Successful Program to Lower Cesarean-Section Rates," *The New England Journal of Medicine*. Vol. 319, No. 23 (December 8, 1988).

National Cancer Institute. "Skin Cancers, Basal Cell and Squamous Cell Carcinomas. Research Report" National Institutes of Health Publication No. 91-2977. Bethesda, Maryland: National Cancer Institute; Revised, September 1990.

National Cancer Institute. "What You Need to Know About Skin Cancer" National Institutes of Health Publication No. 92-1564. Bethesda, Maryland: National Cancer Institute; Revised, February, 1992.

National Institutes of Health. "Older and Wiser, The Baltimore Longitudinal Study of Aging." Rockville, Maryland: Public Health Service; September 1989.

National Institutes of Health. "Sunlight, Ultraviolet Radiation, and the Skin." Bethesda, Maryland: U.S. Department of Health and Human Services, Public Health Service, Office of Medical Applications of Research; Volume 7, Number 8, May 8–10, 1989.

National Institute of Mental Health. "A Consumers Guide to Mental Health Services," U.S. Department of Health and Human Services, Public Health Service, Alcohol, Drug Abuse, and Mental Health Administration, DHHS Publication No. 87-214, Rockville, Maryland: Public Health Service; 1987.

National Academy of Sciences. "Diet and Health: Implications For Reducing Chronic Disease Risk," Washington, DC: National Academy Press; 1989.

Notzon, Francis C. "International Differences in the Use of Obstetric Interventions," *Journal of the American Medical Association*. Vol. 263, No. 24 (June 27, 1990).

O'Connor, Gerald T., Stephen K. Plume, Elaine M. Olmstead, et al. "A Regional Prospective Study of In-hospital Mortality Associated With Coronary Artery Bypass Grafting." *Journal of the American Medical Association*. Vol. 266, No. 6 (August 14, 1991).

Office of Technology Assessment, Congress of the United States. "The Quality of Medical Care," Washington. D.C.: U.S. Government Printing Office; 1988.

Office of Technology Assessment, Congress of the United States. "Special Care Units for People With Alzheimer's and Other Dementias: Consumer Education, Research, Regulatory, and Reimbursement Issues." GPO 052-003-01296-1. (1992) Washington, D.C.: U.S. Government Printing Office.

Office of Technology Assessment, Congress of the United States. "Home Drug Infusion Therapy Under Medicare" OTA Report Brief. (May, 1992) Washington, D.C.: Office of Technology Assessment.

Park, R. E., Robert H. Brook, Jacqueline Kosecoff, et al. "Explaining Variations in Hospital Death Rates." *Journal of the American Medical Association*. Vol. 264, No. 4 (July 25, 1990).

Parks, C. Murry. "Terminal Care: Home, Hospital, or Hospice?" *The Lancet*. Vol. 1 for 1985, No. 8421 (January 19, 1985).

Pekkanen, John. M.D.—Doctors Talk About Themselves. New York: Delacorte Press; 1988.

Pepine, Carl J., Hugh D. Allen, Thomas M. Bashore, et al. "ACC/AHA Guidelines for Cardiac Catheterization and Cardiac Catheterization Laboratories." *Journal of the American College of Cardiology*. Vol. 18, No. 5 (November 1, 1991).

Poon, Leonard W., Peter Martin, Gloria M. Clayton, et al. "The Influences of Cognitive Resources on Adaptation and Old Age." *International Journal of Aging and Human Development*. Vol. 34, No. 1 (1992a).

Poon, Leonard W., Gloria M. Clayton, Peter Martin, et al. "The Georgia Centenarian Study." *International Journal of Aging and Human Development*. Vol. 34, No. 1 (1992b).

Public Health Service. "1991 Report of Center-Specific Graft and Patient Survival Rates." U.S. Department of Health and Human Services, Health Resources and Services Administration (undated, released September 1992).

Regier, Darrel A., Jeffrey H. Boyd, Jack D. Burke Jr., et al. "One-Month Prevalence of Mental Disorders in the United States." *Archives of General Psychiatry*. Vol. 45, 977–986 (November, 1988).

Regier, Darrel A., William E. Narrow, Donald S. Rae, et al. "The de Facto US Mental and Addictive Disorders Service System." *Archives of General Psychiatry*. Vol. 50, 85–94 (February, 1993).

Rhymes, Jill. "Hospice Care in America," *Journal of the American Medical Association*. 1990, Vol. 264, No. 3 (July 18, 1990).

Quill, Timothy E., C.K. Cassel and D.E. Meier. "Care of the Hopelessly Ill." *The New England Journal of Medicine*. 1992; Vol. 327, No. 19 (November 5, 1992).

Quill, Timothy E. "Doctor, I Want to Die. Will You Help Me?" *Journal of the American Medical Association.* Vol. 270, No. 7 (August 18, 1993).

Regier, Darrel A., Jeffrey H. Boyd, Jack D. Burke, et al. "One-Month Prevalence of Mental Disorders in the United States." *Archives of General Psychiatry.* Vol. 45, (November, 1988).

Regier, Darrel A., William E. Narrow, Donald S. Rae, et al. "The de Facto Mental and Addictive Disorders Service System." *Archives of General Psychiatry.* Vol. 50, (February, 1993).

Rooks, Judith P., Norman L. Weatherby, Eunice K.M. Ernst, et al. "Outcomes of Care in Birth Centers: The National Birth Center Study," *The New England Journal of Medicine.* Vol. 321, No. 26 (December 28, 1989).

Rosenblatt, Roger A. "Specialists or Generalists—On Whom Should We Base the American Health Care System." *Journal of the American Medical Association.* Vol. 267, No. 12 (March 25, 1992). A

Rovner, Barry W., Pearl S. German, Larry J. Brant, et al. "Depression and Mortality in Nursing Homes." *Journal of the American Medical Association.* Vol. 265, No. 8 (February 27, 1991).

Rubin, Haya R., Barbara Gandek, William H. Rogers, et al. "Patients' Ratings of Outpatient Visits in Different Practice Settings." *Journal of the American Medical Association.* Vol. 270, No. 7 (August 18, 1993).

Schoenbaum, Stephen C. "Toward Fewer Procedures and Better Outcomes." *Journal of the American Medical Association.* Vol. 269, No. 6 (February 10, 1993).

Schapira, David V., James Studnicki, Douglas D. Bradham, et al. "Intensive Care, Survival, and Expense of Treating Critically Ill Cancer Patients." *Journal of the American Medical Association.* Vol. 269, No. 6 (February 10, 1993).

Shapiro, Martin F. and Sheldon Greenfield. "Experience and Outcomes in AIDS." *The Journal of the American Medical Association.* Vol. 268; No. 19 (November 18, 1992).

Showstack, Jonathan A, Kenneth E. Rosenfeld, Deborah W. Garnick, et al. "Association of Volume with Outcome of Coronary Artery Bypass Graft Surgery," *Journal of the American Medical Association.* Vol. 257, No. 6 (February 13, 1987).

Skoog, Ingmar, Lars Nilsson, Bo Palmertz, et al. "A Population-Based Study of Dementia in 85-Year-Olds." *The New England Journal of Medicine.* Vol. 328, No 3. (January 21, 1993).

Sloan, Frank A., Paula M. Mergenhagen, W. Bradley Burfield, et al. "Medical Malpractice Experience of Physicians, Predictable or Haphazard?" *Journal of the American Medical Association.* Vol. 262. No. 23 (December 15, 1989).

Soffel, D., Harold S. Luft. "Anatomy of Health Care Reform Proposals." *Western Journal of Medicine.* Vol. 159, pp. 494–500 (1993).

Solomon, Mildred Z., Lydia O'Donnell, Bruce Jennings, et al. "Decisions Near the End of Life: Professional Views on Life-Sustaining Treatments." *American Journal of Public Health.* Vol. 83, No. 1 (January, 1993).

Spector, William D. and Hitomi A. Takada. "Characteristics of Nursing Homes that Affect Resident Outcomes." *Journal of Aging and Health.* Vol. 3, No. 4. (November, 1991).

Stafford, Randall S. "Alternative Strategies for Controlling Rising Cesarean Section Rates," *Journal of the American Medical Association.* Vol. 263, No. 5 (February 2, 1990).

Stafford, Randall S. "The Impact of Nonclinical Factors on Repeat Cesarean Section." *Journal of the American Medical Association.* Vol. 265, No. 1 (January 2, 1991).

Stone, Valerie E., George R. Seage, Thomas Hertz, and Arnold M. Epstein. "The Relation Between Hospital Experience and Mortality for Patients With Aids." *Journal of the American Medical Association.* Vol. 268, No. 19 (November 18, 1992).

Tomchik, Robert S., Mary T. Russell, Alina M. Szmant, and Nancy A. Black. "Clinical Perspectives on Seabather's Eruption, Also Known as 'Sea Lice'." *Journal of the American Medical Association.* Vol. 269, No. 13 (April 7, 1993).

Turner, Barbara J. and Judy K. Ball. "Variations in Inpatient Mortality for AIDS in a National Sample of Hospitals." *Journal of Acquired Immune Deficiency Syndromes.* Vol. 5, No. 10 (October, 1992).

U. S. General Accounting Office. "Medicare: Assuring the Quality of Home Health Services" GAO/HRD-90-7. Washington, D.C.: U.S. General Accounting Office; October, 1989.

U. S. General Accounting Office. "Medicare: Improvements Needed in the Identification of Inappropriate Hospital Care." GAO/PEMD-90-7. Washington, D.C.: U.S. General Accounting Office; December, 1989.

U.S. General Accounting Office. "Medical Malpractice—Alternatives to Litigation." GAO/HRD-92-28. Washington, D.C.: U.S. General Accounting Office; January, 1992.

Weiler, Paul C., Joseph P. Newhouse, Howard H. Hiatt. "Proposal for Medical Liability Reform." *Journal of the American Medical Association.* Vol. 267, No. 17 (May 6, 1992).

Wennberg, John E., Jean L. Freeman, and William J. Culp "Are Hospital Services Rationed in New Haven or Over-Utilized in Boston?" *The Lancet.* Vol. 1 for 1987, No. 8543 (May 23, 1987).

Williams, S.V., David B. Nash and Neil Goldfarb. "Differences in Mortality From Coronary Artery Bypass Graft Surgery at Five Teaching Hospitals." *Journal of the American Medical Association.* Vol. 266, No. 6 (August 14, 1991).

Winslow, Constance M., Jacqueline B. Kosecoff, Mark Chassin, et al. "The Appropriateness of Performing Coronary Artery bypass Surgery." *Journal of the American Medical Association.* Vol. 260, No. 4 (July 22/29, 1988).

Wood, Bonnie S. "Hospice Care Under Medicare, Part II." *Corecare Registry.* Vol. 3, No. 1 (August/September, 1993).

Woolhandler, Steffie and David U. Himmelstein. "The Deteriorating Administrative Efficiency of the U.S. Health Care System." *New England Journal of Medicine.* Vol. 324, No. 18 (May 2, 1991).

Appendix A
1991 Hospital statistical tables

This appendix contains statistical information on Florida's hospitals. The data in the tables in this appendix indicate hospitals that:
- Offer the greatest range of medical and surgical services;
- Have the highest overall patient utilization;
- Have the highest utilization by Medicare patients;
- Have the largest physician staffs;
- Have the most types of physician specialists on their staffs; and
- Treat the most severely ill patients.

Hospitals are grouped into 11 districts:

District	Counties
District 1	Escambia, Okaloosa, Santa Rosa, Walton
District 2	Bay, Calhoun, Franklin, Gadsden, Gulf, Holmes, Jackson, Jefferson, Leon, Liberty, Madison, Taylor, Wakulla, Washington
District 3	Alachua, Bradford, Citrus, Columbia, Dixie, Gilchrist, Hamilton, Hernando, Lafayette, Lake, Levy, Marion, Putnam, Sumter, Suwannee, Union
District 4	Baker, Clay, Duval, Flagler, Nassau, St. Johns, Volusia
District 5	Pasco, Pinellas
District 6	Hardee, Highlands, Hillsborough, Manatee, Polk
District 7	Brevard, Orange, Osceola, Seminole
District 8	Charlotte, Collier, DeSoto, Glades, Hendry, Lee, Sarasota
District 9	Indian River, Martin, Okeechobee, Palm Beach, St. Lucie
District 10	Broward
District 11	Dade, Monroe

The following charts include columns specifying:

County code "CY"—The first column is a numerical code for each county. Florida has 67 counties, thus the codes range from 1 to 67. Counties are coded in alphabetical order, with Alachua having a code of 1, and Washington having a code of 67. The county codes are given at the beginning of each table. Eight sparsely populated rural counties do not have hospitals: Dixie, Gilchrist, Glades, Jefferson, Lafayette, Liberty, Sumter, and Wakulla.

Type of hospital "T"—Hospitals are divided into two categories: profit (P) and non-profit (NP).

Name of hospital—The names of hospitals are often abbreviated. The most common abbreviation is MC for Medical Center.

Beds—This is the total number of licensed operational beds in the hospital. The total includes acute care beds, psychiatric beds, substance abuse beds, rehabilitation beds, neonatal intensive care beds, intensive care beds for patients with severe burns, and skilled nursing beds.

Service index—Each of 30 medical services is assigned a score, with the most sophisticated services having the highest scores. For example, open heart surgery, burn intensive care, and neonatal intensive care each have a score of 5, while speech-language pathology has a score of 1.8. The scores for each of the 30 services are totaled and this total is the Service Index. The maximum score that can be obtained is 85.2.

Census—The census is the average number of patients that received care in the hospital on any given day. Simply stated, a hospital with a census of 123.7 had an average of 123.7 patients each day during the year.

Medicare—This reflects the percentage of patients that were admitted under Medicare. For example, if Medicare patients stayed 1,000 days during the year, and if all patients stayed a total of 2,000 days, the percent Medicare variable would be 50 percent.

Number of physicians—This is the total number of active physicians on the medical staff of the hospital.

Physician mix—This indicates how many different types of physician specialists there are on the hospital staff. Hospitals receive one point for each of 26 different physician specialists they have on staff. For example, a hospital with 15 different physician specialists would have a physician mix score of 15. The higher the number, the more varied the physician staff.

Case mix—This is the most complex variable, and a variable that should be evaluated with caution. Case mix measures how severely ill patients are and the complexity of procedures performed. The higher the score, the more complex the illness treated and the more sophisticated the surgeries and procedures. Each hospital's case mix score is computed by multiplying discharges for each Diagnostic Related Group (DRG) by a weight assigned each DRG, summing the product for all DRGs, and dividing by the hospital's total discharges. A DRG is a classification for an illness, surgery or procedure. There are close to 500 DRGs.

In viewing the case mix index score, it is important to note that hospitals with high proportions of Medicare patients (elderly patients) will tend to have high case mix scores because of the severe nature of many medical problems at advanced age. Hospitals that have lower proportions of the elderly tend to have lower case mix scores.

A single asterisk (*)—This indicates that the hospital changed its name after 1991 when the data were reported. The data given for these hospitals is for the hospital as it operated under another name at the same address. For example, in Levy County (District 3), Nature Coast Hospital is the new name for Williston Memorial Hospital. The data given for Nature Coast Hospital was reported while the hospital was named Williston Memorial Hospital.

IRTF—Is the acronym for Intensive Residential Treatment Facility. These residential mental health treatment facilities are licensed as psychiatric hospitals.

The hospital statistical tables include data from : the *1991 Hospital Groupings Report* for 1994 Budget Reviews (March 1993) which reports the service index, census, percent Medicare, physician mix, and case mix; the *1991 Hospital Financial Data Report* (April, 1993) which shows the number of physicians; and, the *Licensed Hospital Beds and Operational Regulated Services by Facility Report* (January, 1993) which shows the number of beds and type of hospital. These reports contain data reported by hospitals to the Agency for Health Care Administration and may be obtained from the agency or examined in a State of Florida depository library. Unless otherwise noted, all data is for the 1991 hospital fiscal year (except for physician mix data for the six statutory teaching hospitals).

1991 HOSPITAL STATISTICS

District 1

County Codes: Escambia (17), Okaloosa (46), Santa Rosa (57), and Walton (66).

ACUTE CARE GENERAL HOSPITALS

CY	T	Name	#Beds	Service Index	Census	Medi-care	Physicians: Number	Mix	Case Mix
17	NP	Baptist Hospital	520	60.8	219.9	48.1	141	23	1.265
17	NP	Sacred Heart	389	56.8	291.0	37.9	386	23	1.183
17	P	West Fla Regional MC	547	60.5	229.5	54.0	152	24	1.453
46	P	HCA Twin Cities	75	22.0	20.4	64.1	29	13	1.168
46	P	Humana, Destin	50	19.3	16.3	51.4	25	12	1.039
46	P	Humana, Ft Walton	247	42.4	129.4	48.3	106	22	1.156
46	P	N Okaloosa MC	110	22.3	37.2	63.0	21	12	1.275
57	NP	Gulf Breeze	60	26.7	21.8	58.0	63	19	1.207
57	NP	Jay Hospital	55	18.2	12.6	59.9	11	5	.890
57	P	Santa Rosa MC	129	27.0	39.2	48.8	56	18	1.074
66	NP	Walton Regional	50	19.2	15.0	70.3	5	2	.980

SHORT-TERM PSYCHIATRIC HOSPITALS

CY	T	Name	#Beds
17	P	Lakeview Center (IRTF)	24
17	P	Baptist Hospital-Univ.	26
46	P	Harbor Oaks Hosp	79

District 2

County Codes: Bay (3), Calhoun (7), Franklin (19), Gadsden (20), Gulf (23), Holmes (30), Jackson (32), Jefferson, Leon (37), Liberty, Madison (40), Taylor (62), Wakulla, and Washington (67). Counties without codes, except for Calhoun County, do not have hospitals. Calhoun Hospital did not report data to the Health Care Cost Containment Board.

ACUTE CARE GENERAL HOSPITALS

CY	T	Name	#Beds	Service Index	Census	Medi-care	Physicians: Number	Mix	Case Mix
3	NP	Bay Medical Center	302	59.2	231.0	53.9	132	22	1.224
3	P	HCA Gulf Coast Comm.	176	36.2	120.3	53.0	151	22	1.045
7	NP	Calhoun Gen Hospital	36	4.6	8.9	52.6	N/A	4	.906
19	P	Emerald Coast Hospital	29	12.5	6.1	48.5	4	2	.785
20	NP	Gadsden Memorial	51	20.3	10.2	48.6	6	3	.904
23	P	Gulf Pines Hospital	45	14.5	11.6	51.9	5	2	.805
30	P	Doctors Mem, Bonifay	34	18.6	16.9	63.9	10	6	1.102
32	NP	Campbellton-Graceville	50	11.1	6.8	65.3	N/A	-	.890
32	MP	Jackson Hospital	107	27.0	57.8	52.7	24	11	.966
37	P	HCA Tallahassee Com	180	44.7	100.8	51.8	175	21	1.249
37	NP	Tallahassee Mem RMC	771	65.3	383.2	37.6	296	24	1.200
40	NP	Madison Memorial	42	19.0	14.7	54.5	N/A	6	.951
62	NP	Doctors, Perry	48	18.3	12.4	48.2	N/A	7	.902
67	NP	NW Fla Community	81	25.5	23.8	69.6	4	2	.969

COMPREHENSIVE REHABILITATION HOSPITALS

37	P	Capitol Rehabilitation	40

SHORT-TERM PSYCHIATRIC HOSPITALS

17	P	Rivendale of Bay	80
37	NP	Eastside Psychiatric	24

LONG-TERM PSYCHIATRIC HOSPITALS

37	NP	Wateroak Hospital	16
19	NP	The Shores	190

District 3

County Codes: Alachua (1), Bradford (4), Citrus (9), Columbia (12), Dixie, Gilchrist, Hamilton (24), Hernando (27), Lafayette, Lake (35), Levy (38), Marion (42), Putnam (54), Sumter, Suwannee (61) and Union (63). Counties without codes do not have hospitals.

ACUTE CARE GENERAL HOSPITALS

CY	T	Name	#Beds	Service Index	Census	Medi-care	Physicians: Number	Mix	Case Mix
1	NP	Alachua General	506	60.0	199.1	49.0	277	24	1.210
1	P	North Fla Reg MC	267	48.0	188.5	55.7	220	24	1.351
1	NP	Shands Hospital	556	75.7	412.7	23.5	372	25	1.337
4	NP	Bradford Hospital	54	15.3	11.1	65.7	9	5	.920
9	NP	Citrus Memorial	171	25.0	104.5	63.7	77	22	1.158
9	P	Seven Rivers Comm	128	35.1	69.4	75.7	66	18	1.193
12	P	Lake City MC	75	23.4	33.9	51.6	19	14	.926
12	NP	Lake Shore Hospital	128	27.0	34.7	44.7	24	12	.950
24	NP	Hamilton County	42	16.5	7.1	63.9	3	2	1.010
27	NP	Brooksville Regional	91	37.4	76.8	68.6	66	19	1.233
27	P	HCA Oak Hill Community	150	29.8	127.1	79.8	128	22	1.323
27	NP	Spring Hill Regional	75	—	—	—	—	—	—
35	NP	Leesburg Reg MC*	294	35.2	123.2	68.3	90	18	1.141
35	NP	South Lake Memorial	68	26.7	30.8	61.8	11	6	1.227
35	NP	Waterman MC	182	37.8	82.2	69.5	65	17	1.171
38	NP	Nature Coast Regional*	40	18.0	9.8	73.2	11	7	1.007
42	P	Marion Community	190	37.2	161.9	74.8	203	24	1.577
42	NP	Munroe Regional MC	293	51.0	199.8	56.1	131	23	1.351
54	P	HCA Putnam Comm	161	36.2	86.7	61.3	63	16	1.095
61	NP	Suwannee Hospital	30	17.1	8.6	60.7	5	4	.968
63	P	Ramadan Hand Institute	27	16.2	5.0	33.3	8	7	.958

SHORT-TERM PSYCHIATRIC HOSPITALS

27	P	Greenbrier Hospital	50
35	NP	Lake Sumter CMHC	40
42	P	Charter Springs	92

LONG-TERM PSYCHIATRIC HOSPITALS

9	P	Heritage, Beverly Hills	88

COMPREHENSIVE REHABILITATION HOSPITALS

01	NP	Upreach Pavilion	40

SPECIALTY HOSPITALS

35	NP	Fla. Elks Children's	100

District 4

County Codes: Baker (2), Clay (10), Duval (16), Flagler (18), Nassau (45), St. Johns (55), and Volusia (64).

ACUTE CARE GENERAL HOSPITALS

CY	T	Name	#Beds	Service Index	Census	Medi-care	Physicians: Number	Mix	Case Mix
2	NP	Ed Fraser Memorial	25	13.3	9.1	43.5	N/A	6	.835
10	P	Humana, Orange Park	224	49.5	127.3	52.7	146	24	1.103
16	NP	Baptist MC of the Beach	82	23.8	33.7	62.8	52	17	1.186
16	NP	Baptist Med Center	601	68.0	341.2	31.5	483	24	1.122
16	NP	Memorial Medical Cntr	353	52.8	249.0	49.7	821	24	1.332
16	NP	Methodist Medical Cntr	244	46.0	121.1	69.0	132	22	1.320
16	NP	Riverside Hospital	183	43.4	50.7	65.3	90	20	1.158
16	NP	St. Luke's Hospital	289	47.6	157.1	63.9	192	23	1.593
16	NP	St. Vincent's MC	528	65.7	353.5	54.2	231	24	1.354
16	NP	University Medical Cntr	517	68.0	358.7	18.9	219	26	1.121
18	NP	Memorial Hosp, Flagler	81	22.0	18.5	61.0	24	12	1.084
45	NP	Nassau General	54	25.0	22.0	54.2	15	8	.918
55	NP	Flagler Hospital	115	24.0	71.3	54.2	61	19	1.043
55	NP	Flagler Hospital, West*	115	22.3	35.0	65.1	34	16	1.260
64	NP	Fish Memorial, Deland	97	24.3	26.3	74.2	79	16	1.106
64	NP	Fish Memorial, N Smyrna	116	25.4	49.0	59.5	34	15	1.222
64	NP	Halifax Medical Center	545	52.6	280.8	47.9	233	22	1.191
64	P	Humana, Daytona	214	38.2	85.4	75.5	148	21	1.367
64	NP	Memorial, Ormond Beach	205	35.1	104.8	70.4	132	21	1.841
64	P	Peninsula Medical Cntr	119	24.3	71.4	53.9	53	14	1.272
64	NP	West Volusia Mem	156	33.6	92.4	49.2	90	18	1.107

SHORT-TERM PSYCHIATRIC HOSPITALS

CY	T	Name	#Beds
16	P	Charter Hospital	64
16	NP	Daniel Memorial (IRTF)	63
16	NP	Methodist Pathway	25
16	P	St. Johns River	99
18	P	St Augustine Psych Cntr	50
64	P	HSA Atlantic Shores	50

COMPREHENSIVE REHABILITATION HOSPITALS
16 NP Memorial Reg Rehab 110

SPECIALTY REHABILITATION HOSPITALS
16 NP Jacksonville MC 107

SPECIALTY HEALTH CARE FACILITIES
16 Mayo Outpatient Clinic

District 5

County Codes: Pasco (51) and Pinellas (52).

ACUTE CARE GENERAL HOSPITALS

CY	T	Name	#Beds	Service Index	Census	Medi-care	Physicians: Number	Mix	Case Mix
51	P	Bayonet Pt/Hudson	200	48.4	162.9	75.6	236	24	1.701
51	NP	East Pasco MC	85	37.8	67.3	67.8	72	20	1.160
51	P	HCA N Port Richey Hosp	414	43.2	267.7	85.3	207	22	1.304
51	P	Humana Hospital, Pasco	120	25.3	46.6	73.4	37	15	1.120
51	P	Riverside Hospital	122	31.1	67.5	59.8	161	20	1.073
52	NP	Bayfront Med Center	518	60.5	258.0	41.7	236	24	1.277
52	P	Clearwater Community	133	30.5	67.1	60.6	257	22	1.240
52	P	Edward White Hospital	167	27.8	66.9	78.4	280	20	1.380
52	P	Gulf Coast Hospital*	200	30.0	57.9	83.4	N/A	14	1.342
52	P	HCA Med Center, Largo	256	52.1	168.8	70.9	247	22	1.550
52	NP	Helen Ellis Hospital	150	40.7	99.9	78.0	82	20	1.268
52	P	Humana, Northside	301	40.7	119.0	76.0	104	22	1.331
52	P	Humana, St Petersburg	219	36.6	105.0	78.7	111	18	1.286
52	NP	Mease, Countryside	100	30.5	69.5	67.5	227	23	1.144
52	NP	Mease, Dunedin	278	57.0	137.5	60.2	227	23	1.139
52	NP	Metropolitan General	154	24.0	50.8	68.5	114	18	1.212
52	NP	Morton Plant Hospital	750	65.7	378.1	61.8	227	24	1.331
52	P	Palms of Pasadena	310	36.6	163.8	72.4	99	21	1.400
52	NP	St. Anthony's	434	52.1	214.5	72.0	230	24	1.293
52	NP	Sun Coast Hospital	300	36.4	110.8	61.6	94	21	1.147
52	P	University Gen Hosp	140	24.3	52.6	67.2	37	13	1.221
52	P	Women's Hosp/Med Cntr	99	14.9	15.3	5.8	49	13	.843

SHORT-TERM PSYCHIATRIC HOSPITALS
51	P	Charter of Pasco	72
52	P	Horizon Hospital	200
52	P	Medfield Center	64

LONG-TERM PSYCHIATRIC HOSPITALS
52	P	The Manors	130
52	P	Bay Harbor IRTF	40

COMPREHENSIVE REHABILITATION HOSPITALS
52	P	Healthsouth Rehab Cntr	40

OTHER SPECIALTY HOSPITALS
52	NP	All Children's	168

District 6

County Codes: Hardee (25), Highlands (28), Hillsborough (29), Manatee (41), and Polk (53).

ACUTE CARE GENERAL HOSPITALS

CY	T	Name	#Beds	Service Index	Census	Medi-care	Physicians: Number	Mix	Case Mix
28	P	Highlands Regional MC	126	30.0	69.7	76.9	59	16	1.237
28	NP	Walker Memorial	151	30.8	102.3	58.4	30	14	1.010
29	P	AMI Town & Country	201	37.9	76.8	43.0	146	22	1.124
29	P	Centurion Hospital	120	24.3	48.4	69.4	146	21	1.217
29	P	Doctors' Hospital/Tampa	102	27.0	35.0	62.9	N/A	24	1.075
29	P	Humana, Brandon	250	48.1	180.2	50.0	120	20	1.178
29	P	Memorial Hospital/Tampa	174	33.4	103.0	62.2	174	23	1.250
29	P	South Bay Hospital	112	31.8	53.0	80.6	48	15	1.353
29	NP	South Fla Baptist Hosp	147	34.8	57.4	62.2	53	17	1.161
29	NP	St. Joseph's Hospital	649	58.8	418.2	50.6	426	24	1.457
29	NP	Tampa General	995	75.7	530.9	30.1	435	23	1.530
29	NP	University Community	404	56.1	196.3	47.8	349	24	1.387
41	P	L.W. Blake Memorial	383	52.4	208.5	77.2	215	24	1.473
41	NP	Manatee Memorial	512	61.5	284.1	53.8	232	24	1.313
53	NP	Bartow Memorial	56	25.0	17.6	49.4	34	13	.930
53	NP	Lake Wales Hospital	154	27.3	31.1	60.6	16	10	1.117
53	NP	Lakeland Regional MC	897	63.4	382.4	57.8	217	23	1.309
53	NP	Mid Florida Hlth Cntrs*	51	20.3	16.4	74.8	12	7	1.045
53	NP	Morrow Memorial	40	13.7	12.7	2.4	22	10	1.301
53	NP	Polk General	180	29.3	68.9	20.0	16	11	.874
53	NP	Winter Haven Hospital	579	56.3	234.9	53.4	195	20	1.147

SHORT-TERM PSYCHIATRIC HOSPITALS

CY	T	Name	#Beds
29	P	Charter Tampa Bay	146
29	P	Glenbeigh of Tampa	100
29	NP	Northside Center	32
29	NP	U of S Fla Psych	114
41	P	Charter Hosp, Bradenton	60
41	NP	Glen Oaks Hospital	27
53	P	Palmview	66

SHORT-TERM PSYCHIATRIC HOSPITALS

CY	T	Name	#Beds
41	P	Manatee Palms (IRTF)	60

SPECIALTY HOSPITALS

CY	T	Name	#Beds
29	NP	Moffit Cancer Center	162
29	P	Humana Women's	234
29	NP	Shriners Children's	60
29	P	Vencor Hospital, Tampa	73

District 7

County Codes: Brevard (5), Orange (48), Osceola (49), and Seminole (59).

ACUTE CARE GENERAL HOSPITALS

CY	T	Name	#Beds	Service Index	Census	Medi-care	Physicians: Number	Mix	Case Mix
5	NP	Cape Canaveral	150	35.5	86.5	53.3	88	22	1.089
5	NP	Holmes Regional MC	468	61.1	354.7	59.4	230	24	1.282
5	NP	Parrish Medical Center	210	37.5	125.3	51.7	96	22	1.016
5	NP	Wuesthoff Memorial	303	48.9	173.4	55.1	131	22	1.096
48	NP	Florida Hospital**	1342	72.0	848.2	50.4	675	24	1.429
48	P	Humana, Lucerne	267	57.4	149.0	57.7	332	23	1.328
48	NP	Orlando Regional MC***	780	73.0	555.5	29.2	384	26	1.276
48	NP	Princeton Hospital	153	32.2	73.7	32.0	137	22	1.015
48	NP	West Orange Mem	141	32.3	36.7	55.5	36	12	.988
48	NP	Winter Park Mem	301	39.4	166.6	52.0	348	24	1.062
49	P	Humana, Kissimmee	169	35.1	104.2	50.3	75	19	1.093
49	P	Kissimmee Memorial	120	25.0	45.5	64.3	87	20	1.138
49	NP	St. Cloud Hospital	84	28.1	45.9	68.7	53	17	1.138
59	P	Central Fla Regional	226	34.9	130.4	61.0	106	19	1.241
59	P	South Seminole MC	126	28.5	48.9	62.8	147	20	1.275

** Florida Hospital reported combined data for: Apopka (50 beds); Orlando (805 beds); East Orlando (197 beds); and Altamonte Springs (290 beds).

***Orlando Regional MC data are combined for ORMC-Orlando (598 beds), and ORMC-Sand Lake (182 beds).

SHORT-TERM PSYCHIATRIC HOSPITALS

5	NP	Circles of Care	72
5	P	CPC Palm Bay	60
5	NP	Devereux Hospital	100
48	P	Crossroads Univ.	100
48	P	Glenbeigh Hospital	80
48	P	La Amistad (IRTF)	40
48	P	Laurel Oaks Hospital	80
48	P	Laurel Oaks (IRTF)	40
49	P	Charter, Orlando South	60
59	P	HCA West Lake	80
59	NP	Winter Park Pavilion	52

LONG-TERM PSYCHIATRIC HOSPITALS

48	P	Laurel Oaks (IRTF)	40

COMPREHENSIVE REHABILITATION HOSPITALS

5	P	Sea Pines Rehab	80

SPECIALTY HOSPITALS

28	NP	Palmer Children & Womens	255

(Affiliated with Orlando Regional Medical Center)

District 8

County Codes: Charlotte (8), Collier (11), Glades, Desoto (14), Hendry (26), Lee (36), and Sarasota (58). Glades County does not have a hospital.

ACUTE CARE GENERAL HOSPITALS

CY	T	Name	#Beds	Service Index	Census	Medi- care	Physicians: Number	Mix	Case Mix
8	P	Fawcett Memorial	254	36.0	113.3	79.6	164	22	1.243
8	NP	Medical Center Hospital	208	48.2	90.1	68.3	162	22	1.443
8	NP	St. Joseph's Hospital	212	35.0	114.2	61.9	83	20	1.088
11	NP	Naples Community**	434	49.9	308.2	56.9	194	23	1.098
14	NP	Desoto Memorial	82	32.5	31.4	50.3	11	9	.880
26	NP	Hendry General	66	19.3	16.9	42.6	10	7	.946
36	NP	Cape Coral Hospital	201	45.7	141.3	68.7	120	19	1.216
36	P	East Pointe Hospital	88	17.3	51.4	74.3	43	14	1.172
36	P	Gulf Coast, Ft Myers	120	26.1	30.8	67.0	320	20	1.144
36	NP	Lee Memorial***	627	58.5	331.8	46.7	554	21	1.253
36	P	SW Fla Regional MC	400	46.7	223.9	66.4	384	24	1.531
58	P	Doctors, Sarasota	168	36.2	88.2	71.9	255	22	1.349
58	P	Englewood Community	100	25.8	52.1	78.5	101	21	1.193
58	NP	Sarasota Memorial	863	61.5	463.0	62.8	395	23	1.456
58	NP	Venice Hospital	342	38.8	171.9	79.9	137	22	1.259

**Naples Community Hospital reported combined data for the Naples and North Collier hospitals.

***Lee Memorial Hospital reported combined data for the Cleveland (407 beds) and HealthPark (220 beds) hospitals.

SHORT-TERM PSYCHIATRIC HOSPITALS
11	P	The Willough	64
36	P	Charter Glade	104
36	P	The Glade Center	50
58	P	Sarasota Palms	125

COMPREHENSIVE REHABILITATION HOSPITALS
58	P	Rehab Inst of Sarasota	60

District 9

County Codes: Indian River (31), Martin (43), Okeechobee (47), Palm Beach (50), and St. Lucie (56).

ACUTE CARE GENERAL HOSPITALS

CY	T	Name	#Beds	Service Index	Census	Medi-care	Physicians: Number	Mix	Case Mix
31	P	Humana Sebastian	133	35.3	61.0	68.9	113	21	1.097
31	NP	Indian River Mem	347	44.0	195.2	64.5	169	24	1.196
43	NP	Martin Memorial**	336	58.2	212.2	61.9	185	24	1.207
47	P	HCA Raulerson Memorial	101	22.3	50.6	72.1	24	12	1.280
50	P	AMI Palm Beach Gardens	204	54.0	127.6	56.7	268	23	1.621
50	NP	Bethesda Memorial	362	56.7	195.6	49.1	125	19	1.094
50	NP	Boca Raton Comm	394	38.9	248.9	72.4	261	24	1.187
50	P	Delray Community	211	42.6	141.9	81.9	203	22	1.620
50	NP	Everglades Memorial	63	25.3	38.7	16.6	52	13	.878
50	NP	Glades General	73	24.0	35.6	22.4	21	10	1.014
50	NP	Good Samaritan	341	46.1	164.8	40.6	442	24	1.138
50	P	Humana, Palm Beach	250	34.8	120.5	72.1	175	20	1.255
50	NP	JFK Medical Center	369	56.8	199.0	68.0	206	22	1.518
50	NP	Jupiter Hospital	156	34.4	87.4	65.7	174	24	1.265
50	P	Palm Beach Regional	200	39.0	95.3	76.8	171	23	1.340
50	P	Palms West Hospital	117	28.5	44.5	35.5	161	22	1.018
50	NP	St. Mary's Hospital	430	55.5	283.9	36.7	448	23	1.085
50	P	Wellington Regional MC	120	34.3	45.2	40.6	312	23	1.173
50	P	West Boca Med Center	185	39.9	97.8	45.6	149	21	.981
56	P	HCA MC Port St. Lucie	150	22.0	83.4	72.2	101	19	1.262
56	P	Lawnwood Regional MC	335	45.5	203.7	50.3	168	23	1.042

**Combined data were reported for Martin Memorial Medical Center (236 beds) and Martin Memorial Hospital South (100 beds).

SHORT-TERM PSYCHIATRIC HOSPITALS

43	P	Sandypines	60
50	P	Charter, W Palm Beach	60
50	NP	45th St Mental Hth	44
50	P	Glenbeigh	60
50	P	Fair Oaks	102
56	P	Savannas Hospital	70

COMPREHENSIVE REHABILITATION HOSPITALS

31	P	Treasure Coast Rehab	70
50	P	Pinecrest Rehab	60

District 10

County Code: Broward County (6)

ACUTE CARE GENERAL HOSPITALS

CY	T	Name	#Beds	Service Index	Census	Medi-care	Physicians: Number	Mix	Case Mix
6	NP	Broward General MC	744	62.0	434.7	26.8	295	24	1.250
6	NP	Coral Springs MC	200	46.8	111.4	31.4	314	23	1.052
6	P	Doctors Hosp, Hollywood	124	24.1	46.7	62.8	131	21	1.064
6	P	Florida Medical Ctr	459	53.8	266.2	65.9	335	23	1.587
6	P	HCA Northwest Regional	150	39.9	73.3	69.0	303	23	1.183
6	P	Hollywood Medical Ctr	334	31.5	102.2	58.9	466	22	1.195
6	NP	Holy Cross Hospital	597	55.5	250.4	66.8	338	24	1.488
6	P	Humana, Bennett	204	31.3	140.2	58.3	419	22	1.076
6	P	Humana, Cypress	273	38.0	112.5	79.2	152	21	1.161
6	P	Humana, Pembroke Pines	301	37.5	81.6	56.2	161	22	1.138
6	NP	Imperial Point MC	204	41.5	121.6	46.1	552	22	1.176
6	NP	Memorial of Hollywood	646	63.2	529.5	42.5	562	23	1.216
6	NP	Memorial West	100	37.7	26.0	35.0	N/A	24	1.052
6	NP	North Beach Hospital	153	30.2	74.3	65.1	68	18	1.509
6	NP	North Broward MC	419	44.4	188.2	51.9	329	24	1.182
6	P	North Ridge MC	395	45.7	149.9	72.4	250	20	1.897
6	P	Plantation General	264	41.9	152.3	30.0	587	24	1.006
6	P	Universal Medical Ctr	202	24.0	52.3	72.6	102	17	1.195
6	P	University Hospital	269	30.3	123.4	76.7	253	22	1.203

SHORT-TERM PSYCHIATRIC HOSPITALS

6	P	Coral Ridge Psychiatric	86
6	P	CPC Ft. Lauderdale	100
6	P	Hollywood Pavilion	46
6	P	Retreat Psychiatric	100
6	P	University Pavilion	60

COMPREHENSIVE REHABILITATION HOSPITALS

| 6 | NP | St. John's Rehab | 20 |
| 6 | P | Sunrise Rehabilitation | 108 |

SPECIALTY REHABILITATION HOSPITALS

| 6 | P | Manor Oaks | 116 |
| 6 | p | Vencor Hospital | 64 |

OTHER SPECIALTY FACILITIES

| 6 | P | Cleveland Outpatient Clinic |

District 11

County Codes: Dade (11) and Monroe (44).

ACUTE CARE GENERAL HOSPITALS

CY	T	Name	#Beds	Service Index	Census	Medi-care	Physicians: Number	Mix	Case Mix
11	P	Kendall Regional MC	412	44.0	142.4	64.5	180	22	1.337
11	P	AMI Palmetto General	360	47.1	216.3	37.6	857	23	1.029
11	NP	Baptist Hospital	513	56.1	364.3	39.9	402	24	1.283
11	NP	Cedars Medical Cnt	585	58.3	308.8	58.1	162	22	1.323
11	P	Coral Gables Hospital	285	34.0	128.4	69.0	125	20	1.226
11	P	Deering Hospital*	260	43.7	112.3	37.3	325	23	1.173
11	P	Golden Glades RMC	352	28.1	60.2	31.3	388	23	.958
11	P	Healthsouth Doctors	285	35.5	82.9	47.2	257	22	1.141
11	NP	Hialeah Hospital	411	40.3	165.0	42.8	667	23	.980
11	P	Humana, Biscayne	458	45.4	159.6	74.3	324	20	1.111
11	NP	Jackson Memorial**	1567	75.6	1159.9	12.9	547	26	1.214
11	P	Larkin General	112	31.0	44.9	51.6	97	17	1.090
11	NP	Mercy Hospital	532	58.6	277.3	53.9	198	22	1.279
11	NP	Miami Beach Community*	273	51.9	122.9	71.9	351	24	1.372
11	NP	Mt. Sinai Medical Ctr	707	67.9	428.2	67.3	*378*	25	1.445
11	NP	North Shore MC	357	54.0	175.3	40.4	547	24	1.034
11	P	Palm Springs General	247	28.5	114.1	61.1	178	20	1.038
11	NP	Pan American Hospital	146	23.7	100.9	63.8	359	22	1.218
11	P	Parkway Regional MC	412	43.0	187.6	64.2	646	23	1.276
11	NP	SMH Homestead*	120	26.7	61.2	46.7	83	18	.949
11	NP	South Miami Hospital	500	58.3	229.5	41.5	1000	24	1.215
11	NP	South Shore Hospital	178	30.6	116.0	67.4	208	23	1.171
11	NP	Univ of Miami Hospital	40	11.3	17.2	42.7	522	21	1.087
11	P	Victoria Hospital	300	39.8	142.9	44.3	184	21	1.126
11	P	Westchester General	100	33.2	20.0	39.0	137	21	.873
44	NP	Health Systems DePoo	49	26.8	35.6	46.9	N/A	18	1.058
44	P	Fishermen's Hospital	58	24.0	20.2	64.1	31	13	1.190
44	NP	Health Systems Fla Keys	120	N/A	N/A	N/A	N/A	N/A	N/A
44	NP	Mariner's Hospital	42	22.3	16.9	68.2	13	9	1.101

**Data includes Jackson Memorial (1,498 beds and Jackson Memorial North (69 beds).

Note: 1990 data were used for the number of physicians at Mt. Sinai Medical Center.

District 11 (continued)

County Codes: Dade (11) and Monroe (44).

SHORT-TERM PSYCHIATRIC HOSPITALS

CY	T	Name	#Beds
11	P	Charter Hosp-Miami	8
11	P	Glenbeigh Hospital	100
11	P	Grant Center	140
11	P	Harbor View Hospital	94
11	P	Southern Winds	60

SPECIALTY HOSPITALS

CY	T	Name	#Beds
11	NP	Ann Leach Eye Hospital	100
11	NP	Miami Childrens	208
11	NP	Miami Heart Institute	258

COMPREHENSIVE REHABILITATION HOSPITALS

CY	T	Name	#Beds
11	NP	Bon Secours Hospital	60
11	P	West Gables Rehab	27

SPECIALTY REHABILITATION HOSPITALS

CY	T	Name	#Beds
11	NP	Douglas Gardens (geriatric)	32
11	P	Vencor Hospital	53

APPENDIX B
1992 Hospital cesarean section rates

This appendix contains cesarean section (c-section) rates and numbers of deliveries reported by Florida hospitals during calendar year 1992. Every hospital completes quarterly diagnostic related group (DRG) patient discharge reports. These reports contain the number of patients that had c-section and vaginal deliveries. The c-section rate is derived by adding DRGs 370 and 371 (these are the c-section DRGs) and dividing this number by the total number of discharges for all DRGs related to delivery (the total for DRGs 370, 371, 372, 373, 374, and 375).

There are three c-section rates; an overall rate, a primary rate, and a repeat rate. The overall rate is the percentage of all patients who delivered by c-section. The primary rate is the percentage of women who have never delivered previously by c-section of all women who delivered. The repeat rate is the percentage of women who delivered by c-section who delivered an earlier child by c-section.

The statewide c-section rate for all deliveries in Florida hospitals in 1992 was 25.1 percent, essentially the same as the 1991 rate of 25.2 percent. There were, however, sharp differences in c-section rates for patients with commercial insurance versus patients covered by Medicaid. For example, during 1992 the statewide c-section rate for patients in commercial HMOs was 31.2 percent, while the rate was only 20.7 percent for patients in Medicaid HMOs. For patients not in HMOs or PPOs, the average rate for persons with commercial insurance was 29.7 percent, compared with 22.1 percent for patients covered by Medicaid.

The disparity between the Medicaid and commercial insurance rates can be partially explained by differences in age. As a group, Medicaid recipients are substantially younger than commercially insured patients. As age increases, so does the probability of a c-section. Except in the early teen years, maternal age is positively correlated with the incidence of c-sections.

Commercial HMO patients accounted for 12.3 percent of deliveries; commercial insurance, 19.7 percent; commercial PPOs, 11.3 percent; Medicaid, 40.2 percent; Medicaid HMOs, 1.9 percent; Self-insured and uninsured, 10.8 percent; and other patients comprised the remaining 3.8 percent.

The Obstetrical section of Chapter 3 contains a discussion of research studies that have examined c-section rates. In examining hospital c-section rates, there are several factors that are important to keep in mind:
- It is the physicians on the hospital's medical staff who perform c-sections, not the hospital itself.
- The hospital's average c-section rate is the average of all physicians on staff who deliver; individual physicians may have higher or lower rates.
- Patient income is related to the c-section rate; c-section rates increase as income increases.

- Cesarean section rates increase as the age of the patient increases.
- Hospital c-section rates vary widely. During 1992 they ranged from a low of 12.8 percent at the University Medical Center in Jacksonville, to a high of 44.2 percent in Hialeah Hospital in Miami. These same two hospitals had the lowest and highest rates during 1991.
- In 1992, the average hospital stay for a patient who delivered by c-section was 4.1 days, compared with 2.1 days for a vaginal delivery.
- The average hospital charge for a cesarean delivery was $6,981 in 1992, more than twice the average charge of $3,247 for a vaginal delivery.
- The average primary cesarean rate during 1992 was 16.0 percent; the average repeat cesarean rate was 9.3 percent; and the vaginal birth after previous cesarean rate was 27.3 percent.
- Primary cesarean rates, repeat cesarean rates, and vaginal birth after previous cesarean rates vary widely among hospitals. During 1992, the primary cesarean rate ranged from a low of 5.7 percent to a high of 28.5 percent; the repeat cesarean rate ranged from a low of 3.2 percent to a high of 20.0 percent; and the vaginal birth after cesarean rate ranged from a low of 0.9 percent to a high of 61.4 percent.

Hospital Deliveries and Cesarean Section Rates
In Hospitals With at Least 10 Deliveries
1992

	Total Number Deliveries	All Patients Cesarean Section Rate
District 1		
Baptist Hospital, Pensacola	1616	23.2
Fort Walton Beach Hospital	1024	24.5
Sacred Heart Hospital, Pensacola	2591	24.8
Santa Rosa Medical Center	616	25.5
HCA West Florida Reg Med Cntr	746	25.5
District 2		
HCA Tallahassee Community	1210	21.2
Tallahassee Memorial Reg Med Cntr	3344	21.4
Jackson Hospital, Marianna	634	27.4
Gulf Coast Hospital	1468	31.5
Bay Medical Center	771	33.6
District 3		
HCA Putnam Community Hospital	463	13.2
Leesburg Regional Medical Cntr	1004	16.8
Munroe Regional Medical Cntr	1908	17.2
HCA North Florida Reg. MC	1492	18.8
Shands Teaching Hospital & Clinics	3654	20.1
Lakeshore Hospital	161	20.5
Citrus Memorial Hospital	705	22.8
Waterman Medical Center	717	25.9
Alachua General Hospital	615	26.0
Brooksville Regional Hospital	148	29.1
Seven Rivers Community	213	29.6
Springhill Regional Hospital	378	29.9
District 4		
University Medical Center	4875	12.8
Flagler Hospital	548	16.8
Halifax Hospital Medical Center	2666	18.3
Riverside Hospital, Jacksonville	366	18.6
St. Vincent's Medical Center	1595	19.2
Nassau General Hospital	1539	24.3
West Volusia Memorial Hospital	1142	24.3
Flagler Hospital West	181	24.9
Baptist Medical Cntr, Jacksonville	3737	25.9
Memorial Medical Cntr, Jacksonville	2521	26.6
Orange Park Medical Center	1030	31.0

	Total Number Deliveries	All Patients Cesarean Section Rate

District 5

Sun Coast Hospital	496	17.7
Morton F. Plant Hospital	2351	18.1
Women's Medical Center	893	24.4
Mease Hospital & Clinics	1646	25.1
St. Petersburg General Hospital	570	26.8
Dade City Hospital	403	26.8
Bayfront Medical Center	3782	27.3
East Pasco Medical Center	481	33.7
Riverside Hospital, Pasco	1141	36.1
St. Anthony's Hospital	374	36.4

District 6

Polk General Hospital	2265	15.5
Tampa General Hospital	5164	15.7
Walker Memorial Hospital	1105	17.5
Lakeland Regional Medical Center	2046	18.6
Winter Haven Hospital	1238	21.6
Manatee Memorial Hospital	1799	22.1
Lake Wales Hospital	191	23.6
Bartow Memorial Hospital	244	25.4
Brandon Hospital	1902	29.0
St. Joseph's Women's	4927	29.9
HCA Blake Memorial Hospital	562	31.1
University Community Hosp, Tampa	1459	36.4

District 7

Florida Hospital	6033	20.8
Central Fla Regional Hospital	680	21.5
J.E. Holmes Regional Medical Center	2341	22.9
Osceola Regional Hospital	1699	23.0
South Seminole Medical Center	465	23.2
West Orange Memorial Hospital	329	23.7
Orlando Regional Medical Center	5644	24.1
Winter Park Memorial Hospital	1862	24.3
Wuesthoff Memorial Hospital	994	26.0
Cape Canaveral Hospital	1041	27.3
Princeton Hospital	930	32.0
Lucerne Hospital	915	33.4
Parrish Medical Center	771	35.3

District 8

Desoto Memorial Hospital	463	15.8
Cape Coral Hospital	1153	18.3
Lee Memorial Hospital	3195	18.7
Sarasota Memorial Hospital	2805	21.1
East Pointe Hospital	209	21.5
St. Joseph Hosp, Port Charlotte	940	22.0
Naples Community Hospital	2200	26.1

	Total Number Deliveries	All Patients Cesarean Section Rate
District 9		
St. Mary's Hospital	4574	21.1
Wellington Reg Medical Center	165	21.8
Martin Memorial Hospital	1425	22.3
Palms West Hospital	561	24.1
Indian River Memorial Hospital	1000	24.3
West Boca Medical Center	1811	26.7
Bethesda Memorial Hospital	2703	26.8
Sebastian Hospital	78	28.2
HCA Lawnwood Reg Medical Center	1506	28.2
Everglades Memorial Hospital	1258	28.6
Good Samaritan Hospital	1547	31.4
AMI Palm Beach Gardens Med Center	599	33.9
HCA Medical Center, Port St. Lucie	195	34.4
District 10		
Memorial Hospital, Hollywood	3931	25.1
Broward General Medical Center	3865	27.9
Coral Springs Medical Center	2041	28.1
Memorial Hospital, West	591	28.6
Holy Cross Hospital	2377	30.8
HCA Northwest Regional Hospital	1281	32.4
Pembroke Pines Hospital	200	36.5
Westside Regional Medical Center	938	39.3
Plantation General Hospital	2730	41.4
District 11		
Hialeah Hospital	2582	44.2
South Miami Hospital	3016	39.2
Mercy Hospital	1407	38.7
AMI Palmetto General	1845	37.3
Mount Sinai Medical Center	1737	34.5
North Shore Medical Center	2379	33.0
Baptist Hospital of Miami	3278	31.5
Parkway Regional Medical Center	1538	30.0
Miami Beach Community Hospital	403	29.3
Health System Depoo	773	25.7
Healthsouth Doctors'	842	24.6
SMH Homestead Hospital	1013	23.2
Jackson Memorial Hospital	12694	21.4
Statewide	182,269*	25.1

*This table includes hospitals that reported at least 10 deliveries during 1992. The total number of deliveries statewide was 182,299; there were 30 births in hospitals not included in this table.

Source: Hospital patient data reported to the Agency for Health Care Administration. "Cesarean Deliveries in Florida Hospitals, 1990–1992—1994 Annual Report," Agency for Health Care Administration, State Center for Health Statistics, January 1, 1994.

Appendix C
1993 Hospital open heart surgery programs

For a discussion of open heart surgery and research findings see Chapter 1 and the "Selecting a Hospital" and "Open Heart Surgery" sections of Chapter 3. Utilization data are reported to the local health councils by hospitals. Local health councils are listed in Chapter 11.

ADULT OPEN HEART SURGERY HOSPITAL UTILIZATION DATA
October 1, 1992–September 30, 1993

	Oct–Dec 1992	Jan–Mar 1993	Apr–Jun 1993	Jul–Sep 1993	Total
District 1					
Sacred Heart Hospital	97	98	96	117	408
HCA West Florida Regional MC	136	110	93	108	447
District 2					
Bay Medical Center	61	72	61	57	251
Tallahassee Memorial Regional MC	101	127	121	123	472
Tallahassee Community Hospital	42	30	45	32	149
District 3					
Alachua General Hospital	42	40	45	36	163
Shands Teaching Hospital	50	105	86	77	318
North Florida Regional MC	92	102	117	114	425
Marion Community/Munroe Reg MC	213	263	275	214	965
District 4					
University Medical Center	46	46	38	42	172
St. Vincent's Medical Center	212	211	194	207	824
Baptist Medical Center	78	73	69	83	303
St. Luke's Hospital	97	102	87	69	355
Memorial Med Center—Jacksonville	98	115	118	123	454
Memorial Hospital—Ormond Beach	139	157	140	126	562
District 5					
Morton Plant Hospital	151	158	146	134	589
HCA Largo Medical Center	129	176	140	118	563
All Children's/Bayfront MC	104	110	75	85	374
HCA Bayonet Point/Hudson MC	245	273	234	188	940

	Oct–Dec 1992	Jan–Mar 1993	Apr–Jun 1993	Jul–Sep 1993	Total
District 6					
St. Joseph's Hospital, Tampa	147	149	136	122	554
Tampa General Hospital	205	178	167	163	713
University Community Hospital	113	141	146	119	519
Manatee Memorial Hospital	80	90	61	56	287
HCA L.W. Blake Memorial	74	78	58	46	256
Lakeland Regional Medical Cntr	114	149	125	114	502
District 7					
J.E. Holmes Regional MC	97	113	123	110	443
Wuesthoff Memorial Hospital	62	90	71	72	295
Lucerne Medical Center	63	46	53	34	196
Florida Hospital, Orlando	519	609	544	500	2172
Orlando Regional Medical Center	150	187	152	131	620
Central Florida Regional Hosp.	0	0	0	19	19
District 8					
Southwest Florida Regional MC	258	239	159	117	773
Lee Memorial Hospital	124	162	119	99	504
Medical Center Hospital	67	99	62	63	291
Sarasota Memorial Hospital	287	350	231	183	1051
District 9					
AMI Palm Beach Gardens MC	102	146	121	115	484
J.F. Kennedy Medical Center	79	117	73	90	359
Delray Community Hospital	122	140	98	98	458
District 10					
Memorial Hospital, Hollywood	148	128	117	154	547
Broward General Medical Center	136	158	179	97	570
Holy Cross Hospital	94	129	121	96	440
Florida Medical Center Hosp	152	132	131	126	541
North Ridge Medical Center	246	256	233	155	890
District 11					
Baptist Hospital of Miami	71	79	68	85	303
Cedars Medical Center	72	69	53	66	260
Jackson Memorial Hospital	65	56	57	56	234
Mount Sinai Medical Center	185	270	227	228	910
Miami Beach Community Hospital	29	13	0	0	42
Miami Heart Institute	110	123	174	113	520
Mercy Hospital	84	90	70	73	317
South Miami Hospital	38	21	23	40	122
Kendall Regional MC	58	42	45	62	207
State Adult Totals	**6284**	**7017**	**6177**	**5655**	**25133**

Source: "Florida Need Projections, Adult Inpatient Cardiac Catheterization and Open Heart Surgery Programs, Pediatric Cardiac Catheterization and Open Heart Surgery Programs, July 1996 Planning Horizon Background Information" (January 26, 1994). This publication, which contains data reported to local health councils by hospitals, may be obtained from the Agency for Health Care Administration or reviewed in a State of Florida depository library.

PEDIATRIC OPEN HEART SURGERY HOSPITAL UTILIZATION DATA
October 1, 1992 to September 30, 1993

	Oct–Dec 1992	Jan–Mar 1993	Apr–Jun 1993	Jul–Sep 1993	Total
Shands Hospital, Alachua	23	29	26	33	111
University Medical Cntr, Duval	11	23	18	29	81
All Children's, Pinellas	37	35	43	49	164
St. Joseph's, Hillsborough	12	16	12	3	43
Orlando Regional MC, Orange	32	28	7	6	73
Memorial Hospital—Hollywood	1	0	0	1	2
Jackson Memorial Hospital, Dade	20	21	28	21	90
Miami Children's Hospital, Dade	32	38	42	57	169
Totals	**168**	**190**	**176**	**199**	**733**

Source: "Florida Need Projections, Adult Inpatient Cardiac Catheterization and Open Heart Surgery Programs, Pediatric Cardiac Catheterization and Open Heart Surgery Programs, July 1996 Planning Horizon Background Information" (January 26, 1994). This publication, which contains data reported to local health councils by hospitals, may be obtained from the Agency for Health Care Administration or reviewed in a State of Florida depository library.

Appendix D
1993 Hospital cardiac catheterization programs

For a discussion of cardiac catheterization and research findings see Chapter 1 and the "Selecting a Hospital" and "Cardiac Catheterization" sections of Chapter 3. Utilization data are reported to the local health councils by hospitals. Local health councils are listed at the end of Chapter 11.

ADULT CARDIAC CATHETERIZATION HOSPITAL UTILIZATION DATA
October 1, 1992–September 30, 1993

	Oct–Dec 1992	Jan–Mar 1993	Apr–Jun 1993	Jul–Sep 1993	Total
District 1					
Sacred Heart Hospital	545	504	509	611	2169
Baptist Hospital	358	297	249	316	1220
HCA West Fla Reg Medical Cntr	454	475	269	462	0
Ft Walton Beach Hospital	101	120	106	118	445
District 2					
Bay Medical Center	401	586	440	346	1773
HCA Gulf Coast Hospital	71	97	60	69	297
Tallahassee Memorial Regional MC	686	710	669	706	2771
Tallahassee Community Hospital	272	215	280	271	1038
District 3					
Alachua General	292	254	254	289	1089
Shands Teaching Hospital	491	472	446	419	1828
North Fla Regional Medical Cntr	498	558	583	508	2147
Leesburg Regional Medical Cntr	165	230	182	205	782
Brooksville Regional Hospital	121	92	76	60	349
Marion Comm/Munroe Regional MC	1200	1324	1088	961	4573
Citrus Memorial Hospital	94	91	79	101	365
Seven Rivers Community Hospital	0	79	70	86	235
HCA Oak Hill Hospital	0	0	0	180	180
District 4					
University Medical Center	349	357	375	360	1441
Methodist Hospital	62	84	72	62	280
St. Vincent's Hospital	685	770	816	738	3009
Baptist Medical Center	488	492	532	673	2185
St. Luke's Hospital	387	404	363	315	1469
Memorial Medical Ctr-Jacksonville	617	644	594	584	2439
Riverside Hospital- Jacksonville	30	51	45	43	169
Orange Park Medical Center	202	216	177	194	789
Daytona Beach Medical Center	124	113	125	109	471
Halifax Memorial	303	374	303	284	1264
Memorial Hospital—Ormond Beach	582	711	628	646	2567
Flagler Hospital—East	29	99	87	89	304

	Oct–Dec 1992	Jan–Mar 1993	Apr–Jun 1993	Jul–Sep 1993	Total
District 5					
HCA Bayonet Point/Hudson MC	745	826	794	653	3018
Morton F. Plant Hospital	700	792	668	592	2752
HCA Largo Medical Center	495	518	456	487	1956
St. Anthony's Health Care Center	127	130	129	111	497
Northside Hospital	206	291	180	153	830
All Children's/Bayfront MC	344	325	312	284	1265
Mease Hospital	169	184	156	193	702
Palms of Pasadena	101	112	115	107	435
Helen Ellis Memorial	127	143	219	194	683
New Port Richey Hospital	0	0	113	434	547
District 6					
St. Joseph's Hospital	465	490	520	537	2012
Tampa General Hospital	975	1019	960	1022	3976
University Community Hospital	550	634	622	520	2326
Brandon Hospital	229	231	233	181	874
Manatee Memorial Hospital	322	414	275	237	1248
HCA L.W. Blake Memorial	248	291	226	201	966
Winter Haven Hospital	263	346	240	267	1116
Lakeland Regional Medical Cntr	557	649	562	570	2338
Memorial Hospital of Tampa	60	45	47	78	230
Walker Memorial Hospital	35	55	35	32	157
District 7					
J.E. Holmes Regional MC	1004	1166	1100	1085	4355
Parrish Medical Center	86	134	79	141	440
Wuesthoff Memorial	202	226	340	339	1107
Cape Canaveral Hospital	58	94	88	83	323
Orlando Regional Medical Cntr	834	819	756	661	3070
Florida Hospital—East Orlando	44	68	58	63	233
Princeton Hospital	33	29	37	35	134
Winter Park Memorial	94	87	98	91	370
Lucerne Medical Center	261	339	268	398	1266
Florida Hospital, Orlando	1322	1546	1821	1683	6372
Osceola Regional Hospital	152	233	69	70	524
Central Florida Regional	83	105	106	128	422
Florida Hospital—Altamonte	82	147	89	71	389
District 8					
Medical Center Hospital	284	338	367	416	1405
Fawcett Memorial Hospital	120	126	86	101	433
Naples/N. Collier Community	156	184	136	114	590
Lee Memorial Hospital-Cleveland	93	61	72	40	266
Lee Memorial Hospital—Healthpark	406	532	362	319	1619
Southwest Florida Regional MC	669	842	679	587	2777
Cape Coral Hospital	165	168	149	139	621
Venice Hospital	191	278	191	141	801
Sarasota Memorial	807	940	681	650	3078
HCA Doctors Hospital of Sarasota	38	45	123	77	283
St. Joseph's—Port Charlotte	104	151	92	91	438

	Oct–Dec 1992	Jan–Mar 1993	Apr–Jun 1993	Jul–Sep 1993	Total
District 9					
Martin Memorial Hospital	198	206	209	209	822
St. Mary's Hospital	97	90	85	69	341
AMI Palm Beach Gardens MC	468	503	427	349	1747
JFK Medical Center	633	705	583	536	2457
Boca Raton Community Hospital	138	185	138	89	550
Delray Community Hospital	508	565	476	424	1973
Bethesda Memorial Hospital	55	106	67	69	297
Indian River Memorial Hospital	112	137	131	106	486
District 10					
Memorial Hospital, Hollywood	535	599	498	480	2112
Broward General Medical Center	350	381	334	359	1424
Holy Cross Hospital	348	475	463	397	1683
North Broward Medical Center	124	112	118	105	459
Plantation General Hospital	85	85	78	81	329
Imperial Point Medical Center	77	54	62	52	245
Florida Medical Center Hospital	651	702	626	747	2726
North Ridge Medical Center	787	1003	711	780	3281
Westside Regional Medical Center	106	92	108	132	438
Pembroke Pines Hospital	70	95	66	73	304
Pompano Beach Medical Center	76	74	86	51	287
Memorial West Hospital			43	82	125
District 11					
Baptist Hospital of Miami	470	504	477	462	1913
Cedars Medical Center	305	393	412	380	1490
HealthSouth Doctors' Hospital	46	48	39	25	158
Aventura Hospital	36	45	40	32	153
Jackson Memorial Hospital	621	560	786	866	2833
Mount Sinai Medical Center	724	920	798	872	3314
Miami Beach Community Hospital	180	170	8	0	358
Miami Heart Institute	655	710	677	682	2724
Mercy Hospital	378	344	304	318	1344
South Miami Hospital	323	337	298	338	1296
Kendall Regional MC	227	193	229	298	947
Palmetto General Hospital	76	89	84	119	368
Parkway Regional Medical Center	53	60	39	36	188
State Adult Totals	**33125**	**37114**	**33686**	**33799**	**137724**

Source: "Florida Need Projections, Adult Inpatient Cardiac Catheterization and Open Heart Surgery Programs, Pediatric Cardiac Catheterization and Open Heart Surgery Programs, July 1996 Planning Horizon Background Information" (January 26, 1994). This publication, which contains data reported to local health councils by hospitals, may be obtained from the Agency for Health Care Administration or reviewed in a State of Florida depository library.

PEDIATRIC CARDIAC CATHETERIZATION
HOSPITAL UTILIZATION DATA
October 1, 1992–September 30, 1993

	Oct–Dec 1992	Jan–Mar 1993	Apr–Jun 1993	Jul–Sep 1993	Total
Shands Hospital, Alachua	79	9	28	711	1369
University Medical Cntr, Duval	42	45	35	53	175
All Children's/Bayfront, Pinellas	83	80	73	78	314
St. Joseph's, Hillsborough	18	16	15	10	59
Orlando Regional MC, Orange	56	56	39	33	184
Memorial Hospital-Hollywood	1	4	1	3	9
Jackson Memorial, Dade	101	145	155	159	560
Miami Children's Hospital, Dade	41	51	45	12	149
State Totals	**421**	**489**	**450**	**459**	**1819**

Source: "Florida Need Projections, Adult Inpatient Cardiac Catheterization and Open Heart Surgery Programs, Pediatric Cardiac Catheterization and Open Heart Surgery Programs, July 1996 Planning Horizon Background Information" (January 26, 1994). This publication, which contains data reported to local health councils by hospitals, may be obtained from the Agency for Health Care Administration or reviewed in a State of Florida depository library.

Appendix E
1992 Nursing home statistics

All of the information in this appendix is from the *1993 Directory of Nursing Home Facilities and Annual Report* published by the Division of Quality Assurance in the Agency for Health Care Administration (AHCA). This publication may be obtained from AHCA or reviewed in a State of Florida depository library. The *Directory* notes that AHCA "does not endorse the institutions included in this directory [and recommends] that the user contact the institutions of interest to gather the most up-to-date information." Readers should verify information in this directory with individual nursing homes, as errors do occur. The *Directory* notes that "AHCA should be informed of incorrect information [and that] revisions will be made in directories issued after such notification." The *Directory* includes information available as of December, 1992 for 597 licensed nursing homes in Florida.

Codes

Beds	total number of beds
Private	number of private rooms
Semi-private	number of semi-private rooms with two or more beds
Medicare	accepts reimbursement from Medicare
Medicaid	accepts reimbursement from Medicaid

Ratings

See Chapter 4 for help in interpreting these ratings and for a discussion of nursing home selection. Ratings are those available as of December, 1992 and are subject to periodic change.

Superior	The facility EXCEEDED minimum standards at the time of the AHCA survey.
Standard	The facility MET the minimum standards at the time of the AHCA survey.
Conditional	The facility DID NOT MEET minimum standards at the time of the AHCA survey.

ALACHUA

Alachua Convalescent Ctr 1000 Southwest 16th Ave Gainesville, FL 32601 (904) 376-2461	Beds: 120 Private: 2 Medicaid, Medicare Rating:	Semiprivate: 11 Superior
Gainesville Nursing Center 4000 Southwest 20th Avenue Gainesville, FL 32608 (904) 377-1981	Beds: 120 Private: 16 Medicaid, Medicare Rating:	Semiprivate: 52 Superior
North Florida Special Care Center 6700 N.W. 10th Place Gainesville, FL 32605 (904) 372-3111	Beds: 120 Private: 16 Medicaid, Medicare Rating:	Semiprivate: 52 Superior
Oaks Residential & Rehabilitation Cntr 3250 Southwest 41st Place Gainesville, FL 32608 (904) 378-1558	Beds: 179 Private: 1 Medicaid, Medicare Rating:	Semiprivate: 70 Superior
Palm Garden 222 S.W. 62nd Boulevard Gainesville, FL 32607 (904) 332-0601	Beds: 120 Private: 4 Medicaid, Medicare Rating:	Semiprivate: 58 Superior
University Nursing Care Center 1311 Southwest 16th St. Gainesville, FL 32608 (904) 376-8821	Beds: 180 Private: 6 Medicaid, Medicare Rating:	Semiprivate: 87 Superior

BAKER

Heritage Health Care Center PO Box 525 MacClenny, FL 32063 (904) 259-4873	Beds: 60 Private: 2 Medicaid, Medicare Rating:	Semiprivate: 29 Superior
W. Frank Wells Nursing Home 159 North Third Street MacClenny, FL 32063 (904) 259-6168	Beds: 68 Private: 2 Medicaid, Medicare Rating:	Semiprivate: 15 Superior

BAY

Bay Convalescent Center 1336 St. Andrews Boulevard Panama City, FL 32405 (904) 763-3911	Beds: 160 Private: 28 Medicaid, Medicare Rating:	Semiprivate: 46 Standard
Glencove Nursing Pavilion 1027 East Business 98 Panama City, FL 32401 (904) 872-1438	Beds: 115 Private: 11 Rating:	Semiprivate: 52 Standard
Gulf Coast Convalescent Center 1937 Jenks Avenue Panama City, FL 32405 (904) 769-7686	Beds: 120 Private: 4 Medicaid, Medicare Rating:	Semiprivate: 43 Superior

Lelah G. Wagner Nursing Home 3409 West 19th Street Panama City, FL 32406 (904) 785-0239	Beds: 66 Private: 10 Medicaid, Medicare Rating:	Semiprivate: 6 Superior
Lisenby on Lake Caroline 1400 W. 11th Street Panama City, FL 32401 (904) 785-6121	Beds: 66 Private: 22 Medicaid, Medicare Rating:	Semiprivate: 4 Standard
National Healthcare Center of Panama City 2100 Jenks Avenue Panama City, FL 32406 (904) 763-0446	Beds: 120 Private: 4 Medicaid, Medicare Rating:	Semiprivate: 58 Superior
Panama City Nursing Center 924 West Thirteenth Street Panama City, FL 32402 (904) 763-8463	Beds: 120 Private: 5 Medicaid, Medicare Rating:	Semiprivate: 12 Superior

BRADFORD

Whispering Pines Care Center 808 South Colley Road Starke, FL 32091 (904) 964-6220	Beds: 120 Private: 8 Medicaid, Medicare Rating:	Semiprivate: 56 Standard
Windsor Manor 602 E. Laura Street Starke, FL 32091 (904) 964-3383	Beds: 120 Private: 4 Medicaid, Medicare Rating:	Semiprivate: 58 Standard

BREVARD

Adare Medical Center 1175 Huntington Lane Rockledge, FL 32955 (407) 632-7341	Beds: 100 Private: 20 Medicaid, Medicare Rating:	Semiprivate: 40 Superior
Carnegie Gardens Nursing Home 1415 South Hickory Street Melbourne, FL 32901 (407) 723-1321	Beds: 138 Private: 6 Medicaid, Medicare Rating:	Semiprivate: 25 Superior
Courtenay Springs Nursing Home 1100 South Courtenay Parkway Merritt Island, FL 32952 (407) 452-1233	Beds: 96 Private: 16 Medicaid, Medicare Rating:	Semiprivate: 40 Superior
Holmes Regional Nursing Center 606 East Sheridan Road Melbourne, FL 32901 (407) 727-0984	Beds: 120 Private: 8 Medicaid, Medicare Rating:	Semiprivate: 56 Superior
Medic Home Health Center 1420 South Oak Street Melbourne, FL 32901 (407) 723-3215	Beds: 110 Private: 2 Medicaid, Medicare Rating:	Semiprivate: 30 Superior

Melbourne Terrace 251 Florida Avenue Melbourne, FL 32901 (407) 725-3990	Beds: 120 Private: 8 Medicaid, Medicare Rating:	Semiprivate: 56 Superior
Meridian Nursing Center 7201 Greensboro Drive West Melbourne, FL 32901 (407) 727-0990	Beds: 120 Private: 12 Medicaid, Medicare Rating:	Semiprivate: 54 Superior
Merritt Manor Nursing Home 125 Alma Boulevard Merritt Island, FL 32952 (407) 453-0202	Beds: 120 Private: 6 Medicaid, Medicare Rating:	Semiprivate: 57 Superior
National Healthcare Center 500 Crockett Blvd. Merritt Island, FL 32952 (407) 454-4035	Beds: 120 Private: 4 Medicare Rating:	Semiprivate: 58 Superior
Palm Bay Care Center 1515 NE Port Malabar Blvd. Palm Bay, FL 32905 (407) 727-2841	Beds: 120 Private: 6 Medicaid, Medicare Rating:	Semiprivate: 57 Superior
Sunny Pines Convalescent Center 587 Barton Boulevard Rockledge, FL 32955 (407) 632-6300	Beds: 75 Private: 3 Medicaid, Medicare Rating:	Semiprivate: 29 Superior
Titusville Nursing & Convalescent Ctr 1705 Jess Parrish Court Titusville, FL 32796 (407) 269-5720	Beds: 157 Private: 5 Medicaid, Medicare Rating:	Semiprivate: 52 Superior
Vista Manor 1550 Jess Parish Court Titusville, FL 32796 (407) 269-2200	Beds: 120 Private: 20 Medicaid, Medicare Rating:	Semiprivate: 50 Superior
West Melbourne Health Care Center 2125 West New Haven Avenue West Melbourne, FL 32904 (407) 725-7360	Beds: 180 Private: 12 Medicaid, Medicare Rating:	Semiprivate: 84 Conditional

BROWARD

Avenel Nursing & Rehab. Center 7751 West Broward Blvd. Plantation, FL 33324 (305) 473-8040	Beds: 120 Private: 8 Medicaid, Medicare Rating:	Semiprivate: 32 Standard
Beacon Pointe Nursing Center 9711 West Oakland Park Blvd. Sunrise, FL 33351 (305) 572-4000	Beds: 120 Private: 12 Medicare Rating:	Semiprivate: 54 Standard
Beverly Manor of Margate 5951 Colonial Drive Margate, FL 33063 (904) 979-6401	Beds: 120 Private: 22 Medicaid, Medicare Rating:	Semiprivate: 49 Superior

Broward Children's Center 200 S.E. 19th Avenue Pompano Beach, FL 33072 (904) 943-7638	Beds: 35 Private: 0 Rating:	Semiprivate: 10 Standard
Broward Convalescent Home 1330 South Andrews Avenue Ft. Lauderdale, FL 33316 (305) 524-5587	Beds: 198 Private: 27 Medicaid, Medicare Rating:	Semiprivate: 76 Conditional
Colonial Palms East 401 E. Sample Road Pompano Beach, FL 33064 (305) 941-4100	Beds: 194 Private: 7 Medicaid, Medicare Rating:	Semiprivate: 74 Standard
Colonial Palms West 51 West Sample Road Pompano Beach, FL 33064 (305) 942-5530	Beds: 127 Private: 1 Medicaid, Medicare Rating:	Semiprivate: 60 Superior
Colonnade Medical Center 3370 N.W. 47th Terrace Lauderdale Lakes, FL 33319 (305) 733-0655	Beds: 120 Private: 8 Medicaid, Medicare Rating:	Semiprivate: 44 Standard
Court at Palm Aire, The 2701 North Course Dr. Pompano Beach, FL 33069 (305) 975-8900	Beds: 60 Private: 8 Medicare Rating:	Semiprivate: 26 Standard
Covenant Village Care Center 9201 W. Broward Blvd. Plantation, FL 33324 (305) 427-8290	Beds: 60 Private: 6 Medicaid, Medicare Rating:	Semiprivate: 27 Superior
Dania Nursing Home 440 Phippen Road Dania, FL 33004 (305) 927-0508	Beds: 88 Private: 1 Medicaid, Medicare Rating:	Semiprivate: 22 Superior
Forum at Deer Creek, The 3001 Deer Creek Country Club Deerfield Beach, FL 33442 (305) 698-9004	Beds: 60 Private: 10 Medicare Rating:	Semiprivate: 25 Conditional
Golfcrest Nursing Home 600 N. 17th Avenue Hollywood, FL 33020 (305) 927-2531	Beds: 67 Private: 1 Medicaid, Medicare Rating:	Semiprivate: 12 Standard
Hallandale Rehabilitation Center 2400 E. Hallandale Beach Bvd Hallandale, FL 33009 (305) 457-9717	Beds: 149 Private: 25 Medicaid, Medicare Rating:	Semiprivate: 62 Superior
Harbor Beach Convalescent Home 1615 South Miami Road Ft. Lauderdale, FL 33315 (305) 523-5673	Beds: 59 Private: 3 Medicaid, Medicare Rating:	Semiprivate: 24 Standard

Heartland Health Care Center 2599 N.W. 55th Avenue Lauderhill, FL 33313 (305) 485-8873	Beds: 85 Private: 3 Medicaid, Medicare Rating:	Semiprivate: 41 Superior
Heartland of Tamarac 5901 79th Avenue Tamarac, FL 32321 (305) 722-7001	Beds: 101 Private: 5 Medicaid, Medicare Rating:	Semiprivate: 48 Superior
Hollywood Hills Nursing Home 1200 N. 35th Avenue Hollywood, FL 33021 (305) 981-5511	Beds: 152 Private: 5 Medicaid, Medicare Rating:	Semiprivate: 45 Superior
John Knox Village Med. Center 631 S.W. 6th Street Pompano Beach, FL 33060 (305) 782-1300	Beds: 120 Private: 6 Medicaid, Medicare Rating:	Semiprivate: 47 Superior
Manor Care of Plantation 6931 West Sunrise Blvd. Plantation, FL 33313 (305) 583-6200	Beds: 120 Private: 40 Medicaid, Medicare Rating:	Semiprivate: 34 Conditional
Manor Pines Convalescent Center 1701 N.E. 26th Street Ft. Lauderdale, FL 33305 (305) 566-8353	Beds: 206 Private: 4 Medicare Rating:	Semiprivate: 101 Superior
Memorial Manor 1701 North Federal Hwy Ft. Lauderdale, FL 33305 (305) 431-1100	Beds: 85 Private: 13 Medicaid, Medicare Rating:	Semiprivate: 32 Superior
Monticello Manor Nursing Home 1701 North Federal Hwy Ft. Lauderdale, FL 33305 (305) 564-3237	Beds: 34 Private: 10 Rating:	Semiprivate: 10 Conditional
Mount Vernon Manor 2331 N.E. 53rd Street Ft. Lauderdale, FL 33308 (305) 771-0739	Beds: 29 Private: 17 Rating:	Semiprivate: 6 Superior
National Healthcare Center 2000 East Commercial Blvd. Ft. Lauderdale, FL 33308 (305) 771-2300	Beds: 253 Private: 14 Medicaid, Medicare Rating:	Semiprivate: 38 Standard
Palm Court Nursing & Rehabilitation 2657 North Andrews Avenue Ft. Lauderdale, FL 33311 (305) 563-5711	Beds: 118 Private: 6 Medicaid, Medicare Rating:	Semiprivate: 56 Standard
Park Summit 8500 Royal Palm Blvd. Coral Springs, FL 33065 (305) 752-9500	Beds: 35 Private: 19 Medicaid, Medicare Rating:	Semiprivate: 8 Superior

Pinehurst Convalescent Center 2401 N.E. 2nd Street Pompano Beach, FL 33062 (305) 943-5100	Beds: 83 Private: 4 Medicaid, Medicare Rating:	Semiprivate: 31 Standard
Plantation Nursing & Rehabilitation Center 4250 N.W. 5th Street Plantation, FL 33317 (305) 587-3296	Beds: 152 Private: 2 Medicaid, Medicare Rating:	Semiprivate: 63 Standard
Springtree Walk Nursing Center 4251 Springtree Drive Sunrise, FL 33351-6119 (305) 572-4251	Beds: 85 Private: 43 Medicaid, Medicare Rating:	Semiprivate: 21 Superior
St. Johns Health Care Center 3075 N.W. 35th Avenue Lauderdale Lakes, FL 33311 (305) 739-6233	Beds: 160 Private: 16 Medicare Rating:	Semiprivate: 72 Superior
Sunrise Health Center 4800 Nob Hill Road Sunrise, FL 33351 (305) 748-3400	Beds: 325 Private: 35 Medicaid, Medicare Rating:	Semiprivate: 145 Standard
Tamarac Convalescent Center 7901 N.W. 88th Avenue Tamarac, FL 33321 (305) 722-9330	Beds: 120 Private: 0 Medicaid, Medicare Rating:	Semiprivate: 60 Superior
Washington Manor Nursing and Rehabilitation Center 4200 Washington Street Hollywood, FL 33021 (305) 981-6300	Beds: 240 Private: 12 Medicaid, Medicare Rating:	Semiprivate: 71 Conditional

CALHOUN

Apalachicola Valley Nursing Center 1510 Crozier Street Blountstown, FL 32424 (904) 674-5464	Beds: 150 Private: 10 Medicaid, Medicare Rating:	Semiprivate: 62 Standard

CHARLOTTE

Bon Secours/St. Joseph Nursing Care Center 2370 Harbor Blvd. Port Charlotte, FL 34252 (813) 624-5966	Beds: 104 Private: 4 Medicaid, Medicare Rating:	Semiprivate: 50 Superior
Englewood Health Care Center 1111 Drury Lane Englewood, FL 34224 (813) 474-9371	Beds: 120 Private: 24 Medicaid, Medicare Rating:	Semiprivate: 48 Standard
Life Care Center of Punta Gorda 450 Shreve Street Punta Gorda, FL 33950 (813) 639-8771	Beds: 180 Private: 16 Medicaid, Medicare Rating:	Semiprivate: 82 Superior

Palm View Healthcare Center 25325 Rampart Blvd. Port Charlotte, FL 33954 (813) 629-7466	Beds: 120 Private: 4 Medicaid, Medicare Rating:	Semiprivate: 58 Superior
Port Charlotte Care Center 4033 Beaver Lane Port Charlotte, FL 33952 (813) 625-3200	Beds: 164 Private: 22 Medicaid, Medicare Rating:	Semiprivate: 71 Standard
South Port Nursing Center 23013 Westchester Blvd. Port Charlotte, FL 33948 (813) 625-1100	Beds: 120 Private: 24 Medicaid, Medicare Rating:	Semiprivate: 48 Standard

CITRUS

Avante at Inverness 304 South Citrus Avenue Inverness, FL 32652 (904) 726-3141	Beds: 104 Private: 1 Medicaid, Medicare Rating:	Semiprivate: 19 Standard
Crystal River Geriatric Center 136 N.E. 12th Avenue Crystal River, FL 32629 (904) 795-5044	Beds: 150 Private: 14 Medicaid, Medicare Rating:	Semiprivate: 68 Superior
Cypress Cove Care Center 700 S.E. Eighth Ave Crystal River, FL 32629 (904) 795-5044	Beds: 120 Private: 2 Medicaid, Medicare Rating:	Semiprivate: 59 Superior
Health Care of Brentwood 2333 N. Brentwood Circle Lecanto, FL 32661 (904) 746-6611	Beds: 60 Private: 14 Medicaid, Medicare Rating:	Semiprivate: 23 Superior
Heritage Health Care Center 611 Turner Camp Road Inverness, FL 32651 (904) 637-1130	Beds: 116 Private: 4 Medicaid, Medicare Rating:	Semiprivate: 56 Superior
Surrey Place Convalescent Center 2730 W. Marc Knighton Ct Lecanto, FL 32661 (904) 746-9500	Beds: 60 Private: 4 Medicaid, Medicare Rating:	Semiprivate: 28 Superior

CLAY

Arbors at Orange Park 1215 Kingsley Avenue Orange Park, FL 32073 (904) 284-5606	Beds: 120 Private: 8 Medicaid, Medicare Rating:	Semiprivate: 56 Superior
Green Cove Springs Geriatric Center 803 Oak Street Green Cove Springs, FL 32043 (904) 284-5606	Beds: 120 Private: 12 Medicaid, Medicare Rating:	Semiprivate: 54 Superior

Heartland Health Care Center 570 Wells Road Orange Park, FL 32073 (904) 264-3912	Beds: 120 Private: 4 Medicaid, Medicare Rating:	Semiprivate: 58 Superior
Holly Point Manor 833 Kingsley Avenue Orange Park, FL 32703 (904) 269-2610	Beds: 120 Private: 12 Medicaid, Medicare Rating:	Semiprivate: 54 Superior
Mary M. Olin Clinic Lewis Avenue Penney Farms, FL 32079 (904) 284-8578	Beds: 40 Private: 16 Rating:	Semiprivate: 12 Standard
Moosehaven Health Center 1700 Park Avenue (Hwy 17) Orange Park, FL 32073 (904) 278-1200	Beds: 170 Private: 42 Rating:	Semiprivate: 56 Superior
Orange Park Care Center 2029 Professional Center Drive Orange Park, FL 32073 (904) 272-6194	Beds: 105 Private: 15 Medicare Rating:	Semiprivate: 45 Standard

COLLIER

Bentley Village 875 Retreat Drive Naples, FL 33963 (813) 598-3153	Beds: 93 Private: 27 Rating:	Semiprivate: 33 Standard
Heritage Healthcare Center 777 Ninth Street, North Naples, FL 33940 (813) 261-8126	Beds: 97 Private: 11 Medicaid, Medicare Rating:	Semiprivate: 28 Superior
Lakeside Plantation 2900 12th Street, North Naples, FL 33940 (813) 261-2554	Beds: 120 Private: 2 Medicaid, Medicare Rating:	Semiprivate: 59 Superior
Lely Palms of Naples Health Care Center 1000 Lely Palms Drive Naples, FL 33962 (813) 793-2762	Beds: 97 Private: 23 Medicaid, Medicare Rating:	Semiprivate: 37 Standard
Manor Care Nursing & Rehabilitation Center 3601 Lakewood Blvd. Naples, FL 33962 (813) 775-7757	Beds: 120 Private: 14 Medicaid, Medicare Rating:	Semiprivate: 35 Superior
Moorings Park, The 120 Moorings Park Drive Naples, FL 33942 (813) 261-1616	Beds: 60 Private: 26 Medicare Rating:	Semiprivate: 17 Superior

Renaissance 900 Imperial Golf Course Blvd. Naples, FL 33942 (813) 591-4800	Beds: 60 Private: 14 Medicaid, Medicare Rating:	Semiprivate: 23 Standard

COLUMBIA

Palm Garden 920 McFarlane Avenue Lake City, FL 32055 (904) 758-4777	Beds: 60 Private: 2 Medicaid, Medicare Rating:	Semiprivate: 29 Standard
Tanglewood Care Convalescent Center 2400 South First Street Lake City, FL 32055 (904) 752-7500	Beds: 95 Private: 1 Medicaid, Medicare Rating:	Semiprivate: 33 Superior

DADE

Anderson Health Center 8401 N.W. 27th Avenue Miami, FL 33147 (305) 691-8052	Beds: 40 Private: 6 Medicaid, Medicare Rating:	Semiprivate: 2 Standard
Arch Creek Nursing Home 12505 N.E. 16th Avenue North Miami, FL 33161 (305) 891-1710	Beds: 118 Private: 0 Medicaid, Medicare Rating:	Semiprivate: 54 Conditional
Ashley Manor Care Center 8785 N.W. 32nd Avenue Miami, FL 33147 (305) 691-5711	Beds: 120 Private: 0 Medicaid, Medicare Rating:	Semiprivate: 24 Standard
Bayshore Convalescent Center 16650 West Dixie Highway No Miami Beach, FL 33160 (305) 945-7447	Beds: 150 Private: 5 Medicaid, Medicare Rating:	Semiprivate: 60 Superior
Brookwood Gardens Convalescent Center 1990 North Canal Drive Homestead, FL 33035 (305) 246-1200	Beds: 120 Private: 8 Medicaid, Medicare Rating:	Semiprivate: 56 Superior
Claridge House 13900 N.E. 3rd Court North Miami, FL 33161 (305) 893-2288	Beds: 240 Private: 8 Medicaid, Medicare Rating:	Semiprivate: 100 Superior
Coral Gables Convalescent Home 7060 S.W. 8th Street Miami, FL 33144 (305) 261-1363	Beds: 87 Private: 3 Medicaid, Medicare Rating:	Semiprivate: 7 Superior
East Ridge Retirement Village 19301 S.W. 87th Avenue Miami, FL 33157 (305) 238-2623	Beds: 60 Private: 0 Medicare Rating:	Semiprivate: 30 Superior

El Ponce De Leon Convalescent Center 335 S.W. 12th Avenue Miami, FL 33130 (305) 545-5417	Beds: 147 Private: 6 Medicaid, Medicare Rating:	Semiprivate: 36 Standard
Fair Havens Center 201 Curtis Parkway Miami Springs, FL 33166-5291 (305) 887-1565	Beds: 269 Private: 10 Medicaid, Medicare Rating:	Semiprivate: 43 Superior
Florida Club Care Center 220 Sierra Drive Miami, FL 33179 (305) 653-8427	Beds: 180 Private: 12 Medicaid, Medicare Rating:	Semiprivate: 84 Superior
Floridean Nursing Home 47 N.W. 32nd Place Miami, FL 33125 (305) 649-2911	Beds: 52 Private: 3 Medicaid Rating:	Semiprivate: 23 Superior
Fountainhead Nursing/Convalescent Home 390 N.E. 135th Street North Miami, FL 33161 (305) 893-0660	Beds: 146 Private: 3 Medicaid, Medicare Rating;	Semiprivate: 39 Superior
Gem Care Center 550 9th Street Miami Beach, FL 33139 (305) 531-3321	Beds: 196 Private: 4 Medicaid, Medicare Rating:	Semiprivate: 80 Standard
Gramercy Park Nursing Center 17475 South Dixie Highway South Miami, FL 33157 (305) 255-1045	Beds: 180 Private: 12 Medicaid, Medicare Rating:	Semiprivate: 84 Conditional
Greenbriar Rehab. & Comp. Care Center 9820 North Kendall Drive Miami, FL 33176 (305) 271-6311	Beds: 203 Private: 7 Medicare Rating:	Semiprivate: 96 Superior
Greynolds Park Manor 17400 West Dixie Hwy North Miami Beach, FL 33160 (305) 944-2361	Beds: 324 Private: 3 Medicaid, Medicare Rating:	Semiprivate: 1 Superior
Hampton Court Nursing & Rehab. Center 16100 N.W. 2nd Avenue North Miami Beach, FL 33169 (305) 354-8800	Beds: 120 Private: 4 Medicaid, Medicare Rating:	Semiprivate: 58 Conditional
Healthsouth Reg Rehab Center 20601 Old Cutler Road Miami, FL 33189 (305) 251-3800	Beds: 180 Private: 6 Medicaid, Medicare Rating:	Semiprivate: 87 Superior
Heartland Health Care Center 9400 S.W. 137th Avenue Kendall, FL 33186 (305) 385-8290	Beds: 120 Private: 4 Medicaid, Medicare Rating:	Semiprivate: 58 Superior

Heartland Health Care Center Kensington Manor 5725 N.W. 186 Street Hialeah, FL 33015 (305) 625-9857	Beds: 120 Private: 4 Medicaid, Medicare Rating:	Semiprivate: 58 Superior
Hebrew Home for the Aged, North Dade 1800 N.E. 168th Street North Miami Beach, FL 33162 (305) 947-3445	Beds: 75 Private: 1 Medicaid, Medicare Rating:	Semiprivate: 13 Conditional
Heritage Nursing & Rehab Center 2201 N.E. 170th Street N. Miami Beach, FL 33160 (305) 945-1401	Beds: 99 Private: 6 Medicaid, Medicare Rating:	Semiprivate: 31 Conditional
Hialeah Convalescent Home 190 West 28th Street Hialeah, FL 33010 (305) 885-2437	Beds: 276 Private: 1 Medicaid, Medicare Rating:	Semiprivate: 14 Superior
Homestead Manor 1330 N.W. First Avenue Homestead, FL 33030 (305) 248-0271	Beds: 54 Private: 2 Medicaid, Medicare Rating:	Semiprivate: 26 Superior
Human Resources Health Center 2500 N.W. 22nd Avenue Miami, FL 33142 (305) 638-6661	Beds: 150 Private: 7 Medicaid, Medicare Rating:	Semiprivate: 64 Standard
Jackson Heights Nursing Home 1404 N.W. 22nd Avenue Miami, FL 33142 (305) 325-1050	Beds: 298 Private: 28 Medicaid, Medicare Rating:	Semiprivate: 67 Conditional
Jackson Manor Nursing Home 1861 N.W. 8th Avenue Miami, FL 33136 (305) 324-0280	Beds: 174 Private: 6 Medicaid, Medicare Rating:	Semiprivate: 84 Conditional
La Posada Convalescent Home 5271 S.W. 8th Street Miami, FL 33134 (305) 448-4963	Beds: 54 Private: 4 Medicaid, Medicare Rating:	Semiprivate: 19 Conditional
Meadowbrook Manor/N. Miami 1255 N.E. 135th Street North Miami, FL 33161 (305) 891-6850	Beds: 245 Private: 3 Medicaid, Medicare Rating:	Semiprivate: 29 Standard
Miami Beach Hebrew Home For the Aged 320 Collins Avenue Miami Beach, FL 33139 (305) 672-6464	Beds: 104 Private: 0 Medicaid, Medicare Rating:	Semiprivate: 24 Standard

Miami Gardens Care Center 190 N.E. 191st Street Miami, FL 33179 (305) 651-6960	Beds: 120 Private: 4 Medicaid, Medicare Rating:	Semiprivate: 58 Conditional
Miami Jewish Home & Hospital for Aged 5200 NE 2nd Avenue Miami, FL 33137 (305) 751-8626	Beds: 454 Private: 181 Medicaid, Medicare Rating:	Semiprivate: 122 Superior
New Riveria Health Resort 6901 Yumuri Street Coral Gables, FL 33146 (305) 661-0078	Beds: 52 Private: 6 Medicaid, Medicare Rating:	Semiprivate: 23 Conditional
North Shore Nursing Home 9380 N.W. 7th Avenue Miami, FL 33150 (305) 759-8711	Beds: 99 Private: 1 Medicaid, Medicare Rating:	Semiprivate: 49 Standard
Oakwood Terrace 18905 N.E. 25th Avenue Miami, FL 33180 (305) 932-6360	Beds: 180 Private: 7 Medicare, Medicaid Rating:	Semiprivate: 67 Superior
Palace at Kendall Nursing & Rehab Center 11215 S.W. 84th Street Miami, FL 33173 (305) 271-2225	Beds: 180 Private: 14 Medicaid, Medicare Rating:	Semiprivate: 83 Superior
Palm Garden 21251 East Dixie Highway N. Miami Beach, FL 33180 (305) 935-4827	Beds: 120 Private: 4 Medicaid, Medicare Rating:	Semiprivate: 58 Superior
Palmetto Rehab Center 6750 West 22nd Court Hialeah, FL 33016 (305) 823-3119	Beds: 90 Private: 8 Medicaid, Medicare Rating:	Semiprivate: 41 Superior
Perdue Medical Center 19590 Old Cutler Road Miami, FL 33157 (305) 233-8931	Beds: 163 Private: 1 Medicaid, Medicare Rating:	Semiprivate: 73 Conditional
Pinecrest Convalescent Home 13650 N.E. Third Court North Miami, FL 33161 (305) 893-1170	Beds: 100 Medicare, Medicaid Medicaid, Medicare Rating:	Semiprivate: 42 Standard
Pines Nursing Home 301 N.E. 141st Street Miami, FL 33161 (305) 893-1102	Beds: 46 Private: 1 Medicaid, Medicare Rating:	Semiprivate: 18 Standard
Plaza Nursing & Rehab. Center 14601 N.E. 16th Avenue Miami, FL 33161 (305) 945-7631	Beds: 85 Private: 1 Medicaid, Medicare Rating:	Semiprivate: 36 Standard

Riverside Care Center 899 N.W. 47th Street Miami, FL 33128 (305) 326-1236	Beds: 80 Private: 2 Medicaid, Medicare Rating:	Semiprivate: 28 Superior
Snapper Creek Nursing Home 9200 S.W. 87th Avenue Miami, FL 33176 (305) 271-1313	Beds: 115 Private: 1 Medicaid, Medicare Rating:	Semiprivate: 47 Conditional
Southpoint Manor 42 Collins Avenue Miami, FL 33139 (305) 672-1771	Beds: 230 Private: 2 Medicaid, Medicare Rating:	Semiprivate: 82 Superior
St. Anne's Nursing Center 11855 Quail Roost Drive Miami, FL 33177 (305) 252-4000	Beds: 180 Private: 0 Medicaid, Medicare Rating:	Semiprivate: 90 Superior
St. Francis Barry Nursing & Rehab Center 201 N.E. 112 Street Miami, FL 33161 (305) 899-4700	Beds: 150 Private: 38 Medicaid, Medicare Rating:	Semiprivate: 56 Conditional
Susanna Wesley Health Center 5300 West 16th Avenue Hialeah, FL 33012 (305) 556-5654	Beds: 120 Private: 12 Medicaid, Medicare Rating:	Semiprivate: 54 Superior
Treasure Isle Convalescent Home 1735 North Treasure Dr. N. Bay Village, FL 33141 (305) 865-2383	Beds: 176 Private: 0 Medicaid, Medicare Rating:	Semiprivate: 13 Standard
Villa Maria Nursing Center 1050 N.E. 125th Street North Miami, FL 33161 (305) 891-8850	Beds: 212 Private: 22 Medicaid, Medicare Rating:	Semiprivate: 75 1989 Superior
Waterford Convalescent Center, The 8333 W. Okeechobee Road Hialeah Gardens, FL 33016 (305) 556-9900	Beds: 180 Private: 18 Medicaid, Medicare Rating:	Semiprivate: 81 Superior
West Gables Rehabilitation Hospital & Healthcare Center 2525 S.W. 75th Avenue Miami, FL 262-6800	Beds: 180 Private: 18 Medicaid, Medicare Rating:	Semiprivate: 81 Conditional

DESOTO

DeSoto Manor Nursing Home 1002 North Brevard Ave. Arcadia, FL 33821 (813) 494-5766	Beds: 98 Private: 24 Medicaid, Medicare Rating:	Semiprivate: 37 Standard

DUVAL

All Saints Catholic Nursing Home 2040 Riverside Avenue Jacksonville, FL 32204 (904) 389-4671	Beds: 120 Private: 12 Medicaid, Medicare Rating:	Semiprivate: 54 Superior
Arlington Manor Care Center 7723 Jasper Avenue Jacksonville, FL 32211 (904) 725-8044	Beds: 100 Private: 4 Medicaid, Medicare Rating:	Semiprivate: 19 Standard
Avante Villa at Jacksonville Beach 1504 Seabreeze Avenue Jacksonville Beach, Fl 32250 (904) 249-7421	Beds: 120 Private: 10 Medicaid, Medicare Rating:	Semiprivate: 47 Superior
Beauclerc Manor 9355 San Jose Blvd. Jacksonville, FL 32357 (904) 739-0877	Beds: 120 Private: 20 Medicaid, Medicare Rating:	Semiprivate: 50 Superior
Cathedral Convalescent Center 333 East Ashley Street Jacksonville, FL 32202 (904) 798-5300	Beds: 120 Private: 28 Medicaid, Medicare Rating:	Semiprivate: 46 Superior
Cedar Hills Nursing Center 2061 Hyde Park Road Jacksonville, FL 32210 (904) 786-7331	Beds: 180 Private: 0 Medicaid, Medicare Rating:	Semiprivate: 26 Standard
Central Park Lodge 1650 Fouraker Road Jacksonville, FL 32221 (904) 786-8668	Beds: 120 Private: 12 Medicaid, Medicare Rating:	Semiprivate: 54 Superior
Cypress Village 4600 Middleton Park Circle West Jacksonville, FL 32224 (904) 223-6185	Beds: 60 Private: 2 Medicaid, Medicare Rating:	Semiprivate: 29 Superior
Eagle Crest Nursing Center 2802 Parental Home Road Jacksonville, FL 32216 (904) 721-0088	Beds: 240 Private: 5 Medicaid, Medicare Rating:	Semiprivate: 70 Superior
Eartha M.M. White Nursing Home 5377 Moncrief Road Jacksonville, FL 32209 (904) 768-1506	Beds: 120 Private: 4 Medicaid, Medicare Rating:	Semiprivate: 10 Superior
Fannie E. Taylor Home/Aged 3937 Spring Park Road Jacksonville, FL 33204 (904) 737-6777	Beds: 24 Private: 0 Medicaid, Medicare Rating:	Semiprivate: 12 Standard
Fleet Landing One Fleet Landing Blvd. Atlantic Beach, FL 32233 (904) 246-3457	Beds: 42 Private: 10 Rating:	Semiprivate: 16 Standard

Florida Christian Health Center 1827 Stockton Street Jacksonville, FL 33204 (904) 384-3457	Beds: 128 Private: 1 Medicaid, Medicare Rating:	Semiprivate: 35 Superior
Heartland Health Care Center 8495 Normandy Blvd. Jacksonville, FL 33204 (904) 783-3749	Beds: 120 Private: 4 Medicaid, Medicare Rating:	Semiprivate: 58 Superior
Jacksonville Convalescent Center 730 College Street Jacksonville, FL 32204 (904) 354-5589	Beds: 104 Private: 0 Medicaid, Medicare Rating:	Semiprivate: 40 Superior
Lake Forest Health Care Center 1771 Edgewood Avenue West Jacksonville, FL 32208 (904) 766-7436	Beds: 60 Private: 2 Medicaid, Medicare Rating:	Semiprivate: 29 Standard
Lanier Manor 12740 Lanier Road Jacksonville, FL 32218 (904) 757-0600	Beds: 120 Private: 8 Medicaid, Medicare Rating:	Semiprivate: 50 Superior
Mandarin Manor 10680 Old St Augustine Rd Jacksonville, FL 32223 (904) 268-4953	Beds: 120 Private: 8 Medicaid, Medicare Rating:	Semiprivate: 56 Superior
Manor Care Nursing/Rehab Center 3648 University Blvd. South Jacksonville, FL 32216 (904) 733-7440	Beds: 120 Private: 4 Medicaid, Medicare Rating:	Semiprivate: 46 Superior
Methodist Regional Nursing Center 4134 Dunn Avenue Jacksonville, FL 32218 (904) 751-6954	Beds: 100 Private: 8 Medicaid, Medicare Rating:	Semiprivate: 46 Standard
Palm Garden 5725 Spring Park Road Jacksonville, FL 32216 (904) 733-6954	Beds: 106 Private: 10 Medicaid, Medicare Rating:	Semiprivate: 48 Superior
Regents Park/Jacksonville 7130 Southside Blvd. Jacksonville, FL 32216 (904) 642-7300	Beds: 120 Private: 4 Medicaid, Medicare Rating:	Semiprivate: 58 Superior
River Garden Hebrew Home for the Aged 11401 Old St Augustine Rd Jacksonville, FL 32258 (904) 260-1818	Beds: 180 Private: 140 Medicaid, Medicare Rating:	Semiprivate: 20 Superior
Southside Nursing Center 40 Acme Street Jacksonville, FL 32211 (904) 724-5933	Beds: 119 Private: 1 Rating:	Semiprivate: 31 Standard

St. Catherine Laboure Manor 1717 Barrs Street Jacksonville, FL 32204 (904) 387-0587	Beds: 232 Private: 24 Medicaid, Medicare Rating:	Semiprivate: 104 Superior
Taylor Care Center 6535 Chester Avenue Jacksonville, FL 32217 (904) 731-8230	Beds: 120 Private: 8 Medicaid, Medicare Rating:	Semiprivate: 56 Superior
Turtle Creek Health Care Center 11565 Harts Road Jacksonville, FL 32218 (904) 751-1834	Beds: 180 Private: 14 Medicaid, Medicare Rating:	Semiprivate: 83 Superior
Wesley Manor Nursing Home SR 13 at Julington Creek Rd Jacksonville, FL 32223 (904) 262-7300	Beds: 57 Private: 13 Rating:	Semiprivate: 23 Superior

ESCAMBIA

Azalea Trace 10100 Hillview Road Pensacola, FL 32514 (904) 474-0610	Beds: 106 Private: 30 Medicaid, Medicare Rating:	Semiprivate: 38 Superior
Baptist Manor 10095 Hillview Road Pensacola, FL 32514 (904) 479-4000	Beds: 170 Private: 4 Medicaid, Medicare Rating:	Semiprivate: 83 Superior
Bluffs Nursing Home, The 4343 Langley Avenue Pensacola, FL 32504 (904) 477-4550	Beds: 120 Private: 8 Medicaid, Medicare Rating:	Semiprivate: 56 Conditional
Cross Creek Health Care Center 10040 Hillview Road Pensacola, FL 32514 (904) 474-0570	Beds: 120 Private: 16 Medicaid, Medicare Rating:	Semiprivate: 52 Standard
Escambia County Nursing Home 3107 North <169>H<170> Street Pensacola, FL 32501 (904) 436-9300	Beds: 155 Private: 7 Medicaid, Medicare Rating:	Semiprivate: 18 Standard
Haven of Our Lady of Peace 5203 North 9th Avenue Pensacola, FL 32904 (904) 477-0531	Beds: 89 Private: 39 Medicaid Rating:	Semiprivate: 25 Standard
Magnolia Nursing & Convalescent Center 600 West Gregory Street Pensacola, FL 32501 (904) 438-2000	Beds: 210 Private: 0 Medicare Rating:	Semiprivate: 100 Standard
Mayfair Manor 6984 Pine Forest Road Pensacola, FL 32526 (904) 477-4550	Beds: 120 Private: 4 Medicare Rating:	Semiprivate: 54 Standard

| Palm Garden
8475 University Parkway
Pensacola, FL 32514
(904) 474-1252 | Beds: 120
Private: 4
Medicare
Rating: | Semiprivate: 58

Superior |
| Pensacola Health Care Facility
1717 West Avery Street
Pensacola, FL 32501
(904) 434-2355 | Beds: 118
Private: 6
Medicaid, Medicare
Rating: | Semiprivate: 56

Standard |

FLAGLER

| Meadowbrook Manor/Flagler
300 South Lemon Street
Bunnell, FL 32010
(904) 437-4168 | Beds: 120
Private: 32
Medicaid, Medicare
Rating: | Semiprivate: 44

Superior |

FRANKLIN

| Apalachicola Health Care Center
150 Tenth Street
Apalachicola, FL 32320
(904) 653-8844 | Beds: 60
Private: 4
Medicaid, Medicare
Rating: | Semiprivate: 28

Superior |
| Bay St. George Care Center
Highway 98 West
East Pointe, FL 32328
(904) 670-8571 | Beds: 90
Private: 2
Medicaid, Medicare
Rating: | Semiprivate: 17

Standard |

GADSDEN

| Gadsden Nursing Home
1021 Experiment Sta. Rd
Quincy, FL 32351
(904) 627-9276 | Beds: 60
Private: 2
Medicaid, Medicare
Rating: | Semiprivate: 29

Superior |
| Meadowbrook Manor/Quincy
Strong Rd., Rt 6, Bx 1000
Quincy, FL 32351
(904) 875-3711 | Beds: 120
Private: 12
Medicaid, Medicare
Rating: | Semiprivate: 54

Superior |

GILCHRIST

| Medic-Ayers Nursing Center
606 N.E. 7th Street
Trenton, FL 32693
(904) 463-7101 | Beds: 120
Private: 4
Medicaid, Medicare
Rating: | Semiprivate: 58

Superior |
| Tri-County Nursing Home
Route 1, Box 1030
Trenton, FL 1030
(904) 463-1222 | Beds: 60
Private: 17
Medicaid, Medicare
Rating: | Semiprivate: 15

Standard |

GULF

| Bay St. Joseph Care Center
220 Ninth Street
Port St. Joe, FL 32445
(904) 229-8244 | Beds: 120
Private: 2
Medicaid, Medicare
Rating: | Semiprivate: 59

Superior |

HAMILTON

| Suwannee Valley Nursing Home
427 N.W. 15th Avenue
Jasper, FL 32502
(904) 792-1868 | Beds: 60
Private: 2
Medicaid, Medicare
Rating: | Semiprivate: 25

Superior |

HARDEE

| Hardee Manor Care Center
401 Orange Place
Wachula, FL 33873
(813) 773-3231 | Beds: 79
Private: 5
Medicaid, Medicare
Rating: | Semiprivate: 37

Standard |

HENDRY

| Clewiston Health Care Center
301 South Gloria Street
Clewiston, FL 33440
(813) 983-5123 | Beds: 120
Private: 2
Medicaid, Medicare
Rating: | Semiprivate: 59

Superior |

| Meadowbrook Manor/LaBelle
250 Broward Avenue
LaBelle, FL 33935
(813) 675-1440 | Beds: 93
Private: 3
Medicaid, Medicare
Rating: | Semiprivate: 30

Superior |

HERNANDO

| Brooksville Nursing Manor
1114 Chatman Blvd.
Brooksville, FL 34601
(904) 796-6701 | Beds: 180
Private: 2
Medicaid, Medicare
Rating: | Semiprivate: 81

Superior |

| Eastbrooke Health Care Center
10295 N. Howell Avenue
Brooksville, FL 34601
(904) 799-1451 | Beds: 120
Private: 8
Medicaid, Medicare
Rating: | Semiprivate: 56

Superior |

| Evergreen Woods
7045 Evergreen Woods Tr
Spring Hill, FL 34608
(904) 596-8371 | Beds: 120
Private: 4
Medicaid, Medicare
Rating: | Semiprivate: 58

Superior |

| Heartland of Brooksville
575 Lamar Avenue
Brooksville, FL 33512
(904) 799-2226 | Beds: 120
Private: 4
Medicaid, Medicare
Rating: | Semiprivate: 58

Superior |

HIGHLANDS

| Avon Park Nursing Center
1010 U.S. 27 North
Avon Park, FL 33825
(813) 453-5200 | Beds: 88
Private: 88

Rating: | Semiprivate: 0

Standard |

| Hillcrest Nursing Home
1281 Stratford Road
Avon Park, FL 33825
(813) 453-6674 | Beds: 90
Private: 3
Medicaid, Medicare
Rating: | Semiprivate: 12

Standard |

Lake Placid Health Care Center 125 Tomoka Blvd. Lake Placid, FL 33852 (813) 465-7200	Beds: 120 Private: 18 Medicaid, Medicare Rating:	Semiprivate: 51 Superior
Palms Health Care Center 725 South Pine Street Sebring, FL 33870 (813) 385-0161	Beds: 120 Private: 4 Medicaid, Medicare Rating:	Semiprivate: 58 Superior
Sebring Care Center 3011 Kenilworth Blvd. Sebring, FL 33870 (813) 382-2153	Beds: 104 Private: 16 Medicaid, Medicare Rating:	Semiprivate: 44 Conditional

HILLSBOROUGH

Ambrosia Home 1709 Taliaferro Ave. Tampa, FL 33602 (813) 223-4623	Beds: 80 Private: 2 Medicaid, Medicare Rating:	Semiprivate: 7 Superior
Bay to Bay Nursing Center 3405 Bay to Bay Blvd. Tampa, FL 33629 (813) 839-5325	Beds: 75 Private: 0 Medicaid, Medicare Rating:	Semiprivate: 12 Superior
Brian Center Nursing Care/Tampa 1818 E. Fletcher Avenue Tampa, FL 33612 (813) 971-2383	Beds: 266 Private: 2 Medicaid, Medicare Rating:	Semiprivate: 96 Standard
Cambridge Convalescent Center 9709 North Nebraska Ave. Tampa, FL 33612 (813) 935-2101	Beds: 70 Private: 0 Medicaid, Medicare Rating:	Semiprivate: 25 Standard
Canterbury Tower Health Center 3501 Bayshore Blvd. Tampa, FL 33629 (813) 837-1083	Beds: 60 Private: 18 Medicare Rating:	Semiprivate: 21 Superior
Carrollwood Care Center 15002 Hutchinson Road Tampa, FL 33625 (813) 960-1969	Beds: 120 Private: 4 Medicaid, Medicare Rating:	Semiprivate: 58 Superior
Casa Marti Riverside 2730 Ridgewood Avenue Tampa, FL 33602 (813) 223-1303	Beds: 42 Private: 1 Medicaid, Medicare Rating:	Semiprivate: 11 Standard
Central Park Lodges 702 South Kings Avenue Brandon, FL 33511 (813) 651-1818	Beds: 120 Private: 12 Medicaid, Medicare Rating:	Semiprivate: 54 Superior
Community Convalescent Center 2202 West Oak Avenue Plant City, FL 33566 (813) 754-3761	Beds: 120 Private: 0 Medicaid, Medicare Rating:	Semiprivate: 60 Superior

Forest Park Nursing Center 1702 West Oak Avenue Plant City, FL 33566 (813) 752-4129	Beds: 97 Private: 1 Medicaid, Medicare Rating:	Semiprivate: 48 Superior
Hillhaven Rehabilitation Center 4411 N. Habana Avenue Tampa, FL 33614-7299 (813) 872-2771	Beds: 174 Private: 18 Medicaid, Medicare Rating:	Semiprivate: 78 Superior
Home Association, The 1203 22nd Avenue Tampa, FL 33605 (813) 229-6901	Beds: 96 Private: 79 Medicaid, Medicare Rating:	Semiprivate: 2 Superior
John Knox Village Med Center 4100 East Fletcher Ave. Tampa, FL 33613 (813) 971-7038	Beds: 110 Private: 4 Medicaid, Medicare Rating:	Semiprivate: 53 Superior
Lakeshore Villas Health Care Center 16002 Lakeshore Villas Dr Tampa, FL 33613 (813) 968-5093	Beds: 120 Private: 4 Medicaid, Medicare Rating:	Semiprivate: 58 Superior
Manhattan Convalescent Center 4610 South Manhattan Ave. Tampa, FL 33611 (813) 839-5311	Beds: 179 Private: 1 Medicaid, Medicare Rating:	Semiprivate: 59 Superior
Manor Care of Carrollwood 3030 Bears Avenue Tampa, FL 33618 (813) 968-8777	Beds: 120 Private: 30 Medicaid, Medicare Rating:	Semiprivate: 45 Superior
McIntosh Manor 12006 McIntosh Road Thonotosassa, FL 33592 (813) 986-4848	Beds: 180 Private: 1 Medicaid, Medicare Rating:	Semiprivate: 31 Superior
Meadowbrook Manor of Tampa 8720 Jackson Springs Road Tampa, FL 33615 (813) 885-6053	Beds: 120 Private: 4 Medicaid, Medicare Rating:	Semiprivate: 58 Standard
Oakwood Park Su Casa 1514 East Chelsea Street Tampa, FL 33610 (813) 238-6406	Beds: 240 Private: 1 Medicaid, Medicare Rating:	Semiprivate: 16 Standard
Padgett Nursing Home 5010 North 40th Street Tampa, FL 33610 (813) 626-7109	Beds: 100 Private: 2 Medicaid, Medicare Rating:	Semiprivate: 25 Standard
Palm Garden 3612 138th Ave. Tampa, FL 33612 (813) 972-8775	Beds: 120 Private: 20 Medicaid, Medicare Rating:	Semiprivate: 50 Superior

Palm Garden/Sun City 3612 138th Avenue Tampa, FL 33612 (813) 633-2875	Beds: 120 Private: 20 Medicaid, Medicare Rating:	Semiprivate: 50 Standard
Plant City Health Care Center 701 North Wilder Road Plant City, FL 33566 (813) 752-3611	Beds: 120 Private: 8 Medicaid, Medicare Rating:	Semiprivate: 56 Superior
Sun Terrace Health Care Center 101 Trinity Lakes Drive Sun City Center, FL 33570 (813) 634-3324	Beds: 120 Private: 4 Medicaid, Medicare Rating:	Semiprivate: 58 Standard
Tampa Health Care Center 2916 Habana Way Tampa, FL 33614 (813) 876-5141	Beds: 150 Private: 6 Medicaid, Medicare Rating:	Semiprivate: 48 Superior
University Village Nursing Center 12250 North 22nd Street Tampa, FL 33615 (813) 971-0378	Beds: 240 Private: 76 Medicaid, Medicare Rating:	Semiprivate: 82 Superior
Village at Brandon, The 701 Victoria Street Brandon, FL 33511 (813) 681-4220	Beds: 120 Private: 4 Medicaid, Medicare Rating:	Semiprivate: 58 Superior
Wellington Manor 10049 N. Florida Ave. Tampa, FL 33612 (813) 935-3183	Beds: 180 Private: 2 Medicaid, Medicare Rating:	Semiprivate: 89 Superior
Woodlands Nursing Center 13806 North 46th Street Tampa, FL 33613 (813) 977-4214	Beds: 120 Private: 2 Medicaid, Medicare Rating:	Semiprivate: 59 Standard

HOLMES

Bonifay Nursing Home 306 West Brock Avenue Bonifay, FL 32425 (904) 547-9289	Beds: 120 Private: 10 Medicaid, Medicare Rating:	Semiprivate: 55 Superior

INDIAN RIVER

Fla Baptist Retirement Center 1006 33rd Street Vero Beach, FL 32961 (407) 567-5248	Beds: 24 Private: 0 Rating:	Semiprivate: 10 Standard
Indian River Estates Medical Facility 2250 Indian River Creek Bvd West Vero Beach, FL 32966 (407) 562-8700	Beds: 60 Private: 6 Medicare Rating:	Semiprivate: 26 Superior

Indian River Village Care Center	Beds: 120	
1310 37th Street	Private: 12	Semiprivate: 54
Vero Beach, FL 32960	Medicaid, Medicare	
(407) 569-5107	Rating:	Superior

Palm Garden	Beds: 91	
1755 37th St.	Private: 13	Semiprivate: 39
Vero Beach, FL 32960	Medicaid, Medicare	
(407) 567-2443	Rating:	Superior

Royal Palm Convalescent Center	Beds: 72	
2180 Tenth Avenue	Private: 4	Semiprivate: 30
Vero Beach, FL 32960		
(407) 567-5166	Rating:	Superior

Vero Beach Care Center	Beds: 110	
3663 15th Avenue	Private: 12	Semiprivate: 49
Vero Beach, FL 32960	Medicaid, Medicare	
(407) 567-2552	Rating:	Conditional

JACKSON

Jackson County Conv. Center	Beds: 120	
1002 Sanders Avenue	Private: 2	Semiprivate: 44
Graceville, FL 32440	Medicaid, Medicare	
(904) 263-4447	Rating:	Standard

Marianna Convalescent Center	Beds: 180	
P.O. Drawer <169>L<170>	Private: 20	Semiprivate: 80
Marianna, FL 32446	Medicaid, Medicare	
(904) 482-8091	Rating:	Superior

Nursing Pavilion at Chipola Ret. Center	Beds: 60	
7710 3rd Avenue	Private: 2	Semiprivate: 29
Marianna, FL 32446	Medicaid, Medicare	
(904) 526-3191	Rating:	Superior

JEFFERSON

Brynwood Center	Beds: 97	
Route 1, Highway 19 South	Private: 3	Semiprivate: 32
Monticello, FL 32344	Medicaid, Medicare	
(904) 997-1800	Rating:	Superior

Jefferson Nursing Center	Beds: 60	
P.O. Box 477	Private: 0	Semiprivate: 4
Monticello, FL 32344	Medicaid, Medicare	
(904) 997-2313	Rating:	Superior

LAKE

Avante at Leesburg	Beds: 116	
2000 Edgewood Avenue	Private: 2	Semiprivate: 33
Leesburg, FL 32748	Medicaid, Medicare	
(904) 787-3545	Rating:	Superior

Eustis Manor	Beds: 138	
2810 Ruleme Street	Private: 9	Semiprivate: 54
Eustis, FL 32726	Medicaid	
(904) 357-1990	Rating:	Superior

Lake Eustis Care Center 411 West Woodward Ave. Eustis, FL 32726 (904) 357-3565	Beds: 60 Private: 4 Medicaid, Medicare Rating:	Semiprivate: 22 Superior
Lake Highlands Retirement/Nursing Center 151 East Minnehaha Ave. Clermont, FL 32711 (904) 394-2188	Beds: 142 Private: 5 Medicaid, Medicare Rating:	Semiprivate: 43 Standard
Lake Port Nursing Center 701 Lake Port Blvd. Leesburg, FL 32702 (904) 728-8525	Beds: 60 Private: 4 Medicaid, Medicare Rating:	Semiprivate: 28 Superior
Lakeview Terrace Christian Retirement Community Health Care P.O. Drawer 100 Altoona, FL 32702 (904) 669-2133	Beds: 20 Private: 4 Medicaid, Medicare Rating:	Semiprivate: 8 Superior
Leesburg Nursing Center 715 East Dixie Avenue Leesburg, FL 33748 (904) 728-3020	Beds: 120 Private: 6 Medicaid, Medicare Rating:	Semiprivate: 57 Superior
LRMC Nursing Center 700 N. Palmetto St. Leesburg, FL 32748 (904) 365-4766	Beds: 120 Private: 8 Medicaid, Medicare Rating:	Semiprivate: 32 Superior
Mount Dora Healthcare Center 3050 Brown Avenue Mount Dora, FL 32757 (904) 383-4161	Beds: 116 Private: 2 Medicaid, Medicare Rating:	Semiprivate: 33 Superior
Oakwood Nursing Center 301 South Bay Street Eustis, FL 32726 (904) 357-8105	Beds: 120 Private: 0 Medicaid, Medicare Rating:	Semiprivate: 60 Superior

LEE

Beacon-Donegan Manor 8359 Beacon Blvd. Ft. Myers, FL 33907 (813) 936-1300	Beds: 150 Private: 44 Medicaid, Medicare Rating:	Semiprivate: 29 Superior
Calusa Harbour Health Center 2525 East First St. Ft. Myers, FL 33901 (813) 332-3333	Beds: 100 Private: 2 Medicaid, Medicare Rating:	Semiprivate: 32 Standard
Cape Coral Nursing Pavilion 2629 Del Prado Blvd. Cape Coral, FL 33904 (813) 574-4434	Beds: 120 Private: 6 Medicaid, Medicare Rating:	Semiprivate: 57 Superior

Coral Trace Manor 216 Santa Barbara Blvd. Cape Coral, FL 33904 (813) 772-4600	Beds: 120 Private: 12 Medicaid, Medicare Rating:	Semiprivate: 54 Superior
Cross Key Manor 1550 Lee Blvd. Lehigh, FL 33936 (813) 369-2194	Beds: 110 Private: 2 Medicaid, Medicare Rating:	Semiprivate: 54 Superior
Cypress Manor 7173 Cypress Drive S.W. Ft. Myers, FL 33907 (813) 936-0203	Beds: 120 Private: 22 Medicaid, Medicare Rating:	Semiprivate: 49 Superior
Fort Myers Care Center 13755 Golf Club Parkway Ft. Myers, FL 33907 (813) 482-2848	Beds: 107 Private: 13 Medicaid, Medicare Rating:	Semiprivate: 47 Superior
Gulf Coast Village Care Center 1333 Santa Barbara Blvd. Cape Coral, FL 33991 (813) 772-1333	Beds: 60 Private: 2 Medicaid, Medicare Rating:	Semiprivate: 29 Superior
Healthpark Care Center 16131 Roserush Court Ft. Myers, FL 33908 (813) 433-4647	Beds: 90 Private: 8 Rating:	Semiprivate: 41 Standard
Heartland Health Care Center 1600 Matthew Drive Fort Myers, FL 33907 (813) 275-6067	Beds: 108 Private: 24 Medicaid, Medicare Rating:	Semiprivate: 42 Standard
Lee Convalescent Center 2826 Cleveland Avenue Ft. Myers, FL 33901 (813) 334-1091	Beds: 146 Private: 0 Medicaid, Medicare Rating:	Semiprivate: 16 Superior
Pines Village Care Center 991 Pondella Road North Fort Myers, FL 33903 (813) 995-8809	Beds: 120 Private: 12 Medicaid, Medicare Rating:	Semiprivate: 54 Superior
Shady Rest Nursing Home 2300 North Airport Road Fort Myers, FL 33907 (813) 936-6400	Beds: 105 Private: 61 Medicaid, Medicare Rating:	Semiprivate: 0 Superior
Shell Point Village Nursing Pavilion 15000 Shell Point Blvd. Fort Myers, FL 33908 (813) 454-2271	Beds: 180 Private: 6 Rating:	Semiprivate: 84 Superior

LEON

Arbors at Tallahassee 1650 Phillips Road Tallahassee, FL 32308 (904) 656-3876	Beds: 120 Private: 120 Medicaid, Medicare Rating:	Semiprivate: 0 Standard

Capital Health Care Center 3333 Capital Medical Bldg Tallahassee, FL 32308 (904) 877-4115	Beds: 120 Private: 20 Medicaid, Medicare Rating:	Semiprivate: 68 Superior
Centerville Care Center 2255 Centerville Road Tallahassee, FL 32308 (904) 386-4054	Beds: 120 Private: 4 Medicaid, Medicare Rating:	Semiprivate: 58 Standard
Heritage Health Care Center 1815 Ginger Drive Tallahassee, FL 32308 (904) 877-2177	Beds: 120 Private: 14 Medicaid, Medicare Rating:	Semiprivate: 53 Superior
Miracle Hill Nursing and Convalescent Home 1329 Abraham Street Tallahassee, FL 32304 (904) 224-8486	Beds: 60 Private: 0 Medicaid, Medicare Rating:	 Semiprivate: 30 Superior
Tallahassee Convalescent Home 2510 Miccosukee Road Tallahassee, FL 32303 (904) 877-3131	Beds: 72 Private: 1 Medicaid, Medicare Rating:	Semiprivate: 8 Standard
Westminster Oaks Health Center 4449 Meandering Way Tallahassee, FL 32308 (904) 878-1136	Beds: 60 Private: 4 Medicaid, Medicare Rating:	Semiprivate: 28 Superior

LEVY

Oakview Care Center 300 Northwest First St. Williston, FL 32696 (904) 528-3561	Beds: 180 Private: 4 Medicaid, Medicare Rating:	Semiprivate: 76 Superior

MADISON

Madison Nursing Center Route 3, Box 2310 Madison, FL 32340 (904) 973-4880	Beds: 60 Private: 2 Medicaid, Medicare Rating:	Semiprivate: 29 Superior
Pine Lake Nursing Home Hwy 90 East (PO Box 445) Greenville, FL 32331 (904) 948-4601	Beds: 58 Private: 0 Medicaid, Medicare Rating:	Semiprivate: 17 Superior

MANATEE

Freedom Care Pavilion 1902 59th St. West Bradenton, FL 34209 (813) 792-1515	Beds: 240 Private: 8 Medicaid, Medicare Rating:	Semiprivate: 116 Superior
Freedom Village Nursing Center 6410 21st Avenue West Bradenton, FL 34209 (813) 798-8301	Beds: 120 Private: 24 Medicaid Rating:	Semiprivate: 48 Superior

Greenbriar Nursing Center 210 West 21st Avenue Bradenton, FL 34205 (813) 747-3786	Beds: 60 Private: 4 Medicaid, Medicare Rating:	Semiprivate: 28 Superior
Heritage Park of Bradenton 2302 59th Street West Bradenton, FL 34209 (813) 792-8480	Beds: 120 Private: 28 Medicaid, Medicare Rating:	Semiprivate: 46 Superior
Manatee Convalescent Center 302 Manatee Avenue East Bradenton, FL 34208 (813) 746-6131	Beds: 147 Private: 3 Medicaid, Medicare Rating:	Semiprivate: 15 Superior
Meadowbrook Manor of Bradenton 105 Fifteenth Street East Bradenton, FL 34208 (813) 747-8681	Beds: 110 Private: 0 Medicaid, Medicare Rating:	Semiprivate: 3 Standard
Mediplex Rehabilitation, Bradenton 5627 9th Street, East Bradenton, FL 34203 (813) 753-8941	Beds: 120 Private: 4 Medicaid, Medicare Rating:	Semiprivate: 58 Superior
Regency Health Care Center 926 Haben Boulevard Palmetto, FL 34221 (813) 722-0553	Beds: 120 Private: 0 Medicaid, Medicare Rating:	Semiprivate: 60 Superior
Shores Health Center, The 1700 West Third Avenue Bradenton, FL 34205 (813) 748-1700	Beds: 21 Private: 1 Rating:	Semiprivate: 20 Superior
Suncoast Manor Nursing Home 2010 Manatee Avenue East Bradenton, FL 34208 (813) 747-3706	Beds: 208 Private: 15 Medicaid, Medicare Rating:	Semiprivate: 54 Superior
Surrey Place Convalescent Center 5525 21st Avenue West Bradenton, FL 34209 (813) 795-0448	Beds: 60 Private: 4 Medicaid, Medicare Rating:	Semiprivate: 28 Superior
Westminster Asbury Manor 1700 21st Avenue West Bradenton, FL 34205 (813) 748-4161	Beds: 59 Private: 1 Medicaid, Medicare Rating:	Semiprivate: 21 Superior
Westminster Asbury Towers 1533 Fourth Avenue West Bradenton, FL 34205 (813) 747-1881	Beds: 34 Private: 1 Medicaid, Medicare Rating:	Semiprivate: 11 Standard

MARION

Marion House Health Care Center 3930 E. Silver Spring Blvd. Ocala, FL 32670-5506 (904) 236-2626	Beds: 120 Private: 8 Medicaid, Medicare Rating:	Semiprivate: 40 Conditional

New Horizon Rehabilitation Center 635 S.E. 17th St. Ocala, FL 32671 (904) 629-7921	Beds: 89 Private: 3 Medicaid, Medicare Rating:	Semiprivate: 29 Superior
Oakhurst Manor Nursing Center 1501 S.E. 24th Road Ocala, FL 32671 (904) 629-8900	Beds: 120 Private: 10 Medicaid, Medicare Rating:	Semiprivate: 43 Superior
Ocala Geriatric Center 1201 S.W. 24th Street Ocala, FL 32671 (904) 732-2449	Beds: 180 Private: 16 Medicaid, Medicare Rating:	Semiprivate: 82 Standard
Palm Garden 3400 S.W. 27th Ave. Ocala, FL 32674 (904) 854-6262	Beds: 120 Private: 4 Medicaid, Medicare Rating:	Semiprivate: 58 Superior
Stonegate Rehab. & Nursing Center 2021 Southwest First Ave Ocala, FL 32671 (904) 629-0063	Beds: 133 Private: 7 Medicaid, Medicare Rating:	Semiprivate: 18 Superior
Surrey Place Convalescent Center 4100 S.W. 33rd Avenue Ocala, FL 32678 (904) 237-7776	Beds: 120 Private: 64 Medicaid, Medicare Rating:	Semiprivate: 28 Superior
Timberridge Nursing & Rehab. Center 9848 S.W. 110th Street Ocala, FL 32676 (904) 854-8200	Beds: 56 Private: 6 Medicaid, Medicare Rating:	Semiprivate: 25 Superior

MARTIN

Manors at Hobe Sound 9555 S.E. Federal Hwy Hobe Sound, FL 33455 (407) 546-5800	Beds: 120 Private: 7 Medicaid, Medicare Rating:	Semiprivate: 33 Superior
National Health Care Center of Stuart 800 S.E. Central Parkway Stuart, FL 34994 (407) 287-9912	Beds: 104 Private: 16 Medicaid, Medicare Rating:	Semiprivate: 44 Superior
Salerno Bay Manor 4801 S.E. Cove Road Port Salerno, FL 34992 (407) 286-9440	Beds: 120 Private: 24 Medicaid, Medicare Rating:	Semiprivate: 48 Standard
Stuart Convalescent Center 1500 Palm Beach Road Stuart, FL 34994 (407) 283-5887	Beds: 182 Private: 5 Medicaid, Medicare Rating:	Semiprivate: 41 Superior

MONROE

Key West Convalescent Center 5860 W. Junior College Dr Key West, FL 33040 (305) 296-2459	Beds: 120 Private: 2 Medicaid, Medicare Rating:	Semiprivate: 59 Conditional
Marathon Manor Sombrero Beach Rd. Marathon, FL 33050 (305) 743-4466	Beds: 120 Private: 10 Medicaid, Medicare Rating:	Semiprivate: 55 Conditional
Plantation Key Convention Center 48 High Point Road Tavernier, FL 33070 (305) 852-3021	Beds: 120 Private: 2 Medicaid, Medicare Rating:	Semiprivate: 59 Conditional

NASSAU

Hilliard Manor US 1 & 3rd Street Hilliard, FL 32046 (904) 261-0771	Beds: 60 Private: 2 Medicaid, Medicare Rating:	Semiprivate: 29 Superior
Quality Health of Fernandina Beach 1625 Lime Street Fernandina Beach, FL 32034 (904) 261-0771	Beds: 120 Private: 10 Medicaid, Medicare Rating:	Semiprivate: 55 Standard

OKALOOSA

Bay Heritage Nursing and Convalescent Center 115 Hart Street Niceville, FL 32578 (904) 698-6667	Beds: 90 Private: 6 Medicaid, Medicare Rating:	Semiprivate: 42 Standard
Crestview Nursing & Convalescent Center 1849 East First Street Crestview, FL 32536 (904) 682-5322	Beds: 180 Private: 4 Medicaid, Medicare Rating:	Semiprivate: 88 Standard
Fort Walton Beach Care Center 1 LBJ Sr. Drive Ft. Walton Beach, FL 32548 9904) 243-6134	Beds: 120 Private: 2 Medicaid, Medicare Rating:	Semiprivate: 37 Standard
Gulf Convalescent Center 114 East Third Street Ft. Walton Beach, FL 32548 (904) 243-6134	Beds: 120 Private: 2 Medicaid, Medicare Rating:	Semiprivate: 37 Standard
Silvercrest Manor Nursing Home 103 Ruby Lane Crestview, FL 32536 (904) 682-1903	Beds: 60 Private: 2 Medicaid, Medicare Rating:	Semiprivate: 29 Superior
Westwood Healthcare Center 1001 Mar-Walt Drive Ft. Walton Beach, FL 32548 (904) 863-5174	Beds: 60 Private: 6 Medicare Rating:	Semiprivate: 23 Superior

OKEECHOBEE

Okeechobee Health Care Facility 1646 Highway 441 North Okeechobee, FL 33472 (813) 763-2226	Beds: 155 Private: 9 Medicaid, Medicare Rating:	Semiprivate: 61 Standard

ORANGE

Barrington Terrace Nursing Home 215 Annie Street Orlando, FL 32806 (407) 841-4371	Beds: 60 Private: 9 Rating:	Semiprivate: 18 Standard
Central Park Village Health Care Center 9309 South Orange Blossom Trail Orlando, FL 32821 (407) 859-7990	Beds: 120 Private: 12 Medicaid, Medicare Rating:	Semiprivate: 54 Superior
Conway Lakes Nursing Center 5201 Currey Ford Road Orlando, FL 32812 (407) 384-8838	Beds: 120 Private: 8 Medicaid, Medicare Rating:	Semiprivate: 56 Standard
Florida Living Nursing Center 3355 E. Semoran Blvd. Apopka, FL 32703 (407) 862-6263	Beds: 184 Private: 28 Medicaid, Medicare Rating:	Semiprivate: 78 Superior
Florida Manor Nursing Home 830 West 29th Street Orlando, FL 32805 (407) 843-3230	Beds: 420 Private: 2 Medicaid, Medicare Rating:	Semiprivate: 197 Superior
Guardian Care Convalescent Center 2500 West Church Street Orlando, FL 32805 (407) 295-5371	Beds: 120 Private: 2 Medicaid, Medicare Rating:	Semiprivate: 44 Superior
Manor Care Nursing/Rehab Center 2075 Lock Lomond Dr. Winter Park, FL 32792 (407) 628-5418	Beds: 138 Private: 4 Medicaid, Medicare Rating:	Semiprivate: 34 Superior
Mary Lee Depugh Nursing Home 550 West Morse Blvd. Winter Park, FL 32789 (407) 644-6634	Beds: 40 Private: 0 Medicaid, Medicare Rating:	Semiprivate: 7 Conditional
Mayflower Retirement Community, The 1620 Mayflower Court Winter Park, Florida 32792 (407) 672-1620	Beds: 60 Private: 2 Medicare Rating:	Semiprivate: 29 Superior
Ocoee Health Care Center 1556 Maguire Road Ocoee, FL 34761 (407) 877-2272	Beds: 120 Private: 6 Medicaid, Medicare Rating:	Semiprivate: 57 Standard

Orlando Care Center 1900 Mercy Avenue Orlando, FL 32808 (407) 299-5404	Beds: 120 Private: 6 Medicaid, Medicare Rating:	Semiprivate: 57 Standard
Orlando Health Care Center 2000 N. Semoran Blvd. Orlando, FL 32807 (407) 671-5400	Beds: 118 Private: 2 Medicaid, Medicare Rating:	Semiprivate: 34 Standard
Orlando Lutheran Towers 300 E. Church Street Orlando, FL 32779 (407) 425-1033	Beds: 60 Private: 1 Medicaid, Medicare Rating:	Semiprivate: 29 Superior
Orlando Memorial Convalescent Center 1730 Lucerne Terrace Orlando, FL 32806 (407) 423-1612	Beds: 115 Private: 0 Medicaid, Medicare Rating:	Semiprivate: 56 Superior
Palm Garden 654 South Econlockhatchee Trail Orlando, FL 32817 (407) 273-6158	Beds: 60 Private: 2 Medicaid, Medicare Rating:	Semiprivate: 29 Superior
Park Lake Nursing and Rehab. Center 1700 Monroe Avenue Winter Park, FL 32751 (407) 647-2092	Beds: 180 Private: 10 Medicaid, Medicare Rating:	Semiprivate: 85 Superior
Pinar Terrace Manor 7950 Lake Underhill Rd Orlando, FL 32822 (407) 658-2046	Beds: 180 Private: 10 Medicaid, Medicare Rating:	Semiprivate: 85 Superior
Quality Health Care Center/Orange Co. 941 East Highway 50 Winter Garden, FL 32787 (407) 877-6636	Beds: 120 Private: 10 Medicaid, Medicare Rating:	Semiprivate: 55 Superior
Regents Park of Winter Park 558 N. Semoran Blvd. Winter Park, FL 32792 (407) 679-1515	Beds: 120 Private: 2 Medicaid, Medicare Rating:	Semiprivate: 59 Conditional
Rosemont Health Care Center 3920 Rosewood Way Orlando, FL 32808 (407) 298-9335	Beds: 120 Private: 20 Medicaid, Medicare Rating:	Semiprivate: 50 Conditional
Sunbelt Living Center of Orlando 2414 Bedford Road Orlando, FL 32803 (407) 898-5051	Beds: 102 Private: 12 Medicaid, Medicare Rating:	Semiprivate: 43 Superior
West Orange Manor 122 E. Division Street Winter Garden, FL 32787 (407) 656-3810	Beds: 228 Private: 20 Medicaid, Medicare Rating:	Semiprivate: 86 Superior

Westminster Towers 70 West Lucerne Circle Orlando, FL 32801 (407) 841-1310	Beds: 120 Private: 8 Medicaid, Medicare Rating:	Semiprivate: 56 Superior
Winter Garden Health Care Center 1600 West Highway 50 Winter Garden, FL 32787 (407) 877-2394	Beds: 120 Private: 2 Medicare Rating:	Semiprivate: 59 Superior
Winter Park Care Center 2970 Scarlet Road Winter Park, FL 32792 (407) 671-8030	Beds: 103 Private: 17 Medicaid, Medicare Rating:	Semiprivate: 43 Superior
Winter Park Towers 1111 South Lakemont Avenue Winter Park, FL 32792 (407) 647-4083	Beds: 121 Private: 1 Medicaid, Medicare Rating:	Semiprivate: 60 Superior

OSCEOLA

Donegan Health Care & Rehab. Center 1120 West Donegan Ave. Kissimmee, FL 32741 (407) 847-2854	Beds: 149 Private: 23 Medicaid, Medicare Rating:	Semiprivate: 47 Superior
Kissimmee Good Samaritan Health Care Center 1500 Southgate Drive Kissimmee, FL 32741 (407) 846-7201	Beds: 170 Private: 2 Medicaid, Medicare Rating:	Semiprivate: 60 Superior
Oaks of Kissimmee 320 N. Mitchell Street Kissimmee, FL 32741 (407) 847-7200	Beds: 59 Private: 0 Medicaid, Medicare Rating:	Semiprivate: 28 Superior
Osceola Health Care Center 4201 W. New Nolte Road St. Cloud, FL 34772 (407) 957-3341	Beds: 120 Private: 4 Medicaid, Medicare Rating:	Semiprivate: 58 Superior
Southern Oaks Health Care Center 2355 Kissimmee Park Road St. Cloud, FL 34769 (407) 957-2280	Beds: 120 Private: 4 Medicare Rating:	Semiprivate: 58 Standard
St. Cloud Health Care Center 1301 Kansas Avenue St. Cloud, FL 34769 (407) 892-5121	Beds: 131 Private: 7 Medicaid, Medicare Rating:	Semiprivate: 20 Superior

PALM BEACH

American-Finnish Nursing Home 1800 South Drive Lake Worth, FL 33461 (407) 588-4333	Beds: 60 Private: 0 Medicaid, Medicare Rating:	Semiprivate: 18 Superior

Atlantis Nursing Center 6026 Old Congress Road Lantana, FL 33462 (407) 964-4430	Beds: 120 Private: 0 Medicaid, Medicare Rating:	Semiprivate: 60 Superior
Avante at Lake Worth 2501 North A Street Lake Worth, FL 33460 (407) 585-9301	Beds: 162 Private: 4 Medicaid, Medicare Rating:	Semiprivate: 67 Superior
Boca Raton Rehabilitation Center 755 Meadows Road Boca Raton, FL 33432 (407) 391-5200	Beds: 120 Private: 4 Medicaid, Medicare Rating:	Semiprivate: 28 Superior
Boulevard Manor Nursing Center 2839 South Seacrest Blvd. Boynton Beach, FL 33435 (407) 732-2464	Beds: 167 Private: 13 Medicaid, Medicare Rating:	Semiprivate: 55 Superior
Convalescent Center of the Palm Beaches 300 15th Street West Palm Beach, FL 33401 (407) 832-6409	Beds: 99 Private: 1 Medicaid, Medicare Rating:	Semiprivate: 31 Superior
Crest Manor Nursing Home 504 Third Avenue, South Lake Worth, FL 33460 (407) 585-4695	Beds: 71 Private: 3 Medicaid, Medicare Rating:	Semiprivate: 19 Superior
Darcy Hall Nursing Home 2170 Palm Beach Lakes Blvd West Palm Beach, FL 33409 (407) 683-3333	Beds: 220 Private: 10 Medicaid, Medicare Rating:	Semiprivate: 57 Standard
Eason Nursing Home 1711 Sixth Avenue, South Lake Worth, FL 33460 (407) 582-1472	Beds: 99 Private: 3 Medicaid, Medicare Rating:	Semiprivate: 45 Superior
Edgewater Pointe Estates 23305 Blue Water Circle Boca Raton, FL 33433 (407) 368-5600	Beds: 60 Private: 10 Medicare Rating:	Semiprivate: 25 Superior
Fountains Nursing Home, The 3800 North Federal Hwy Boca Raton, FL 33431 (407) 395-7510	Beds: 51 Private: 2 Medicaid, Medicare Rating: ·	Semiprivate: 15 Superior
Glades Health Care Center 230 South Barfield Highway Pahokee, FL 33476 (407) 924-5561	Beds: 120 Private: 4 Medicaid, Medicare Rating:	Semiprivate: 58 Superior
Harbour's Edge 401 E. Linton Blvd. Delray Beach, FL 33483 (407) 272-7979	Beds: 54 Private: 54 Medicaid, Medicare Rating:	Semiprivate: 0 Superior

Haverhill Care Center 5065 Wallis Road West Palm Beach, FL 33415 (407) 689-1799	Beds: 120 Private: 2 Medicaid, Medicare Rating:	Semiprivate: 48 Superior
Health Center at Abbey Delray 2105 S.W. 11th Court Delray Beach, FL 33445 (407) 243-4526	Beds: 100 Private: 2 Medicaid, Medicare Rating:	Semiprivate: 49 Superior
Health Center at Abbey Delray South 1717 Homewood Blvd. Delray Beach, FL 33445-6875 (407) 272-9600	Beds: 60 Private: 10 Medicaid, Medicare Rating:	Semiprivate: 25 Superior
Heartland Health Care Center 3600 Old Boynton Road Boynton Beach, FL 33436 (407) 736-9992	Beds: 120 Private: 2 Medicaid, Medicare Rating:	Semiprivate: 59 Superior
Heartland Health Care—Prosperity Oaks 1375 Prosperity Farms Road Palm Beach Gardens, FL 33410 (407) 624-2179	Beds: 120 Private: 12 Medicare Rating:	Semiprivate: 54 Standard
Helen Wilkes Healthcare Center 750 Bayberry Drive Lake Park, FL 33403 (407) 844-4396	Beds: 85 Private: 1 Medicaid, Medicare Rating:	Semiprivate: 30 Standard
Henry I. Loutitt Healthcare Center 4445 Pine Forest Drive Lake Worth, FL 33463 (407) 965-5954	Beds: 60 Private: 2 Medicare Rating:	Semiprivate: 29 Superior
Hillhaven Convalescent Center 5430 Linton Blvd. Delray Beach, FL 33484 (407) 495-3188	Beds: 120 Private: 12 Medicaid, Medicare Rating:	Semiprivate: 54 Superior
Joseph L. Morse Geriatric Center 4847 Fred Gladstone Drive West Palm Beach, FL 33417 (407) 471-5111	Beds: 280 Private: 74 Medicaid, Medicare Rating:	Semiprivate: 103 Superior
Jupiter Care Center 17781 Yancy Street Jupiter, FL 33458 (407) 746-2998	Beds: 120 Private: 2 Medicare Rating:	Semiprivate: 47 Superior
Jupiter Convalescence Pavilion 1230 South Old Dixie Hwy Jupiter, FL 33458 (407) 744-4444	Beds: 120 Private: 8 Medicaid, Medicare Rating:	Semiprivate: 48 Superior
King David Center at Palm Beach 1101 54th Street West Palm Beach, FL 33407 (407) 844-4343	Beds: 191 Private: 22 Medicaid, Medicare Rating:	Semiprivate: 74 Standard

Lakeside Health Center 2501 Australian Avenue West Palm Beach, FL 33407 (407) 655-7780	Beds: 97 Private: 5 Medicaid, Medicare Rating:	Semiprivate: 45 Superior
Lourdes-Noreen McKeen Res 315 South Flagler Dr. West Palm Beach, FL 33401 (407) 655-8544	Beds: 120 Private: 60 Medicaid, Medicare Rating:	Semiprivate: 30 Superior
Maclen Rehabilitation Center 1201 12th Avenue, S. Lake Worth, FL 33460 (407) 586-7404	Beds: 120 Private: 4 Medicaid, Medicare Rating:	Semiprivate: 58 Superior
Manor Care of Boca Raton 375 N.W. 51st Street Boca Raton, FL 33487 (407) 997-8111	Beds: 180 Private: 30 Medicaid, Medicare Rating:	Semiprivate: 75 Superior
Manor Care of Boynton Beach 3001 South Congress Avenue Boynton Beach, FL 33435 (407) 737-5600	Beds: 180 Private: 60 Medicaid, Medicare Rating:	Semiprivate: 45 Superior
Meadowbrook Manor/Boca Cove 1130 N.W. 15th Street Boca Raton, FL 33432 (407) 394-6282	Beds: 120 Private: 8 Medicaid, Medicare Rating:	Semiprivate: 50 Standard
Medicana Nursing Center 1710 Lucerne Avenue Lake Worth, FL 33460 (407) 582-5331	Beds: 117 Private: 1 Medicaid, Medicare Rating:	Semiprivate: 26 Superior
Mediplex Rehabilitation 6414 13th Road, South West Palm Meach, FL 33415 (407) 478-9900	Beds: 120 Private: 8 Medicaid, Medicare Rating:	Semiprivate: 56 Standard
Menorah House 9945 Central Park Blvd. Boca Raton, FL 33428 (407) 483-0498	Beds: 120 Private: 8 Medicaid Rating:	Semiprivate: 56 Superior
Palm Beach County Home & General Care Facility 1200 45th Street West Palm Beach, FL 33407 (407) 842-6111	Beds: 210 Private: 14 Medicaid, Medicare Rating:	Semiprivate: 48 Superior
Palm Garden 300 Executive Center Dr West Palm Beach, FL 33401 (407) 471-5566	Beds: 120 Private: 4 Medicaid, Medicare Rating:	Semiprivate: 58 Superior
Regency Health Care Center 3599 South Congress Ave Lake Worth, FL 33461 (407) 965-8876	Beds: 168 Private: 1 Medicaid, Medicare Rating:	Semiprivate: 3 Superior

Regents Park of Boca Raton 6363 Verde Trail Boca Raton, FL 33433 (407) 483-9282	Beds: 120 Private: 12 Medicaid, Medicare Rating:	Semiprivate: 54 Superior
Ridge Terrace Health Care Center 2180 Hypoluxo Road Lantana, FL 33462 (407) 582-6711	Beds: 120 Private: 4 Medicaid, Medicare Rating:	Semiprivate: 58 Superior
Royal Manor 100 Bob White Court Royal Palm Beach, FL 33411 (407) 798-3700	Beds: 120 Private: 18 Medicaid, Medicare Rating:	Semiprivate: 51 Superior
St. Andrews Estates Medical Center 6152 North Verde Trail Boca Raton, FL 33433 (407) 487-5200	Beds: 120 Private: 34 Medicaid, Medicare Rating:	Semiprivate: 43 Superior
Sutton Place Convalescent Center 4405 Lakewood Road Lake Worth, FL 33461 (407) 969-1400	Beds: 120 Private: 4 Medicaid, Medicare Rating:	Semiprivate: 58 Conditional
Waterford Health Center 601 South U.S. Hwy 1 Juno Beach, FL 33408 (407) 627-3800	Beds: 60 Private: 8 Medicaid, Medicare Rating:	Semiprivate: 26 Superior
West Palm Beach Village Care Center 1626 Oavis Road West Palm Beach, FL 33406 (407) 439-8897	Beds: 120 Private: 12 Medicaid, Medicare Rating:	Semiprivate: 54 Superior
Whitehall Boca Raton 7300 Del Prado, South Boca Raton, FL 33433 (407) 392-3000	Beds: 73 Private: 13 Medicare Rating:	Semiprivate: 30 Superior

PASCO

Bear Creek Nursing Center 8041 State Road 52 Hudson, FL 34667 (813) 863-5488	Beds: 120 Private: 2 Medicaid, Medicare Rating:	Semiprivate: 59 Superior
Dade City Geriatric Center 805 West Coleman Avenue Dade City, FL 33525 (904) 567-8615	Beds: 120 Private: 10 Medicaid, Medicare Rating:	Semiprivate: 55 Superior
Heartland of Zephyrhills 38220 Henry Drive Zephyrhills, FL 34248 (813) 788-7114	Beds: 120 Private: 4 Medicaid, Medicare Rating:	Semiprivate: 58 Standard
Heather Hill Nursing Home 6630 Kentucky Avenue New Port Richey, FL 33653 (813) 849-6939	Beds: 120 Private: 2 Medicaid, Medicare Rating:	Semiprivate: 59 Superior

National Healthcare Center 7210 Beacon Woods Drive Hudson, FL 34667 (813) 863-1521	Beds: 120 Private: 8 Medicaid, Medicare Rating:	Semiprivate: 56 Superior
Orchard Ridge Nursing Center 4927 Voorhees Road New Port Richey, FL 34653 (813) 848-3578	Beds: 120 Private: 16 Medicaid, Medicare Rating:	Semiprivate: 40 Superior
Park Lake Village Care Center 8417 State Road 54 New Port Richey, FL 34653 (813) 376-1585	Beds: 120 Private: 12 Medicaid, Medicare Rating:	Semiprivate: 54 Standard
Pasco Nursing Center 447 North 5th Street Dade City, FL 33525 (904) 567-1978	Beds: 40 Private: 0 Medicaid, Medicare Rating:	Semiprivate: 5 Standard
Richey Manor Nursing Home 6020 Indiana Avenue New Port Richey, FL 34653 (813) 849-7555	Beds: 119 Private: 3 Medicaid, Medicare Rating:	Semiprivate: 36 Standard
Royal Oak Nursing Resort 700 Royal Oak Lane Dade City, FL 33525 (904) 567-3122	Beds: 120 Private: 2 Medicaid, Medicare Rating:	Semiprivate: 59 Superior
Southern Pines Nursing Center 6140 South Congress Street New Port Richey, FL 34653 (813) 842-8402	Beds: 120 Private: 2 Medicaid, Medicare Rating:	Semiprivate: 34 Superior
Whispering Pines Convalescent Center 8151 Treelet Court New Port Richey, FL 34653 (813) 849-7205	Beds: 56 Private: 10 Medicaid, Medicare Rating:	Semiprivate: 14 Standard
Windsor Woods Convalescent Center 13719 Lakeshore Blvd. Hudson, FL 34667 (813) 862-6795	Beds: 103 Private: 45 Medicaid, Medicare Rating:	Semiprivate: 29 Superior
Zephyr Haven Nursing Home 38250 Avenue A Zephyrhills, FL 33541 (813) 782-5508	Beds: 120 Private: 8 Medicaid, Medicare Rating:	Semiprivate: 52 Superior

PINELLAS

Abbey Nursing Home, The 7101 Ninth Street, N. St. Petersburg, FL 33702 (813) 527-7231	Beds: 152 Private: 1 Medicaid Rating:	Semiprivate: 43 Superior
Alhambra Nursing Home 7501 38th Avenue, North St. Petersburg, FL 33710 (813) 345-9307	Beds: 60 Private: 10 Medicare Rating:	Semiprivate: 22 Standard

Alpine Nursing Center 3456 21st Avenue South St. Petersburg, FL 33711 (813) 327-1988	Beds: 57 Private: 1 Medicaid, Medicare Rating:	Semiprivate: 28 Superior
Arbors at Safety Harbor 1410 4th Street, North Safety Harbor, FL 34695 (813) 867-1104	Beds: Private: Medicaid, Medicare Rating:	Semiprivate: Superior
Bay Pointe Nursing Pavilion 4201 31st Street, South St. Petersburg, FL 33712 (813) 867-1104	Beds: 120 Private: 4 Medicaid, Medicare Rating:	Semiprivate: 58 Standard
Bay Tree Nursing Center 2600 Highlands Blvd., North Palm Harbor, FL 34684 (813) 785-5671	Beds: 120 Private: 10 Medicare Rating:	Semiprivate: 43 Superior
Beach Convalescent Hotel 8008 Blind Pass Road St. Petersburg, FL 33706 (813) 367-7651	Beds: 38 Private: 1 Medicaid, Medicare Rating:	Semiprivate: 16 Standard
Belleair East Healthcare Center 1150 Ponce DeLeon Blvd. Clearwater, FL 34616 (813) 585-5491	Beds: 120 Private: 0 Medicaid, Medicare Rating:	Semiprivate: 60 Conditional
Bon Secours Maria Manor 10300 4th Street, North St. Petersburg, FL 33716 (813) 576-1025	Beds: 274 Private: 6 Medicaid, Medicare Rating:	Semiprivate: 134 Superior
Bruce Manor Nursing Home 1100 Pine Street Clearwater, FL 33516 (813) 442-7106	Beds: 76 Private: 4 Medicaid, Medicare Rating:	Semiprivate: 26 Superior
Carrington Place 10501 Roosevelt Blvd., N. St. Petersburg, FL 33716 (813) 577-3800	Beds: 120 Private: 28 Medicaid, Medicare Rating:	Semiprivate: 46 Standard
Central Park Lodge 900 Beckett Way Tarpon Springs, FL 34689 (813) 934-0876	Beds: 120 Private: 8 Medicaid, Medicare Rating:	Semiprivate: 55 Superior
Central Park Lodge 2055 Palmetto Street Clearwater, FL 34625 (813) 461-6613	Beds: 150 Private: 22 Medicaid, Medicare Rating:	Semiprivate: 58 Superior
Central Park Lodge Nursing Center 8701 49th Street, North Pinellas Park, FL 34666 (813) 546-4661	Beds: 120 Private: 12 Medicaid, Medicare Rating:	Semiprivate: 54 Superior

Clearwater Convalescent Center 1270 Turner Street Clearwater, FL 33516 (813) 443-7639	Beds: 120 Private: 1 Medicaid, Medicare Rating:	Semiprivate: 38 Superior
College Harbor 4600 54th Ave., South St. Petersburg, FL 33711 (813) 866-3124	Beds: 60 Private: 2 Medicare Rating:	Semiprivate: 29 Superior
Colonial Care Center 6300 46th Avenue North St. Petersburg, FL 33709 (813) 544-1444	Beds: 102 Private: 2 Medicaid, Medicare Rating:	Semiprivate: 38 Superior
Concordia Manor 321 13th Avenue North St. Petersburg, FL 33701 (813) 822-3030	Beds: 39 Private: 1 Medicaid Rating:	Semiprivate: 1 Standard
Convalescent Care Center 550 South 62nd Street St. Petersburg, FL 33707-1533 (813) 347-6151	Beds: 120 Private: 2 Medicaid, Medicare Rating:	Semiprivate: 59 Superior
Country Place of Clearwater 905 South Highland Ave. Clearwater, FL 34616 (813) 442-9606	Beds: 103 Private: 1 Medicaid, Medicare Rating:	Semiprivate: 27 Conditional
Countryside Health Care Center 3825 Countryside Blvd. Palm Harbor, FL 34684 (813) 784-2848	Beds: 120 Private: 12 Medicaid, Medicare Rating:	Semiprivate: 54 Standard
Crown Nursing Home 5351 Gulf Blvd. St. Petersburg Beach, FL 33706 (813) 360-5548	Beds: 54 Private: 21 Medicaid, Medicare Rating:	Semiprivate: 12 Standard
Deluxe Care Inn 1820 Shore Dr., South South Pasadena, FL 33707 (813) 384-9300	Beds: 58 Private: 1 Medicare Rating:	Semiprivate: 25 Standard
Drew Village Nursing Home 401 Fairwood Avenue Clearwater, FL 34619 (813) 797-6313	Beds: 120 Private: 4 Medicaid, Medicare Rating:	Semiprivate: 58 Standard
Dunedin Care Center 1351 San Christopher Dr. Dunedin, FL 34698 (813) 736-1421	Beds: 104 Private: 16 Medicaid, Medicare Rating:	Semiprivate: 44 Conditional
East Bay Nursing Center 4470 E. Bay Drive Clearwater, FL 34624 (813) 530-7100	Beds: 120 Private: 4 Medicaid, Medicare Rating:	Semiprivate: 58 Standard

Freedom Square Nursing Center 10801 Johnson Blvd. Seminole, FL 34642 (813) 398-0379	Beds: 120 Private: 24 Rating:	Semiprivate: 48 Superior
Golfview Nursing Home 3636 10th Avenue North St. Petersburg, FL 33713 (813) 323-3611	Beds: 56 Private: 11 Medicaid, Medicare Rating:	Semiprivate: 21 Superior
Good Samaritan Nursing Home 3127 North 57th Avenue St. Petersburg, FL 33714 (813) 527-2171	Beds: 60 Private: 3 Medicaid, Medicare Rating:	Semiprivate: 5 Superior
Greenbrook Nursing Center 1000 North 24th Street St. Petersburg, FL 33713 (813) 323-4711	Beds: 120 Private: 0 Medicaid, Medicare Rating:	Semiprivate: 48 Standard
Gulfport Convalescent Center 1414 South 59th Street Gulfport, FL 33707 (813) 344-4608	Beds: 120 Private: 1 Medicaid, Medicare Rating:	Semiprivate: 38 Standard
Heartland of St. Petersburg 1001 Ninth Street, N. St. Petersburg, FL 33701 (813) 896-8619	Beds: 108 Private: 0 Medicaid, Medicare Rating:	Semiprivate: 47 Superior
Highland Pines Nursing Manor 1111 South Highland Ave. Clearwater, FL 33516 (813) 446-0581	Beds: 120 Private: 12 Medicaid, Medicare Rating:	Semiprivate: 51 Standard
Huber Restorium 521 69th Avenue North St. Petersburg, FL 33701 (813) 526-7000	Beds: 96 Private: 4 Medicare Rating:	Semiprivate: 26 Standard
Jacaranda Manor 4250 66th Street North St. Petersburg, FL 33702 (813) 546-2405	Beds: 299 Private: 1 Medicaid, Medicare Rating:	Semiprivate: 95 Superior
Laurels Rehabilitation Center, The 550 9th Avenue South St. Petersburg, FL 33715 (813) 898-4105	Beds: 258 Private 1 Medicaid, Medicare Rating:	Semiprivate: 106 Superior
Majestic Towers Health Center 1255 Pasadena Avenue, South St. Petersburg, FL 33707 (813) 381-7301	Beds: 150 Private: 2 Medicaid, Medicare Rating:	Semiprivate: 14 Standard
Manor Care Nursing Center 870 Patricia Avenue Dunedin, FL 34698 (813) 734-8861	Beds: 120 Private: 42 Medicare Rating:	Semiprivate: 39 Superior

Manor Care Of Palm Harbor 2851 Tampa Road Palm Harbor, FL 34684 (813) 787-4777	Beds: 180 Private: 54 Medicaid, Medicare Rating:	Semiprivate: 63 Superior
Masonic Home of Florida 3201 1st Street N.E. St. Petersburg, FL 33704 (813) 822-3499	Beds: 85 Private: 5 Rating:	Semiprivate: 27 Standard
Mease Continuing Care 910 New York Avenue Dunedin, FL 34698 (813) 733-2113	Beds: 100 Private: 8 Medicaid, Medicare Rating:	Semiprivate: 46 Standard
Menorah Manor 255 59th Street, N. St. Petersburg, FL 33710 (813) 345-2775	Beds: 120 Private: 48 Medicaid, Medicare Rating:	Semiprivate: 36 Superior
Morton Plant Rehabilitation Center 1250 South Fort Harrison Ave Clearwater, FL 33516-3392 (813) 462-7600	Beds: 126 Private: 1 Medicaid, Medicare Rating:	Semiprivate: 57 Superior
National Healthcare Center 435 42 Avenue South St. Petersburg, FL 33705 (813) 822-1871	Beds: 159 Private: 1 Medicaid, Medicare Rating:	Semiprivate: 65 Standard
North Horizon Health Care Center 1301 16th Street North St. Petersburg, FL 33705 (813) 898-5119	Beds: 49 Private: 1 Medicaid, Medicare Rating:	Semiprivate: 22 Superior
North Shore Center 939 Beach Dr., N.E. St. Petersburg, FL 33701 (813) 823-1571	Beds: 26 Private: 1 Medicaid, Medicare Rating:	Semiprivate: 4 Conditional
Oak Bluffs Nursing Center 420 Bay Avenue Clearwater, FL 33516 (813) 445-4700	Beds: 60 Private: 3 Medicaid, Medicare Rating:	Semiprivate: 9 Standard
Oak Cove Nursing Center 210 South Osceola Ave. Clearwater, FL 34616 (813) 441-3763	Beds: 56 Private: 12 Medicaid, Medicare Rating:	Semiprivate: 7 Standard
Oak Manor Nursing Center 3500 Oak Manor Lane Largo, FL 34644 (813) 581-9427	Beds: 180 Private: 28 Medicaid, Medicare Rating:	Semiprivate: 68 Standard
Osceola Inn 221 N. Osceola Ave. Clearwater, FL 34615 (813) 461-3321	Beds: 13 Private: 1 Rating:	Semiprivate: 2 Conditional

Palm Garden 3480 McMullen-Booth Road Clearwater, FL 34621 (813) 786-6697	Beds: 120 Private: 4 Medicaid, Medicare Rating:	Semiprivate: 58 Superior
Palm Garden 10500 Starkey Road Largo, FL 34647 (813) 397-8166	Beds: 78 Private: 24 Medicaid, Medicare Rating:	Semiprivate: 27 Superior
Palm Garden of Pinellas 200 16th Avenue, S.E. Largo, FL 34641 (813) 894-2102	Beds: 120 Private: 10 Medicaid, Medicare Rating:	Semiprivate: 55 Standard
Palm Shores Retirement Center 830 North Shore Drive St. Petersburg, FL 33701 (813) 894-2102	Beds: 42 Private: 18 Rating:	Semiprivate: 2 Standard
Parkway Nursing Home 7575 North 65th Way Pinellas Park, FL 346655 (813) 544-6673	Beds: 55 Private: 1 Medicaid, Medicare Rating:	Semiprivate: 15 Conditional
Pasadena Manor 1430 Pasadena Ave., South St. Petersburg, FL 33707 (813) 347-1257	Beds: 126 Private: 2 Medicaid, Medicare Rating:	Semiprivate: 60 Superior
Regency Oaks Nursing Center 2770 Regency Oaks Blvd. Clearwater, FL 34619 (813) 791-3381	Beds: 60 Private: 8 Medicaid, Medicare Rating:	Semiprivate: 26 Standard
Rosedale Manor 3479 54th Avenue St. Petersburg, FL 33714 (813) 527-7315	Beds: 189 Private: 1 Medicaid, Medicare Rating:	Semiprivate: 26 Superior
Sabal Palms Health Care Center 499 Alternate Keene Road Largo, FL 34641 (813) 586-4211	Beds: 120 Private: 24 Medicaid, Medicare Rating:	Semiprivate: 48 Superior
Seminole Nursing Pavilion 10800 Temple Terrace Seminole, FL 33542 (813) 398-0123	Beds: 120 Private: 18 Medicaid, Medicare Rating:	Semiprivate: 51 Standard
Shore Acres Nursing & Convalescent Home 4500 Indianapolis St., NE St. Petersburg, FL 33703 (813) 527-5801	Beds: 109 Private: 2 Medicaid, Medicare Rating:	Semiprivate: 48 Standard
South Heritage Nursing Center 718 Lakeview Ave., South St. Petersburg, FL 33705 (813) 894-5125	Beds: 74 Private: 1 Medicaid, Medicare Rating:	Semiprivate: 33 Standard

Spanish Gardens Nursing Center 1061 Virginia Street Dunedin, FL 34698 (813) 733-4189	Beds: 93 Private: 1 Medicaid, Medicare Rating:	Semiprivate: 40 Standard
St. Mark Village 2655 Nebraska Ave. Palm Harbor, FL 34684 (813) 785-2576	Beds: 80 Private: 6 Medicare Rating:	Semiprivate: 37 Standard
Stratford Court of Palm Harbor 45 Katherine Blvd. Palm Harbor, FL 34684 (813) 867-1131	Beds: 60 Private: 4 Medicaid, Medicare Rating:	Semiprivate: 28 Standard
Suncoast Manor Health Center 6909 Ninth St., South St. Petersburg, FL 33705 (813) 867-1131	Beds: 161 Private: 69 Rating:	Semiprivate: 42 Standard
Suncoast Nursing Home 2000 South 17th Avenue St. Petersburg, FL 33712 (813) 821-3544	Beds: 59 Private: 1 Medicaid, Medicare Rating:	Semiprivate: 2 Standard
Sunset Point Nursing Center 1980 Sunset Point Road Clearwater, FL 34625 (813) 443-1580	Beds: 120 Private: 10 Medicaid, Medicare Rating:	Semiprivate: 43 Standard
Sunshine Village Nursing Home 8600 U.S. Hwy 19, N. Pinellas Park, FL 33565 (813) 541-7515	Beds: 120 Private: 14 Medicaid, Medicare Rating:	Semiprivate: 53 Conditional
Swanholm Nursing & Rehabilitation Center 6200 Central Avenue St. Petersburg, FL 33707 (813) 347-5196	Beds: 273 Private: 21 Medicaid, Medicare Rating:	Semiprivate: 89 Standard
T.L.C. St. Petersburg 1735 Ninth Street, South St. Petersburg, FL 33707 (813) 821-8866	Beds: 272 Private: 3 Medicaid, Medicare Rating:	Semiprivate: 95 Standard
Tarpon Health Care Center 501 South Walton Avenue Tarpon Springs, FL 34689 (813) 938-2814	Beds: 120 Private: 8 Medicaid, Medicare Rating:	Semiprivate: 56 Conditional
Tarpon Springs Convalescent Center 515 Chesapeake Drive Tarpon Springs, FL 34689 (813) 934-4629	Beds: 120 Private: 2 Medicaid, Medicare Rating:	Semiprivate: 49 Superior
Tierra Pines Health Care Center 7625 Ulmerton Road Largo, FL 34641 (813) 535-9833	Beds: 120 Private: 2 Medicaid, Medicare Rating:	Beds: 59 Conditional

Tyrone Medical Inn 1100 66th Street North St. Petersburg, FL 33712 (813) 345-9331	Beds: 59 Private: 1 Medicaid, Medicare Rating:	Semiprivate: 27 Standard
Victoria Martin Nursing Home 555 South 31st Street St. Petersburg, FL 33712 (813) 327-0995	Beds: 38 Private: 2 Medicaid, Medicare Rating:	Semiprivate: 8 Conditional
West Bay Nursing Center 400 State Rd 584, West Oldsmar, FL 33557 (813) 855-4661	Beds: 120 Private: 10 Medicaid, Medicare Rating:	Semiprivate: 43 Superior
Westchester Gardens 3301 McMullen Booth Road Clearwater, FL 34621 (813) 785-8335	Beds: 120 Private: 8 Medicaid, Medicare Rating:	Semiprivate: 56 Standard
Westminster Shores 125 South 56th Avenue St. Petersburg, FL 33705 (813) 867-2131	Beds: 120 Private: 8 Medicaid, Medicare Rating:	Semiprivate: 56 Standard
Whitehall Nursing Home 5601 South 31st Street St. Petersburg, FL 33712 (813) 867-6955	Beds: 60 Private: 6 Medicare Rating:	Semiprivate: 27 Superior
William & Mary Nursing Home 811 Jackson Street, North St. Petersburg, FL 33705 (813) 896-3651	Beds: 96 Private: 1 Medicaid, Medicare Rating:	Semiprivate: 47 Standard
Wright's Nursing Home 11300 110th Avenue North Largo, FL 33544 (813) 391-9986	Beds: 60 Private: 1 Rating:	Semiprivate: 19 Standard

POLK

Arbors at Lakeland 2020 W. Lake Parker Drive Lakeland, FL 33805 (813) 682-7580	Beds: 120 Private: 8 Medicaid, Medicare Rating:	Semiprivate: 56 Superior
Bartow Convalescent Center 2055 E. Georgia Street Bartow, FL 33830 (813) 533-0578	Beds: 120 Private: 1 Medicaid, Medicare Rating:	Semiprivate: 38 Superior
Brandywyne Convalescent Center 1801 N. Lake Miriam Drive Winter Haven, FL 33884 (813) 293-1989	Beds: 120 Private: 4 Medicaid, Medicare Rating:	Semiprivate: 58 Standard
Carpenter's Home Manor 1001 Carpenter's Way Lakeland, FL 33809 (813) 859-4249	Beds: 60 Private: 12 Medicaid, Medicare Rating:	Semiprivate: 24 Standard

Central Park Lodge Nursing Center 919 Old Winter Haven Rd Auburndale, FL 33823 (813) 967-4125	Beds: 120 Private: 12 Medicaid, Medicare Rating:	Semiprivate: 54 Superior
Grovemont Nursing & Rehab. Center 202 Avenue O, N.E. Winter Haven, FL 33881 (813) 293-3103	Beds: 144 Private: 16 Medicaid, Medicare Rating:	Semiprivate: 64 Superior
Haines City Health Care 409 South 10th Street Haines City, FL 33844 (813) 422-8656	Beds: 120 Private: 12 Medicaid, Medicare Rating:	Semiprivate: 54 Superior
Imperial Village Care Center 5245 N. Socrum Loop Road Lakeland, FL 33809 (813) 859-1446	Beds: 120 Private: 12 Medicaid, Medicare Rating:	Semiprivate: 54 Superior
Lake Alfred Restorium 350 West Haines Blvd. Lake Alfred, FL 33850 (813) 956-1700	Beds: 31 Private: 3 Medicaid, Medicare Rating:	Semiprivate: 14 Superior
Lake Wales Convalescent Center 730 North Scenic Hwy Lake Wales, FL 33853 (813) 676-1512	Beds: 100 Private: 3 Medicaid Rating:	Semiprivate: 29 Superior
Lake Wales Hospital Extended Care Facility 414 South 11th Street Lake Wales, FL 33853 (813) 676-3481	Beds: 120 Private: 16 Medicaid, Medicare Rating:	Semiprivate: 48 Superior
Lakeland Convalescent Center 610 E. Bella Vista Drive Lakeland, FL 33804 (813) 688-8591	Beds: 120 Private: 1 Medicaid, Medicare Rating:	Semiprivate: 38 Standard
Lakeland Health Care Center 1530 Kennedy Blvd. Lakeland, FL 33809 (813) 858-4402	Beds: 300 Private: 8 Medicaid, Medicare Rating:	Semiprivate: 82 Superior
Meridian Healthcare at Lakeland 4240 Lakeland Highlands Road Lakeland, FL 33813 (813) 646-8699	Beds: 179 Private: 19 Medicaid, Medicare Rating:	Semiprivate: 80 Superior
Oakbridge Village 3110 Oakbridge Blvd., East Lakeland, FL 33801 (813) 648-4800	Beds: 120 Private: 14 Medicaid, Medicare Rating:	Semiprivate: 53 Superior
Palm Garden 1120 Cypress Gardens Blvd. Winter Haven, FL 33880 (813) 293-3100	Beds: 60 Private: 2 Medicaid, Medicare Rating:	Semiprivate: 29 Superior

Presbyterian Nursing Center 1919 Lakeland Hills Blvd Lakeland, FL 33805 (813) 688-5612	Beds: 185 Private: 9 Medicaid, Medicare Rating:	Semiprivate: 88 Superior
Ridge Convalescent Center 512 South 11th Street Lake Wales, FL 33853 (813) 676-8502	Beds: 120 Private: 1 Medicaid, Medicare Rating:	Semiprivate: 38 Superior
Rhor Home, The 2010 E. Georgia St. Bartow, FL 33830 (813) 533-1806	Beds: 60 Private: 0 Medicaid, Medicare Rating:	Semiprivate: 30 Superior
Spring Lake Nursing Center 1540 6th Street, N.W. Winter Haven, FL 33881 (813) 294-3055	Beds: 120 Private: 4 Medicaid, Medicare Rating:	Semiprivate: 58 Standard
William L. Hargrave Health Center 206 West Orange Street Davenport, FL 33837 (813) 422-4961	Beds: 60 Private: 0 Medicaid, Medicare Rating:	Semiprivate: 30 Superior

PUTNAM

Lakeshore Nursing Home 100 Lake Street Crescent City, FL 32112 (904) 698-2222	Beds: 92 Private: 4 Medicaid, Medicare Rating:	Semiprivate: 44 Superior
Palatka Health Care Center 110 Kay Larkin Drive Palatka, FL 32177 (904) 325-0173	Beds: 120 Private: 10 Medicaid, Medicare Rating:	Semiprivate: 55 Superior
Putnam Memorial Nursing Home 510 South Palm Avenue Palatka, FL 32077 (904) 328-1472	Beds: 65 Private: 1 Medicaid, Medicare Rating:	Semiprivate: 32 Superior

SANTA ROSA

Bay Breeze Nursing/Ret Center 3375 Gulf Breeze Parkway Gulf Breeze, FL 32561 (904) 932-9257	Beds: 120 Private: 16 Medicaid, Medicare Rating:	Semiprivate: 52 Superior
Sandy Ridge Care Center 101 Glover Lane Milton, FL 32570 (904) 626-9225	Beds: 60 Private: 2 Medicaid, Medicare Rating:	Semiprivate: 29 Superior
Santa Rosa Convalescent Center 500 Broad Street Milton, FL 32570 (904) 623-4661	Beds: 120 Private: 2 Medicaid, Medicare Rating:	Semiprivate: 57 Superior

SARASOTA

Bay Village of Sarasota 8400 Vamo Road Sarasota, FL 34231 (813) 966-561	Beds: 107 Private: 1 Rating:	Semiprivate: 49 Standard
Beneva Nursing Pavilion 741 South Beneva Road Sarasota, FL 34232 (813) 957-0310	Beds: 120 Private: 20 Medicaid, Medicare Rating:	Semiprivate: 50 Superior
Burzenski Nursing Home 4450 Eighth Street Sarasota, FL 34239 (813) 371-6438	Beds: 60 Private: 9 Medicaid, Medicare Rating:	 Conditional
East Manor Medical Care Center 1524 East Avenue South Sarasota, FL 34239 (813) 365-2422	Beds: 169 Private: 5 Medicaid, Medicare Rating:	Semiprivate: 70 Superior
Heritage Healthcare Center 1026 Albee Farm Road Venice, FL 34292 (813) 484-0425	Beds: 120 Private: 14 Medicaid, Medicare Rating:	Semiprivate: 53 Standard
Hillhaven Convalescent Center 5640 Rand Blvd. Sarasota, FL 34292-5174 (813) 922-8009	Beds: 120 Private: 14 Medicaid, Medicare Rating:	Semiprivate: 53 Superior
J.H. Floyd Sunshine Manor 1755 18th Street Sarasota, FL 34234 (813) 955-4915	Beds: 68 Private: 2 Medicaid, Medicare Rating:	Semiprivate: 21 Superior
Kensington Manor 3250 12th Street Sarasota, FL 34237 (813) 365-4185	Beds: 147 Private: 1 Medicaid, Medicare Rating:	Semiprivate: 52 Superior
Manor Care of Sarasota 5511 Swift Road Sarasota, FL 34231 (813) 921-7462	Beds: 120 Private: 32 Medicaid, Medicare Rating:	Semiprivate: 44 Conditional
Oak Pointe Manor 1507 South Tuttle Ave. Sarasota, FL 34292 (813) 365-2737	Beds: 114 Private: 37 Medicaid Rating:	Semiprivate: 34 Superior
Pinebrook Pl. Healthcare Center 1240 Pinebrook Road Venice, FL 34236 (813) 488-6733	Beds: 120 Private: 4 Medicaid, Medicare Rating:	Semiprivate: 58 Superior
Pines of Sarasota 1501 N. Orange Avenue Sarasota, FL 34292 (813) 365-0250	Beds: 204 Private: 106 Medicaid, Medicare Rating:	Semiprivate: 41 Superior

Plymouth Harbor 700 John Ringling Blvd. Sarasota, FL 34236 (813) 365-2600	Beds: 60 Private: 24 Rating:	Semiprivate: 18 Superior
Quality Health Care Center 6940 Pan American Drive North Port, FL 34287-3499 (813) 426-8411	Beds: 120 Private: 10 Medicaid, Medicare Rating:	Semiprivate: 54 Superior
Regents Park of Sarasota 7848 Beneva Road Sarasota, FL 34238 (813) 923-5694	Beds: 120 Private: 12 Medicaid, Medicare Rating:	Semiprivate: 54 Superior
Sarasota Health Care Center 5157 Park Club Drive Sarasota, FL 34235 (813) 365-2926	Beds: 120 Private: 8 Medicaid, Medicare Rating:	Semiprivate: 56 Conditional
Sarasota Nursing Pavilion 2600 Courtland Street Sarasota, FL 34237 (813) 365-2926	Beds: 180 Private: 18 Medicaid, Medicare Rating:	Semiprivate: 81 Superior
Southwest Fla Retirement Center 910 Tamiami Trail South Venice, FL 34285 (813) 484-9753	Beds: 60 Private: 2 Medicaid, Medicare Rating:	Semiprivate: 29 Superior
Springwood Nursing Center 4602 Northgate Court Sarasota, FL 34234 (813) 355-2913	Beds: 120 Private: 7 Medicaid, Medicare Rating:	Semiprivate: 43 Superior
Sunnyside Nursing Home 5201 Bahia Vista Sarasota, FL 34232 (813) 371-2729	Beds: 60 Private: 1 Medicaid, Medicare Rating:	Semiprivate: 23 Conditional
Venice Nursing Pavilion North 437 South Nokomis Avenue Venice, FL 34285 (813) 488-9696	Beds: 178 Private: 2 Medicaid, Medicare Rating:	Semiprivate: 72 Superior
Venice Nursing Pavilion South 200 Field Avenue, E. Venice, FL 34285 (813) 484-2477	Beds: 120 Private: 2 Medicaid, Medicare Rating:	Semiprivate: 37 Superior
Venice Pines 1131 Jacaranda Blvd Venice, FL 34292 (813) 492-5313	Beds: 120 Private: 16 Medicaid, Medicare Rating:	Semiprivate: 52 Standard

SEMINOLE

Hillhaven Healthcare Center 950 Mellonville Avenue Sanford, FL 32771 (407) 322-8566	Beds: 114 Private: 2 Medicaid, Medicare Rating:	Semiprivate: 34 Conditional

Lakeview Nursing Center 919 East Second Street Sanford, FL 32771 (407) 322-6707	Beds: 105 Private: 7 Medicaid, Medicare Rating:	Semiprivate: 22 Conditional
Life Care Center of Altamonte Springs 989 Orienta Avenue Altamonte Springs, FL 32701 (407) 831-3446	Beds: 240 Private: 10 Medicaid, Medicare Rating:	Semiprivate: 83 Superior
Longwood Health Care Center 1520 South Grant Avenue Longwood, FL 32750 (407) 339-9200	Beds: 120 Private: 8 Medicaid, Medicare Rating:	Semiprivate: 56 Standard
Lutheran Haven 2063 West State Rd 426 Oviedo, FL 32765 (407) 365-3456	Beds: 42 Private: 0 Rating:	Semiprivate: 21 Superior
Meridian Nursing Center 155 Landover Place Longwood, FL 32750 (407) 830-7744	Beds: 119 Private: 13 Medicaid, Medicare Rating:	Semiprivate: 53 Superior
Village on the Green 500 Village Place Longwood, FL 32779 (407) 682-0230	Beds: 60 Private: 2 Medicare Rating:	Semiprivate: 29 Superior

ST. JOHNS

Buckingham-Smith Mem Home 169 Martin Luther King Avenue St. Augustine, FL 32084 (904) 824-3638	Beds: 51 Private: 3 Medicaid, Medicare Rating:	 Superior
Ponce De Leon Care Center 1999 Old Moultrie Road St. Augustine, FL 32086 (904) 824-3311	Beds: 120 Private: 24 Medicaid, Medicare Rating:	Semiprivate: 48 Superior
Regency Health Care Center 200 Mederial Drive St. Augustine, FL 32084 (904) 797-1800	Beds: 120 Private: 10 Medicaid, Medicare Rating:	Semiprivate: 55 Superior
St. Augustine Geriatric Center 51 Sunrise Blvd. St. Augustine, FL 32084 (904) 824-4479	Beds: 120 Private: 12 Medicaid, Medicare Rating:	Semiprivate: 54 Superior
St. Johns County Senior Citizens Home 169 Marine Street St. Augustine, FL 32084 (904) 824-1755	Beds: 51 Private: 1 Medicaid, Medicare Rating:	Semiprivate: 1 Superior

St. Johns Health Care Center 189 San Marco Avenue St. Augustine, FL 32081 (904) 824-3326	Beds: 68 Private: 3 Medicaid, Medicare Rating:	Semiprivate: 13 Standard
Vicar's Landing 1000 Vicars Landing Way Ponte Verda Beach, FL 32082 (904) 285-1055	Beds: 30 Private: 26 Medicare Rating:	Semiprivate: 2 Superior

ST. LUCIE

Abbiejean Russell Care Center 700 South 29th Street Ft. Pierce, FL 34947 (407) 465-7560	Beds: 79 Private: 1 Medicaid, Medicare Rating:	Semiprivate: 39 Superior
Advantage Therapy & Nursing Center 611 South 13th Street Fort Pierce, FL 34950 (407) 464-5262	Beds: 171 Private: 5 Medicaid, Medicare Rating:	Semiprivate: 40 Superior
Fort Pierce Care Center 703 South 29th Street Fort Pierce, FL 34947 (407) 466-3322	Rooms: 107 Private: 13 Medicaid, Medicare Rating:	Semiprivate: 47 Superior
Palm Garden 1751 Hillmoor Drive Port St. Lucie, FL 34952 (407) 335-8844	Beds: 120 Private: 4 Medicaid, Medicare Rating:	Semiprivate: 58 Superior
Port St. Lucie Convalescent Center 7300 Oleander Avenue Port St. Lucie, FL 34952-8299 (407) 466-4100	Beds: 180 Private: 10 Medicaid, Medicare Rating:	Semiprivate: 85 Standard
Savana Cay Manor 1655 S.E. Walton Road Port St. Lucie, FL 34952 (407) 337-1333	Beds: 120 Private: 12 Medicaid, Medicare Rating:	Semiprivate: 54 Superior
We Care Nursing Center 490 South Old Wire Road Wildwood, FL 34785 (904) 748-3322	Beds: 180 Private: 6 Medicaid, Medicare Rating:	Semiprivate: 24 Superior

SUWANNEE

Good Samaritan Center PO Box 4307 Dowling Park, FL 32060 (904) 658-3334	Beds: 161 Private: 22 Medicaid, Medicare Rating:	Semiprivate: 68 Superior
Surrey Place Convalescent Center 110 S.E. Lee Avenue Live Oak, FL 32060 (904) 364-5961	Beds: 60 Private: 4 Medicaid Rating:	Semiprivate: 28 Superior

| Suwannee Health Care Center
1620 E. Helvenston Street
Live Oak, FL 32060
(904) 362-7860 | Beds: 120
Private: 16
Medicaid
Rating: | Semiprivate: 52

Superior |

TAYLOR

| Perry Health Facility
207 Forest Drive
Perry, FL 32347
(904) 584-6334 | Beds: 120
Private: 8
Medicaid, Medicare
Rating: | Semiprivate: 56

Standard |

VOLUSIA

| Alliance Nursing Center
151 W. Winnemissett Ave
Deland, FL 32720
(904) 734-6401 | Beds: 60
Private: 1
Medicaid, Medicare
Rating: | Semiprivate: 14

Superior |

| Bishop's Glen Foundation
900 11th Street
Daytona Beach, FL 32117
(904) 255-9000 | Beds: 60
Private: 4
Medicaid, Medicare
Rating: | Semiprivate: 28

Superior |

| Bowmans Nursing Center
350 South Ridgewood Ave.
Ormond Beach, FL 32174
(904) 677-4545 | Beds: 143
Private: 3
Medicaid, Medicare
Rating: | Semiprivate: 70

Standard |

| Clyatt Quality Care
1001 South Beach Street
Daytona Beach, FL 32114
(904) 258-3334 | Beds: 99
Private: 67
Medicare
Rating: | Semiprivate: 16

Superior |

| Daytona Beach Geriatric Center
1055 Third Street
Daytona Beach, FL 32117
(904) 252-3686 | Beds: 180
Private: 14
Medicaid, Medicare
Rating: | Semiprivate: 83

Superior |

| Daytona Manor Nursing Home
650 Reed Canal Street
So Daytona, FL 32119
(904) 767-4831 | Beds: 65
Private: 1
Medicaid, Medicare
Rating: | Semiprivate: 16

Superior |

| De Bary Manor
60 N. Hwy 17-92
DeBary, FL 32713
(407) 668-4426 | Beds: 120
Private: 40
Medicaid, Medicare
Rating: | Semiprivate: 38

Superior |

| Deland Convalescent Center
451 South Amelia Avenue
Deland, FL 32724
(904) 734-8614 | Beds: 122
Private: 3
Medicare
Rating: | Semiprivate: 58

Superior |

| Deltona Healthcare Center
1851 Elkham Blvd.
Deltona, FL 32725
(904) 789-3769 | Beds: 120
Private: 20
Medicaid, Medicare
Rating: | Semiprivate: 50

Superior |

Fairview Manor 324 Wilder Blvd. Daytona Beach, FL 32114 (904) 252-2600	Beds: 192 Private: 8 Medicaid, Medicare Rating:	Semiprivate: 30 Superior
Fountains Nursing & Rehabilitation Center 1350 S. Nova Road Daytona Beach, FL 32114 (904) 258-5544	Beds: 55 Private: 0 Medicaid, Medicare Rating:	Semiprivate: 5 Standard
Halifax Convalescent Center 820 N. Clyde Morris Blvd. Daytona, FL 32117 (904) 274-4575	Beds: 84 Private: 6 Medicaid, Medicare Rating:	Semiprivate: 57 Superior
Holiday Care Center 1031 South Beach Street Daytona Beach, FL 32114 (904) 255-2453	Beds: 48 Private: 16 Medicaid, Medicare Rating:	Semiprivate: 6 Superior
Huntington Square Convalarium 100 Broadway Daytona Beach, FL 32118-4697 (904) 255-6571	Beds: 60 Private: 2 Medicaid, Medicare Rating:	Semiprivate: 7 Superior
Indigo Manor 595 Williamson Blvd. Daytona Beach, FL 32114 (904) 257-4400	Beds: 120 Private: 4 Medicaid, Medicare Rating:	Semiprivate: 58 Superior
John Knox Village Med Center 101 North Lake Drive Orange City, FL 32763 (904) 775-3840	Beds: 120 Private: 8 Medicare Rating:	Semiprivate: 56 Superior
Meridian Nursing Center 170 North Center Street Ormond Beach, FL 32174 (904) 672-7113	Beds: 120 Private: 120 Medicaid, Medicare Rating:	Semiprivate: 0 Superior
Ocean View Nursing Home 2810 South Atlantic Ave. New Smyrna Beach, FL 32169 (904) 428-6424	Beds: 239 Private: 5 Medicaid, Medicare Rating:	Semiprivate: 100 Superior
Olds Hall Good Samaritan 325 South Segrave Street Daytona Beach, FL 32114 (904) 253-6791	Beds: 119 Private: 17 Medicaid, Medicare Rating:	Semiprivate: 51 Superior
Ormond Beach Health Care Center 170 North Kings Road Ormond Beach, FL 32174 (904) 677-7955	Beds: 133 Private: 7 Medicaid, Medicare Rating:	Semiprivate: 18 Superior
Ormond in the Pines 100 Clyde Morris Blvd. Ormond Beach, FL 32074 (904) 673-0450	Beds: 60 Private: 16 Medicare, Medicaid Rating:	Semiprivate: 22 Superior

Regency Gardens Nursing & Rehab. Center 5600 Victoria Gardens Blvd. Port Orange, FL 32127 (904) 760-7773	Beds: 120 Private: 12 Rating:	Semiprivate: 54 Standard
Regency Park Nursing Center 2810 Enterprise Road De Bary, FL 32713 (407) 668-6200	Beds: 120 Private: 12 Medicaid, Medicare Rating:	Semiprivate: 54 Superior
Ridgecrest Manor 1200 N. Stone St. DeLand, FL 32720 (904) 734-6200	Beds: 134 Private: 2 Medicaid, Medicare Rating:	Semiprivate: 30 Superior
University Convalescent Center East 991 East New York Avenue DeLand, FL 32724 (904) 734-9083	Beds: 60 Private: 1 Medicaid, Medicare Rating:	Semiprivate: 9 Superior
University Convalescent Center West 545 W. Euclid Avenue DeLand, FL 32720 (904) 734-9085	Beds: 60 Private: 1 Medicaid, Medicare Rating:	Semiprivate: 9 Superior

WAKULLA

Wakulla Manor Highway 319 South at Medart Crawfordville, FL 32427 (904) 926-7181	Beds: 120 Private: 10 Medicaid, Medicare Rating:	Semiprivate: 47 Superior

WALTON

Village at Sandestin 5851 Hwy 98 East Destin, FL 32541 (904) 267-2887	Beds: 60 Private: 4 Medicaid, Medicare Rating:	Semiprivate: 28 Standard
Walton County Convalescent Center 614 South 2nd Street DeFuniak Springs, FL 32433 (904) 892-2176	Beds: 60 Private: 2 Medicaid, Medicare Rating:	Semiprivate: 44 Superior

WASHINGTON

Brookwood-Washington County Convalescent Center 805 Usery Road Chipley, FL 32428 (904) 638-4654	Beds: 180 Private: 6 Medicaid, Medicare Rating:	Semiprivate: 75 Superior